Antimicrobial Drug Discovery

Antimicrobial Drug Discovery

Editor: Dylan Lucas

AMERICAN
MEDICAL PUBLISHERS
www.americanmedicalpublishers.com

AMERICAN
MEDICAL PUBLISHERS
www.americanmedicalpublishers.com

Cataloging-in-Publication Data

Antimicrobial drug discovery / edited by Dylan Lucas.
p. cm.
Includes bibliographical references and index.
ISBN 978-1-63927-882-4
1. Anti-infective agents. 2. Drugs--Design. 3. Drug development. 4. Drug resistance.
5. Diseases--Animal models. 6. Pharmacology. I. Lucas, Dylan.
RM267 .A58 2023
615.329--dc23

American Medical Publishers,
41 Flatbush Avenue,
1st Floor, New York,
NY 11217, USA

ISBN 978-1-63927-882-4 (Hardback)

Contents

Preface

Antimicrobial drugs include those medicines which use antimicrobial agents in the prevention and treatment of infections in humans. An antimicrobial agent is a drug used to prevent and treat the pathogenicity of microorganisms. There are different types of antimicrobial drugs, including antibacterial drugs, antifungal drugs, antiviral agent and antiparasitic drugs. There is increased antimicrobial resistance (AMR) in a variety of human pathogenic microorganisms, which includes Enterococcus faecium, Staphylococcus aureus, Klebsiella pneumoniae, Acinetobacter baumannii, Pseudomonas aeruginosa, and Enterobacter spp. The discovery and development of the antimicrobial drugs is aimed at enhancing the pharmacokinetic properties, overcoming pathogen resistance, and extending the spectrum of microorganisms targeted. The five key areas of research in antimicrobial drug discovery are molecular genetics and systems microbiology; synthetic and computational chemistry, and chemoinformatics; high throughput screening (HTS); non-vertebrate model hosts; and light- and nano-based technologies. This book aims to shed light on some of the unexplored aspects of antimicrobial drug discovery. It includes contributions of experts and scientists which will provide innovative insights into this field.

The information shared in this book is based on empirical researches made by veterans in this field of study. The elaborative information provided in this book will help the readers further their scope of knowledge leading to advancements in this field.

Finally, I would like to thank my fellow researchers who gave constructive feedback and my family members who supported me at every step of my research.

Editor

1

Current Insights on Antifungal Therapy: Novel Nanotechnology Approaches for Drug Delivery Systems and New Drugs from Natural Sources

Filipa Sousa [1,*], Domingos Ferreira [1], Salette Reis [2] and Paulo Costa [1,*]

[1] UCIBIO, REQUIMTE, Laboratory of Pharmaceutical Technology, Department of Drug Sciences, Faculty of Pharmacy, University of Porto, Rua Jorge Viterbo Ferreira n° 228, 4050-313 Porto, Portugal; domingos@ff.up.pt

[2] LAQV, REQUIMTE, Department of Chemical Sciences, Faculty of Pharmacy, University of Porto, Rua Jorge Viterbo Ferreira n° 228, 4050-313 Porto, Portugal; shreis@ff.up.pt

* Correspondence: filipambtsousa@gmail.com (F.S.); pccosta@ff.up.pt (P.C.)

Abstract: The high incidence of fungal infections has become a worrisome public health issue, having been aggravated by an increase in host predisposition factors. Despite all the drugs available on the market to treat these diseases, their efficiency is questionable, and their side effects cannot be neglected. Bearing that in mind, it is of upmost importance to synthetize new and innovative carriers for these medicines not only to fight emerging fungal infections but also to avert the increase in drug-resistant strains. Although it has revealed to be a difficult job, new nano-based drug delivery systems and even new cellular targets and compounds with antifungal potential are now being investigated. This article will provide a summary of the state-of-the-art strategies that have been studied in order to improve antifungal therapy and reduce adverse effects of conventional drugs. The bidirectional relationship between Mycology and Nanotechnology will be also explained. Furthermore, the article will focus on new compounds from the marine environment which have a proven antifungal potential and may act as platforms to discover drug-like characteristics, highlighting the challenges of the translation of these natural compounds into the clinical pipeline.

Keywords: nanoparticles; fungi; drug delivery systems; marine; biological synthesis; myconanotechnology

1. Introduction

There is a wide range of fungal infections, from superficial, affecting skin, to systemic infections with invasion of internal organs [1]. Fungal infections affect millions of people every year worldwide. Of these, more or less 1.5 million are invasive fungal infections therefore requiring advanced treatment and hospitalization. Most of these disseminated infections are caused by *Candida, Cryptococcus, Aspergillus,* and *Pneumocystis* species, being the cause of cryptococcosis, candidiasis, aspergillosis, and pneumocystis pneumonia, respectively [2].

Superficial fungal infections are rather common and, despite rarely being life threatening, they can spread to other skin regions and even become widespread. Furthermore, they can be transmitted to other people and may cause secondary bacterial skin infections, harming the quality of a person's life. Skin mycoses are classified according to the causative fungal agents into dermatophytosis, yeast infections, and mold infections [1].

Invasive fungal infections represent a significant burden to healthcare systems, having high morbidity and mortality rates. These rates are most worrisome among immunocompromised patients that are more prone to opportunistic infections, such as patients with Acquired Immune Deficiency Syndrome (AIDS), transplant patients whose immune systems are suppressed to prevent organ rejection, patients with cancer who are taking immunosuppressive chemotherapy or autoimmune patients undergoing immunosuppressive therapy [2,3].

The currently major available agents to treat invasive fungal infections can be grouped into four main classes according to their mechanism of action: polyenes, azoles, allylamines, and echinocandins (Table 1) [4]. They all present drawbacks when it comes to spectrum of activity, drug–drug interactions, pharmacokinetics and pharmacodynamics, resistance mechanisms, and the toxicity of the compounds themselves. Furthermore, there are some limitations in terms of clinical efficacy and efficiency, mainly because of their physical-chemical properties, like their hydrophobic character that leads to a low solubility in water and also selectivity problems deriving from the similarities between fungi and human cells [3,5].

Table 1. Targets of each group of antifungals [6,7].

Class	Target (Mechanism of Action)	Antifungal	
Azoles	Ergosterol (inhibition of lanosterol 14-α-demethylase)	Imidazoles	Miconazole
			Econazole
			Ketoconazole
			Clotrimazole
		Triazoles	Itraconazole
			Fluconazole
			Voriconazole
Allylamines	Ergosterol (inhibition of squalene epoxidase)	Terbinafine	
		Naftifine	
		Butenafine	
Polyenes	Cell membrane (production of ROS)	Amphotericin B	
	Ergosterol (inhibition of lanosterol 14-α-demethylase)	Nystatin	
Echinocandines	Cell wall (block of β-1,3 glucan synthesis)	Caspofungin, Micafungin, Anidulafungin	
Other antifungals	Chelation of polyvalent metal cations	Ciclopirox	
	Microtubules (prevention of the formation of the mitotic spindle)	Griseofulvin	
	Ergosterol (inhibition of D14 reductase and D7-D8 isomerase)	Amorolfine	

Nevertheless, the design and development of new drug delivery systems or even new antifungals is an emerging need, owing to the following facts [8]:

- There are 20–40% mortality rates with invasive mycoses, therefore these figures need to be improved;
- The increase in patients undergoing prolonged antifungal therapies reflects the need to develop better fungicidal drugs and thus reduce the length of the treatments and the costs associated;
- There is still space for improvement in pharmacokinetics and pharmacodynamics, in order to reduce the frequency of drug use;
- More attention needs to be given to the host toxicities and drug–drug interactions of current therapy so that their effects can be eliminated or, at least, minimized;
- New therapy groups with different mechanisms of action are needed; this way, these new drugs may synergize with present ones and allow better responses;
- There is an alarming growth in antifungal resistance in all therapeutic groups [8].

Nanotechnology is an emerging field of science that has shown an undeniable versatility and has boosted a revolution when it comes to medical treatments, quicker diagnosis, cellular regeneration, and drug delivery [9,10]. The material to produce nanoparticles can be divided into three main groups: polymers, lipids, or metals, each one giving rise to a different type of nanoparticle [11]. The main representatives of each of these three different groups of nanoparticles are mentioned in Figure 1 below.

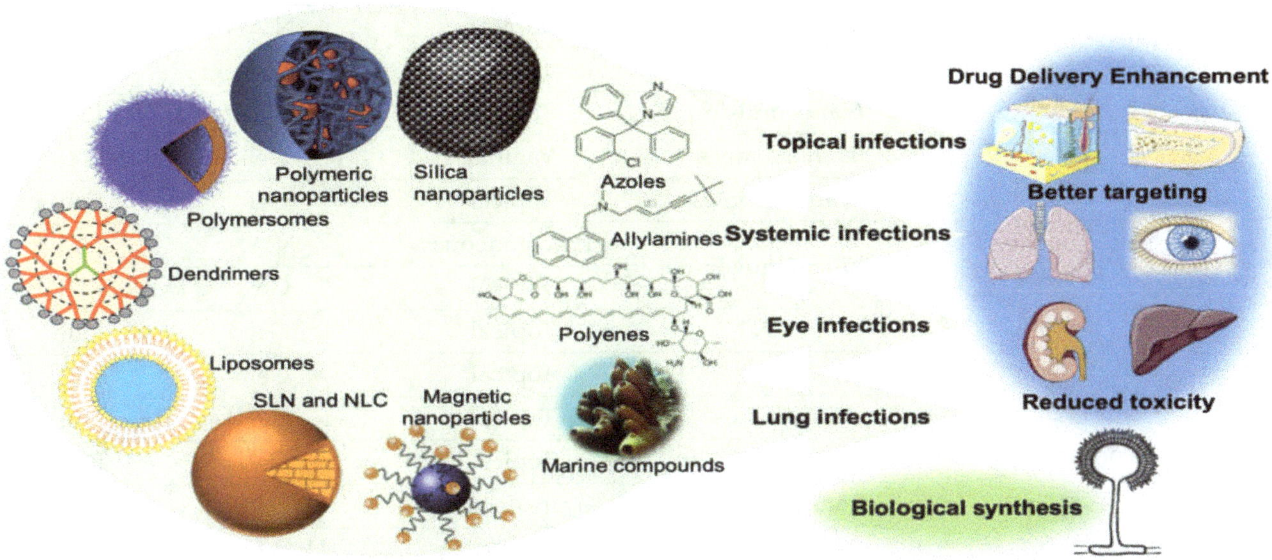

Figure 1. The new drug delivery systems based on nanotechnology that are currently being employed in order to enhance drug delivery, promote a better targeting, and reduce the toxicity of conventional antifungal drugs. It is also important to point out the importance of the production of nanoparticles by fungi (biological synthesis) and the undeniable potential of the sea as a source of new molecules with antifungal activity.

Nanoparticles have been employed in pharmaceutical formulations because of their ability to alter and improve the pharmacokinetic and pharmacodynamic properties of the drugs. This is given to their capability to increase the solubility and stability of the drugs, to allow a controlled release and to exhibit biocompatibility with tissues and cells, which is reflected in an overall improvement on therapeutic efficiency [11,12]. In addition, its subcellular size is compatible with an intravascular injection and its high surface area is amenable to modification so that the drug is released in a specific target, thus reducing the systemic adverse effects and increasing the therapeutic compliance, by decreasing the usual dose and the frequency of administration [13,14]. This targeted-specific action is possible since, at a nanomolecular level, it is possible to incorporate target ligands that allow a preferential binding of certain types of cells, by conjugation with antibodies and peptides on the surface of the transporters [15–17]. Hence, the development of new biopharmaceutical systems, especially nanoparticulate carriers, is a good strategy to improve the therapeutic efficacy, safety, and compliance of conventional antifungal drugs.

In Table 2 an overview of the new antifungal drug delivery systems is presented, and the drug chemical group, their route of administration, and their dosage form provided.

Table 2. Some of the novel drug delivery systems already developed for each antifungal drug.

Antifungal Drugs	Novel Drug Delivery Systems	Routes of Administration	Dosage Forms	References
Miconazole	Niosomes	Transdermal	Gel	[18]
	SLN	Oral	N.A.	[19]
		Topical	Gel	[20]
	Microemulsion	Topical	N.A.	[21]
	Liposomes	Topical	Gel	[22]
	Nanoemulsion	Topical	N.A.	[23]
	Nanosponges	Vaginal	Gel	[24]
	Transfersomes	Topical	Gel	[25]
Econazole	Microemulsion	Percutaneous	N.A.	[26]
		Topical	Gel	[27]
	SLN	Topical	Gel	[28]
	NLC	Topical	Gel	[29]
	Liposomes	Topical	Gel	[30]
	Ethosomes	Topical	Gel	[31]
	Transethosomes	Transdermal	Gel	[32]
	Nanosponges	Topical	Hydrogel	[33]
	Niosomes	Transdermal	Gel	[34]
	Polymeric micelles	Topical	N.A.	[35]
	Nanoemulsion	Topical	N.A.	[36]
Ketoconazole	SLN/NLC	Topical	Gel	[37]
	Niosomes	Topical	Gel	[38]
	Microemulsion	Oral	N.A.	[39]
	Spanlastics	Ocular	N.A.	[40]
	Dendrimers	Topical	Hydrogel	[41]
	Liposomes	Topical	N.A.	[42]
Clotrimazole	Liposomes	Topical	Gel	[43]
	Nanosponges	Topical	Hydrogel	[44]
	Ethosomes	Topical	Gel	[45]
	Niosomes	Topical	Gel	[46]
	Polymeric emulgel	Topical	Gel	[47]
	Polymeric micelles	Topical	N.A.	[35]
	SLN/NLC	Topical	N.A.	[48]
	Microemulsion	Buccal	Gel	[49]
		Vaginal	Gel	[50]
	Transfersomes	Transdermal/Topical	N.A.	[51]
Itraconazole	Transfersomes	Transdermal	N.A.	[52]
	SLN	Ocular	N.A.	[53]
	NLC	Inhalation	N.A.	[54]
	Niosomes	Topical	N.A.	[55]

Table 2. *Cont.*

Antifungal Drugs	Novel Drug Delivery Systems	Routes of Administration	Dosage Forms	References
	Microemulsion	Transdermal	N.A.	[56]
	Liposomes	Topical	N.A.	[57]
	Polymeric nanoparticles	Oral	N.A.	[58]
	Polymersome	Intravenous	N.A.	[54]
	Spanlastics	Ocular	N.A.	[59]
	Silica nanoparticles	Oral	N.A.	[60]
Fluconazole	Microemulsion	Vaginal	Gel	[61]
	Niosomes	Ocular	Gel	[62]
	Liposomes	Intravitral	N.A.	[63]
	SLN	Topical	Gel	[64]
	NLC	Oral	N.A.	[65]
	Microsponges	Topical	Gel	[66]
	Ethosomes	Topical	Gel	[67]
	Spanlastics	Ocular	N.A.	[68]
	Polymeric amphiphilogel	Topical	Gel	[69]
	Polymeric micelles	Topical	N.A.	[35]
Voriconazole	Microemulsion	Ocular	N.A.	[70]
	Polymeric nanoparticles	Ocular	N.A.	[71]
		Pulmonar	N.A.	[72]
	SLN	Topical	Gel	[73]
	Transethosome	Topical	N.A.	[74]
	Ethosome	Topical	N.A.	[75]
Terbinafine	Liposomes	Topical	Gel	[76]
	SLN	Topical	N.A.	[77]
	Transfersomes	Topical	N.A.	[78]
	Spanlastics	Transungual	N.A.	[79]
	Polymeric chitosan nanoparticles	Topical	Hydrogel	[80]
Naftifine	Microemulsion	Topical	N.A.	[81]
	Niosomes	Topical	Gel	[82]
Butenafine	Microemulsion	Topical	Hydrogel	[83]
Amphotericin B	Liposomes	Intravenous	N.A.	[84]
	SLN/NLC	Oral	N.A.	[85]
		Topical	N.A.	[86]
	Magnetic nanoparticles	Nasal instilation	N.A.	[87]
	Nanoemulsion	Topical	N.A.	[88]
	Polymeric nanoparticles	Intravenous	N.A.	[89]
		Oral	N.A.	[90]

Table 2. *Cont.*

Antifungal Drugs	Novel Drug Delivery Systems	Routes of Administration	Dosage Forms	References
	Polymersomes	Oral	N.A.	[91,92]
	Transfersomes	Topical	N.A.	[93]
	Micelles	Intravenous	N.A.	[94]
	Silica nanoparticles	Intravenous	N.A.	[95]
Nystatin	SLN	Topical	N.A.	[96]
	Nanoemulsion	Topical	N.A.	[97]
	Liposomes	Intravenous	N.A.	[98]
	Niosomes	Parenteral	N.A.	[99]
Griseofulvin	Niosomes	Oral	N.A.	[100]
Ciclopirox	Niosomes	Topical	Gel	[101]
Caspofungin, Micafungin, Anidulafungin, Amorolfine	No nano-tech studies yet released			

N.A.: the dosage form is not mentioned in the reference cited; SLN: Solid Lipid Nanoparticles; NLC: Nanostructured Lipid Carriers.

However, the efficacy and human safety of these new therapies remain uncertain in most of the articles found in literature. They generally lack controlled clinical trials and sometimes the suggested routes of administration are less practical, or the production cost may hinder the replacement of the conventional treatment. Nevertheless, in other cases, the opposite is verified, and some options have potential to become a viable first line treatment [102]. Moreover, given the widespread use of antifungal agents and the limited therapeutic offer, fungi have developed resistance mechanisms, like overexpression of efflux pump proteins and formation of biofilms. These mechanisms can mean not only a decrease in a drug's effective concentration, but also changes and subexpression of drug targets and metabolic bypass [6]. It is important to add that resistance is a cross-cutting issue to all of the currently available classes of antifungal agents, therefore overcoming antifungal resistance can be considered as the mainstay for improving therapeutic strategies to treat antifungal infections [2,103].

Despite the uprising of these issues in antifungal therapy, there are several mechanisms by which nanoparticles overcome the development of resistance mechanisms:

- The chemical features and simultaneous multiple mechanisms used by nitric oxide, chitosan, and metallic nanoparticles make the likelihood of resistance development unviable (for example, through the direct reaction of reactive nitrogen oxide intermediates with DNA structure) [104,105];
- The resistance mechanisms can be prevented by packaging multiple antimicrobial drugs within the same nanoparticle, because the likelihood of multiple simultaneous gene mutations in the same cell is low. The most striking examples are the encapsulation of antifungal drugs in chitosan or silver nanoparticles, combining the antifungal properties of both and decreasing the possibility of drug resistance [104,106];
- Some nanoparticles, such as liposomes and dendrimers, are able to overcome the resistance mechanisms of decreased uptake and increased efflux of drug from the microbial cell. Liposomes are able to quickly fuse with the plasma membrane of the microbial cell and release a high concentration of drug into its plasma membrane or cytoplasm, thereby circumventing the decreased uptake mechanism of resistance. This means a faster delivery and avoidance of the transmembrane pumps that catalyze increased efflux of drugs. Dendrimers, on the other hand, are extensively branched molecules, whose surface can be filled with positively charged quaternary ammonium compounds, which bind to negatively charged microbial cell envelopes and increase membrane permeability. This allows the entrance of more dendrimers to the

microbial cell, the flow of its cytoplasmic contents to the exterior, and the ultimate destruction of the microbial cell membrane. This goes to show that dendrimers are also able to surpass the resistance mechanism of decreased uptake of drug [107]. Other nanoparticles, specifically nitric oxide nanoparticles made of silica and zinc oxide nanoparticles are able to overcome biofilm formation by killing the microbes present in already formed biofilms or by inhibiting biofilm formation through the generation of reactive oxygen species, respectively [108,109];

- Nanoparticles have been used to target antifungal drugs to the specific site of infection, allowing the local release of high concentrations of drug, while keeping the total dose of drug administered low. This high local dose is able to destroy the infecting fungi before they can develop resistance, thereby overcoming this worrisome issue and translating into fewer side effects upon the patient [104].

That being said, it is also important that the research done, not only focuses on formulating these systems, but also in overcoming the major challenges that their placing on the market faces: the physical instability of nanoparticles, their small capacity of drug loading, the cytotoxicity/immunogenicity, and the high cost of production and standardization, given the complexity of the formulations. Besides that, there is almost a complete lack of studies in vivo as reaching the therapeutic range needed to perform these studies has proven to be an arduous job. That lies in the fact that, in many cases, there is an anticipated release of the drug, aggregation and precipitation of the nanoparticles, and the accumulation in non-target tissues.

2. Nanotechnology and Mycology

Mycology and Nanotechnology have created a bidirectional relationship throughout the years. This dynamic interface between mycology and nanotechnology led to the creation of the term "myconanotechnology" (Figure 2) [110]. Nanotechnology has proven to be an interesting strategy to increase the potency and efficiency of conventional antifungals, to enable a decrease in toxicity and cost, to avoid an anticipated degradation, to ameliorate the drug distribution, by increasing the circulation time and improving pharmacokinetics, and also to improve drug targeting, with promising in vitro and in vivo results [5]. Furthermore, many metallic nanoparticles have been used against human and plant pathogenic fungi in the light of their intrinsic antifungal activity and a wide spectrum of fungi are able to biosynthesize nanoelemental particles [110].

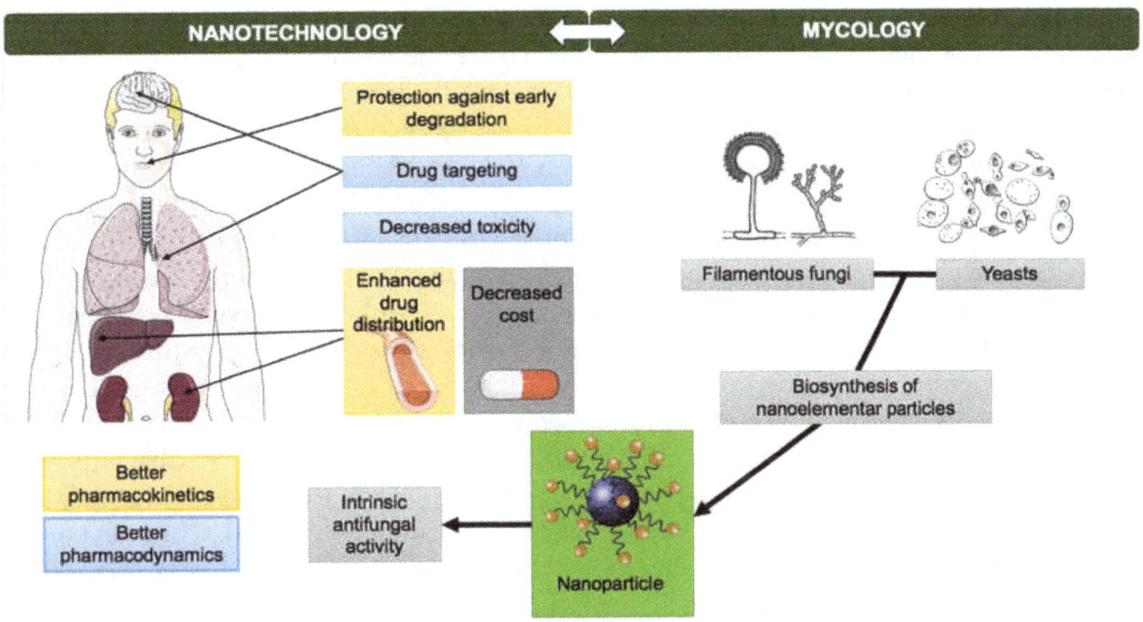

Figure 2. Bidirectional relationship of Nanoparticles and Mycology: nanotechnology has proven to be useful in improving antifungals pharmacokinetics and pharmacodynamics and many fungi have been used to biologically synthetize nanoparticles.

2.1. Antifungal Potential of Nanoparticles

Metallic nanoparticles have been used to eliminate fungi that are pathogenic to Man and to plants, because of their intrinsic antimicrobial activity [110]. The exact mechanisms this activity occurs through are only hypothesized and can be explained through three main pathways: (1) direct uptake of nanoparticles, (2) indirect activity of nanoparticles by production of reactive oxygen species (ROS), (3) impairment of cell wall/membrane through accumulation [111]. It is highly probable that it is the combination of these multiple pathways that is responsible for antimicrobial activity [112].

Nanoparticles undergo dissolution processes thanks to their electrochemical potential [113]. This leads to their separation into ions within the microbial fluid or in the culture medium. These ions also accumulate in the interior or exterior causing an inhibitory answer against microtubules. The accumulation of nanoparticles outside the microtubules causes the formation of layers that block cellular respiratory chain and destroy the microtubules [111].

The electrical charge of the nanoparticle is vital for the interaction that occurs between it and the carried drug. The electrostatic mechanism justifies why the antimicrobial activity was firstly described in silver nanoparticles. It is widely accepted that the positive charge of the silver ion is crucial for the antimicrobial activity of these nanoparticles through electrostatic attraction between the negatively charged cellular membrane of microorganisms and the positively charged membrane of nanoparticles [111]. Ag^+ has high affinity to thiol groups in cysteine of respiratory chain enzymes, therefore it uncouples the synthesis of adenosine triphosphate (ATP). Ag^+ also binds to proteins of transport from the respiratory chain, causing the leak out of protons and thus the collapse of the proton motive force. Furthermore, Ag^+ obstructs the uptake of phosphate and so promotes the efflux of intracellular phosphate [113].

Silver nanoparticles exhibit potent antifungal activity against clinical isolates and ATCC strains of *Trichophyton mentagrophytes* with concentrations of 1–7 μg/mL and a MIC (minimum inhibitory concentration) of 25 μg/mL against *Candida albicans* [114]. Silver nanoparticles also reveal good antifungal activity against *Aspergillus niger*, by inhibiting spore germination and preventing biofilm formation; when combined with simvastatin, there is an additive and synergistic effect that increases the antifungal effect, perhaps because simvastatin, as an ergosterol synthesis inhibitor (see Table 1), disrupts fungal cell membrane, which allows the entry of the nanoparticles [115].

Metals present in nanoparticles can act as catalysts, reacting with biomolecules thanks to their high specific surface area, inducing the direct production of free radicals when exposed to the acidic environment of lysosomes or interacting with oxidative organelles [112,113].

ROS, like superoxide anions, hydroxyl radicals, and hydrogen peroxide, are oxygen-derived by-products formed when a material is exposed to an oxygenated environment, allowing their interaction with biomolecules. This way, they can cause an imbalance between the production of reactive species and the capacity of the biological system to detoxify reactive intermediates or repair damage [111]. Although the antioxidant cell defense prevents the effects of ROS to some extent, excessive ROS production may cause oxidative stress and lipid peroxidation, leading to membrane impairment, mitochondrial dysfunction, and DNA damage. That being a toxic mechanism to human cells, cytotoxicity tests should be performed on nanoparticles that owe their antimicrobial effects to ROS production, therefore avoiding interactions and toxic reactions in human beings [111].

Chitosan and its chemical derivates have been used as building blocks for drug delivery nanoformulations in light of their biocompatibility, biodegradability, and mucoadhesivity, presenting some advantages such as in situ gelling performance, mucoadhesive properties, and ability to prolong the release of low-molecular-weight compounds to macromolecular drugs [116]. Chitosan nanoparticles have proven to exhibit great antimicrobial activity against Candida infections [1]. According to the literature and research already undertaken, this antimicrobial activity is attributed to positively charged amino groups that react with negatively charged groups of lipopolysaccharides and proteins on the surface of the microbial cells, resulting in disintegration of the cell membrane. By doing this, the nanoparticles are able to bind with DNA molecules and inhibit mRNA and protein synthesis.

In the specific case of fungi, chitosan acts by inhibiting the sporulation and germination of spores, by interfering with the activity of the growth-promoting enzymes [1,117].

Zinc oxide nanoparticles (ZnONPs) have also proved antifungal activity against dermatophyte infections and other pathogenic fungi, such as Candida and Aspergillus [1]. Meanwhile, the synergistic antifungal activity of ZnONPs was evaluated along with common antifungal drugs, which revealed that their inhibitory efficiency can be increased in combination with ZnONPs, which could possibly reduce the overuse of these drugs, decrease their toxicity, and increase their antifungal activity [118]. In addition, these nanoparticles might be an interesting and promising alternative to conventional preservatives in cosmetics in the future [119].

In addition to these nanoparticles mentioned above, dendrimers also exhibit antifungal activity and provide the opportunity for complex therapy in which dendrimers are both the drug carrier and the adjunctive component of the dosage form [41].

2.2. Synthesis of Nanoparticles by Fungi

Thanks to their tolerance and ability to bioaccumulate metals, fungi now occupy a central role in the biological production of metallic nanoparticles (Table 3) [10]. They can not only be used to produce the nanomaterials that will make up the nanosystem coating, but also be, themselves, carried by the nanosystem. This way, new ecological processes are developed, which imply a reduced waste of solvents and chemical substances. The biosynthesis methods are simpler and allow size and shape control of nanoparticles. Besides fungi, other organisms are used to synthesize nanoparticles, for instance, bacteria, plants, or plant extracts [110]. Compared to bacteria, fungi produce higher quantity of enzymes, which is translated into a higher yield in the nanoparticles production. Furthermore, their growth, both in laboratory and at an industrial scale, is easier to control [110].

Table 3. Some examples of metallic nanoparticles produced by fungi and their method of synthesis [10,120].

Fungal Species	Nanoparticles Type	Method of Synthesis
Phoma sp.	Silver	Extracellular
Fusarium oxysporum	Gold; Magnetite	Extracellular
Verticillium sp.	Silver	Intracellular
Aspergillus fumigatus	Silver	Extracellular
Aspergillus niger	Silver	Extracellular
Fusarium semitectum	Silver	Extracellular
Trichoderma asperellum	Silver	Extracellular
Phaenerochaete chrysosporium	Silver	Extracellular

The biological synthesis can either be intracellular or extracellular according to the nanoparticles' locations. In intracellular synthesis, the ions are transported to the inner part of microbial cells to form nanoparticles in the presence of an enzyme. The nanoparticles formed inside the organism are of shorter size, when compared to the extracellular ones, because there is nucleation of particles inside the organisms. Extracellular synthesis has more applications than intracellular, as there is no need to join cellular components from the cell. The majority of the fungi produce nanoparticles extracellularly as a result of their secretory components that participate in nanoparticles reduction and capping [10].

Both yeasts and filamentous fungi can be used to synthetize nanoparticles. The process of synthetizing filamentous fungi-mediated nanoparticles is easy and cost-effective, since the mycelia in the biomass has high surface area and high intracellular metal absorption. Moreover, the fungi cell wall has many functional groups that facilitate the absorption to the metals [110].

Silver nanoparticles are the most fundamental among metallic nanoparticles that are involved in biomedical applications, specially cancer diagnosis and antimicrobial therapy [114]. One of the most remarkable examples is the extracellular synthesis of silver nanoparticles from filamentous fungi, like *Fusarium solani*, a pathogenic fungus isolated from infected onions. Ingle et al. [121] believe that, in these cases, the fungus does the "phagocytosis" of the nanoparticles, depositing them in their cellular wall, by binding to their functional groups. Afterwards, the fungus carries the nanoparticles and excretes them through exocytosis. The silver nanoparticles obtained were quite stable in solution because fungus-secreted proteins capped the nanoparticles. The authors argued that the procedure with this fungus could work for other metal nanomaterials such as gold and platinum with countless applications in the medical field [121].

Afterwards, many other scientists were able to optimize the biological production of silver nanoparticles using other fungi, such as *Fusarium oxysporum* [122], *Cochliobolus lunatus, Beauveria bassiana* [123], *Bipolaris maydis* [124], and many others. It was also concluded that some of these biologically synthesized silver nanoparticles showed enhanced antifungal activity with fluconazole against *Phoma glomerata, Phoma herbarum, Fusarium semitectum, Trichoderma* sp., *Phoma glomerata, Phoma herbarum,* and *Candida albicans* [114]. Surprisingly, it was additionally observed that the potential of silver nanoparticles is much wider than the inhibition of human and plant pathogenic fungi, as they also inhibit indoor fungal species such as *Penicillium brevicompactum, Aspergillus fumigatus, Cladosporium cladosporoides, Chaetomium globosum,* and *Stachybotrys chartarum* [125].

Likewise, yeasts can be useful for nanoparticle synthesis, as they produce enzymes responsible for the reduction of metallic salts and their conversion into elementary nanoparticles. Some examples are the biosynthesis of cadmium nanoparticles by *Candida glabrata* and *Schizosaccharomyces pombe* [110] and of selenium and silver nanocompounds by *Saccharomyces cerevisiae* in aerobic conditions [126,127].

2.3. Antifungal Drug Administration

The administration of antifungal drugs is not restricted to oral or parenteral routes. Other routes such as transungual, pulmonary, and ocular have also acquired great importance in the treatment of certain fungal infections. The development of a drug delivery system for attaining therapeutic concentration at these target organs is a challenge that requires a comprehensive understanding of the dynamics and specific features of the nails, lungs, and eyes, respectively.

2.3.1. The Transungual Route

This special topical route acquires singular importance in antifungal therapy, mainly when onychomycosis (*Tinea ungium*) caused by dermatophytes (such as *Trichophyton rubrum*) or yeasts are concerned [128]. These infections affect the nail plate and/or the nail bed and are very frequent [129].

Drug delivery through nails has its own challenges and the use of nail penetration enhancers is compulsory in formulations. The nail plate is composed by cross linked keratin linkages, an extensive bonding network responsible for its rigidity. Although there has been considerable research regarding new approaches for transungual drug delivery, topical permeability was limited by its barrier properties. Therefore, the lookout for novel approaches is important to enhance treatment efficacy and reduce treatment time and relapse rate [128]. There are still no nanotech solutions for this purpose, but medicated nail lacquers loaded with ciclopirox or amorolfine are the most feasible delivery vehicles [130]. The main hurdle in the development of nail lacquers for nail disorders is delivering the therapeutically effective concentrations to the site of infection, which is often under the nail [129].

2.3.2. Pulmonary Delivery

Drug delivery to the lungs is challenging because the availability of therapeutic quantities of antifungal drug at the site of infection is often inadequate on account of high blood flow turnover in the tissue. This can be problematic since a local and prolonged drug release is desirable when targeting this organ.

Developing a nanoparticle-based system and delivering it to the lungs in case of a pulmonary infection may help retain the antifungal in lungs over a prolonged period and may reduce the toxicity compared to the parenteral route [72,131].

A study in which voriconazole was encapsulated within a PLGA nanoparticle revealed that this is a better option to deliver the drug in deep lung tissue at a high concentration for a prolonged period of time and assumedly to provide greater antifungal effect in fungal infections. This was concluded because these nanoparticles were retained for a prolonged time in lungs and showed higher biodistribution when compared to voriconazole alone [72].

2.3.3. The Ocular Route

The eye is a particularly puzzling organ for drug delivery systems. Physical barriers that hinder drug access into the eye limit the drug bioavailability. In addition, physiological processes like blinking and tear drainage reduce the residence time of ocular drug delivery systems and drastically reduce the amount of trans-corneal drug absorption [131,132].

Fungal ocular infections are much less prevalent when compared to bacteria or virus. However, fungal keratitis is considered the second cause of blindness in developing countries and is an important cause of morbidity [133,134]. People with prolonged use of corticosteroids or antibiotics, with diabetes mellitus, with corneal trauma or surgery, and even people wearing contact lenses are at a higher risk of having fungal keratitis [134].

New formulations such as polymer-based nanoparticles, liposomes, dendrimers, SLNs, spanlastics, and niosomes were developed to enhance drug bioavailability to the eye and to minimize antifungal adverse effects [135]. They also have the ability to overcome the disadvantages of conventional eye drops, like short residence time, by prolonging the contact time at the corneal surface and achieving a sustained release of the drug. In addition, the encapsulation into these systems protects antifungals from degradation promoted by the metabolic enzymes on conjunctival and corneal surfaces and in tear fluids [134].

A study assessed the efficacy of a fluconazole liposomal formulation for candidal keratitis that aimed at prolonging the antifungal action by increasing the contact time. The authors reported 86.4% healing observed in rabbits treated with fluconazole encapsulated liposomes, presumably because of higher viscosity and lipid solubility of fluconazole-loaded liposomes [136].

Furthermore, a fluconazole-loaded niosomal gel can also be successfully used as a topical drug delivery system for corneal fungal infections. Ethosomes are known to improve both transcorneal permeability and ocular bioavailability of poorly water-soluble drugs, which is a tremendous improvement in topical ocular drug delivery [137].

Spanlastics also enhance permeability and bioavailability of antifungal drugs and their nano-size makes them able to reach the posterior segment of the eye, when eye drops are used [138]. For instance, an itraconazole-loaded spanlastic proved to be safe and non-irritant to the eyes; moreover, the elasticity of these vesicles serves as a drug deliver for both anterior and posterior eye diseases [59].

2.4. *An Overview of Nanoparticle Types and Their Applicability on Antifungal Therapy*

2.4.1. Lipid Nanoparticles

Albeit the safety and tolerability of systemic antifungal therapy has improved considerably, a rising proportion of immunocompromised patients are receiving systemic antifungal agents for progressively longer treatment courses and that increases the probability of longer-term risks, drug interaction, and other toxicity-related reactions in different organs [139].

Ambisome® was the first successful example of a nanotech antifungal drug and it was manufactured by the Nexatar Company USA in 1990 [84,140]. In this formulation, amphotericin B was incorporated in an unilamellar liposomal bilayer of approximately 45–80 nm. Compared to the conventional formulation, this one showed less toxicity and prolonged circulation time, which suggests a higher distribution rate [84]. Even though Ambisome® circumvented the initial toxicity issues, its daily-basis usage is still limited by its cost [5]. Thus, nanosomal formulations of amphotericin B were latter developed, with a special focus on lipid nanoparticles for intravenous delivery, which showed lower cytotoxicity against human kidney cells and much less hematotoxicity compared to the ones already marketed [141].

Besides amphotericin B, some other drugs have also been incorporated into liposomes with promising results. One good example of that is nystatin, a drug used mainly topically because of its poor oral bioavailability, thus excluded for the treatment of systemic fungal infections [134]. A daily injection of liposomal nystatin, however, showed great efficacy in the treatment of invasive aspergillosis, although with some mild renal toxicity and some infusion-related events [98]. Additionally, a multilamellar liposome gel system containing clotrimazole revealed to be useful in the treatment of vaginal candidiasis, providing a sustained release in the vaginal fluid and a reduced dosing interval [43].

Econazole is a topical antifungal that may be an irritant to the skin when conventional vehicles are employed. Applying a liposomal formulation has revealed to be a good strategy to minimize the irritating potential and to increase the compliance. Bioavailability studies of the liposomal gel revealed a seven-fold increase in the drug concentration in the epidermis, when compared to a control. Thus, the authors proved that it is possible to reduce the amount of drug applied and keep the therapeutic efficacy, minimizing the cutaneous irritation [142].

Transfersomes are generally regarded as an upgrade of liposomes, because they overcome their poor penetration through the stratum corneum, by modifications in the bilayer composition [134]. They are elastic nanovesicles made up from phospholipids and edge activators, most often surfactants or hydrophilic detergents with high mobility.

These particles are essentially studied as carriers for dermal and transdermal delivery, but have also shown to be effective carriers for genetic material and vaccines [143]. Ultradeformable liposomes or transfersomes were tested in a topical delivery system for amphotericin B and were found to enhance the drug penetration towards deep skin layers in a scale 40 times higher than Ambisome®, making this system clinically significant [93].

Ethosomes are essentially a type of transfersome that employs ethanol instead of the edge activator molecules; the main difference lies in the fact that ethanol evaporates once applied on the skin, whereas the edge activator molecules remain on the skin surface after water evaporation from the formulations [144].

Ethanol also plays an essential role in enhancing the delivery of both hydrophilic and lipophilic drugs without impairing their deformability and elastic characteristics, which was a significant disadvantage of transfersomes [143]. Henceforth ethosomes show great potential as topical delivery systems for antifungal drugs [134].

The formulation of an ethosomal gel containing econazole nitrate pointed out the outstanding potential of this system to function as a topical delivery system, since it allowed controlled drug release, increased antifungal activity, and good stability after storage [31].

Fluconazole is used both for local and systemic fungal infections. Despite its worldwide usage, it shows low penetration rate because of its high solubility and low permeability. The preparation of an ethosomal gel for topical delivery of fluconazole has proved to be an efficient way to overcome the issues associated with bioavailability, degradation, stability, and side effects of this therapeutic agent [67].

Although the great potential of ethosomes, when the concentration of ethanol used is above 30–40% w/w, the vesicular membrane tends to become more permeable and leaky, leaking out the entrapped drug, specially hydrophilic/ionized drugs [45,145]. Furthermore, this high ethanolic content may affect the skin causing irritation or contact dermatitis. To solve that, Cavamax W7, a permeation enhancer, was developed so as to improve topical delivery and to reduce the amount of ethanol used therefore reducing the risk of adverse effects [45]. The Cavamax W7 ethosomes were able to reach the last layer of epidermis (stratum basale) which turned them into a very valuable tool in the treatment of deep-seated fungal infections [134]. A clotrimazole encapsulated Cavamax W7 composite ethosome gel presented a more stable and more efficient vesicular system than the conventional ethosomal formulation along with a better antifungal activity against *Candida albicans* and *Aspergillus niger* [45].

Transethosomes are lipid vesicles with irregular shapes that represent a combination of the concepts applied to transfersomes and ethosomes, having a high content of ethanol (up to 30%) along with an edge activator molecule. This combination causes a rearrangement in the lipid bilayer of transethosomes, allowing them to have both higher deformability and skin permeation/penetration than the other deformable molecules. The formulation of these vesicles also presents the advantage of being quite easy to scale up, which constitutes an enormous advantage for industrial purposes [144]. Contrary to other deformable vesicles, transethosomes improve skin delivery of drugs both under occlusive and non-occlusive condition [146]. For these reasons, they are considered the most promising lipid nanoparticles in antifungal therapy.

An econazole nitrate loaded transethosome gel for transdermal delivery has been developed. Comparing it with the marketed cream of econazole nitrate, the authors found out that the former presented less ex vivo penetration, higher ex vivo skin retention, and higher in vitro antifungal activity [32]. Transethosomes containing terbinafine, amphotericin B, ketoconazole also disclosed enhanced permeation [146]. In addition, voriconazole transethosomes significantly enhanced skin permeation and deposition of the drug when compared to conventional liposomes, transfersomes, and ethosomes [74].

Regardless of the fact that transethosomes represent the state-of-the-art in ultradeformable vesicles, they still have some drawbacks that are important to mention such as the solubility that the drugs need to fulfil in both lipophilic and aqueous environment so that they can reach the dermal microcirculation and access the systemic circulation. In addition, the molecular size of the drug needs to be reasonable to make the percutaneous absorption possible (40–200 nm) [146].

Solid Lipid Nanoparticles (SLN) and Nanostructured Lipid Carriers (NLC) have become very attractive options to the development of drugs for cutaneous application and as an alternative to overcome the drawbacks of liposomes. They provide an occlusive effect by virtue of their ability to form a surface film that reduces the transepidermal water loss, which can reduce the atopic eczema symptoms and improve the skin appearance [147]. Besides that, they exhibit an excellent tolerability profile and its reduced size promotes a closer contact with the stratum corneum, intensifying the skin penetration of drugs. These particles are also able to increase the chemical stability of compounds sensitive to light, oxidation, and hydrolysis [148].

One application of SLN and NLC is the incorporation of azoles to treat cutaneous fungal infections. The most common azoles (clotrimazole, miconazole, econazole) are extremely water insoluble, being very difficult to administrate and to release those drugs in infection sites. However, compounds with lipophilic character can be efficiently encapsulated in SLNs [107].

In 2010, a formulation was developed in which the SLN nanoparticles were dispersed in a hydrogel to carry miconazole nitrate (MN), an azole frequently used in cutaneous fungal infections [149]. The studies indicated that this MN-loaded SLN-bearing hydrogel formulation was less prone to cause cutaneous irritation in comparison to the MN hydrogel and MN suspension formulation, showing an even greater efficacy in animal models (male albino rabbits). Furthermore, SLN-bearing hydrogel provided sustained release of miconazole (slow initial release with a lag time of 1 h and a sustained drug release over a 24 h period) with greater drug deposition on the skin. This happens because gels help disperse the matrix carriers evenly, increasing the contact time and the deposition of carriers on the skin, resulting in a higher cutaneous penetration of the drug [16,149].

2.4.2. Polymeric Nanoparticles

Polymeric nanoparticles are produced either from natural or synthetic polymers, in which the drug is dissolved, trapped, or bound to the nanoparticle matrix. Depending upon the composition of the organic phase and the preparation method, nanocapsules (matrix-like structure) or nanospheres (core-shell morphology) can be obtained [110,150].

These nanoparticles are capable of carrying proteins, DNA, and drugs, such as antifungals, for cells and specific target organs, which increases the safety profile. Their nanometric size promotes an effective permeation through the cellular membranes and increases their stability in blood flow.

It is also important to point out the gelling systems that can be used to formulate polymeric carriers: microsponges and nanosponges, amphiphilic gels and emulgels or gellified emulsions, which play an important role in cutaneous drug delivery [143].

Microsponge and nanosponge systems are polymer-based spheres that can encapsulate or suspend many substances and then be incorporated into a dosage form (hydrogel) or be used for oral delivery [44,66,151].

A polymeric microsponge based gel system was successfully produced for the topical delivery of fluconazole, with especially great entrapment efficiency, production yield, and extended drug release, which allows a reduction in application frequency, a feature with great importance in recidivist and prolonged fungal infections [66].

A nanosponge based gel formulation loaded with clotrimazole showed controlled release with reduced side effects, indicating the safe and effective profile of these colloidal carriers for topical use [46]. An econazole nanosponge hydrogel was developed and was found to solubilize poorly soluble drugs and also had the ability of forming a local depot for sustained drug release [33].

Amphiphilic gels are semisolid systems of nonionic nature that can be used as topical/transdermal carriers without promoting irritation of the skin. They aim at delivering the antifungal in a level within the therapeutic window for as long as possible and to avoid fluctuations in plasma drug level [69].

An amphiphilogel of fluconazole was successfully formulated for topical application, presenting overall stability and cumulative drug release within the range expected [69].

Emulgels have dual release control system (emulsion/microemulsion and gel), which increases the overall stability of the antifungal formulations [143]. In comparison to conventional creams or ointments, they exhibit better application properties, faster, and more complete drug release profile and they lack greasiness and residues upon application [47].

Emulgels are suitable solutions to incorporate hydrophobic drugs in water soluble gel bases, for instance the incorporation of clotrimazole in an emulgel formulation prepared using either Carbopol 934 or HMPC 2910 showed good physical properties, stability, and antifungal activity [47].

A formulation with amphotericin B encapsulated in poly(lactic-co-glycolic acid) PLGA in association with ε-caprolactone was developed and proved the potential of polymeric nanoparticles in preventing cytotoxicity, yet preserving the fungicidal efficacy. With this polymeric combination, the authors described an amphotericin B encapsulation efficacy of 84% and a fungicidal effect for *Candida albicans* equal to the free drug, with the advantage of presenting less toxicity and less mortality associated [91].

A nanoformulation of the same drug in PLGA was also developed but, this time, it was functionalized with dimercaptosuccinic acid (DMSA). This acid exhibits tropism to lungs, being appropriate to be included in a formulation in which it is desired a release at this site. In this study an intraperitoneal administration was also tested and verified that the therapeutic effect on paracoccidioidomycosis (PCM) was equivalent to the free drug. The greatest advantage of this formulation was that it only required to be taken every three days, given the slow release of amphotericin B from the nanoparticles, and did not require a daily administration as the currently commercialized formulation [152].

Chitosan is a very versatile polymer owing to the ease presented by their groups to be modified or deacetylated [153]. Some studies have shown that this polymer also possesses antioxidant, antimicrobial, and anti-inflammatory properties, becoming very attractive from a biopharmaceutical viewpoint [154]. Some other studies pointed out that chitosan nanoparticles themselves have a huge potential to become safe and effective antifungal agents [155].

Chitosan nanoparticles containing amphotericin B were initially developed with the aim of avoiding the drug gastrointestinal degradation, increasing the stability and the bioavailability in target organs like the lung, the liver, and the spleen, whilst decreasing renal exposition. The researchers determined that when administered by an oral route, these nanoparticles were effective in treating visceral leishmaniosis, aspergillosis, and candidiasis, showing an efficacy comparable to the parenteral

Ambisome® formulation. Moreover, this natural polysaccharide was also employed in the cutaneous release of amphotericin B in wounds caused by infected burns with *Candida albicans*, promoting better tissue healing and increased antifungal activity, when compared to the conventional formulation [156].

Polymeric micelles present a unique architecture where the hydrophobic core can incorporate hydrophobic drugs, such as antifungals, which leads to a very significant improvement in their aqueous solubility [134]. These systems have attracted attention in drug delivery because their critical micelle concentration (CMC) is several 1000-fold lower (<10 mg/L) than classic micelles, this means that ionic surfactants have greater ease in self-assembling in water to form micelles [157].

Amphotericin B has been incorporated in polymeric micelles to treat brain fungal infections. The system was intended to improve drug solubility and permeability through biological membranes as well as obviate issues like high toxicity and low efficacy against *Candida meningoencephalitis* [94].

Polymersomes are spherical structures composed of an aqueous core surrounded by a polymeric bilayer membrane, being viewed as synthetic analogues to liposomes. They are very versatile structures, which spontaneously self-assemble from amphiphilic diblock copolymers. This capacity increases drug efficacy and enables them to encapsulate both hydrophilic and hydrophobic drugs, including antifungals [158,159]. Furthermore, polymersomes present stimuli-responsive drug release, which means that their physical and chemical properties are mutable in response to certain features (pH, temperature, redox conditions, light, magnetic field, ionic strength, or even concentration). This ability is promising in drug-controlled release, an important feature in antifungal drug therapy [159,160]. In Figure 3 the process by which a polymersome is formed is represented as well as its ability to carry different biological molecules.

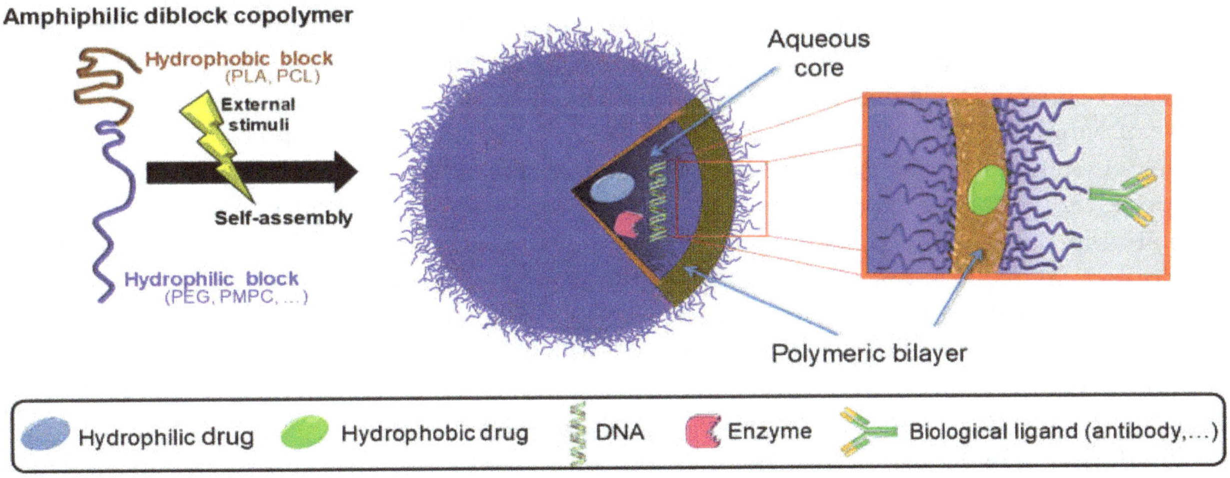

Figure 3. Schematic representation of the formation of a polymersome and its versatile properties. Polymersomes are generally self-assembled from block copolymers, presenting a unique structure that is able to encapsulate different biological molecules.

A research group developed an amphotericin B loaded polymersome by solvent injection method, using $(PEG)_3$-PLA as co-polymer. This formulation was compared with two marketed formulations (Fungizone® and Ambisome®) in terms of release, molecular organization of amphotericin B, and hemolysis. The results were similar to the marketed formulations, which indicated the potential for further in vivo development [92].

Dendrimers are homogenous polymeric tridimensional nanoarchitectures characterized by a highly-branched and symmetrical structure consisting of a central core (a single atom or a group of atoms), building blocks of repeating units emanating from the core (generations), and a high density of water-soluble functional groups on the surface (terminal group) [161–163]. The elements are added through sequential interactive chemical reactions to the central core, the spaces within the voids facilitate the encapsulation of active substances within the dendritic structure, and the terminal functional groups dictate the efficacy of nucleic acid complexation or drug entrapment [164]. Their nano and uniform size structure (2–10 nm in diameter), high degree of branching, water solubility, multivalence, well-defined molecular weight, and available internal cavities makes them extremely valuable as drug delivery systems and as carrier systems for antifungal agents [161,165].

Albeit different types of dendrimers have been described, the most frequently used for antifungal therapy are polyamidoamine (PAMAM) and polypropylene imine (PPI) dendrimers [163]. PAMAM dendrimers containing ketoconazole were shown to improve the solubility and the in vitro release of the drug and also to enhance the antifungal activity of ketoconazole [41].

2.4.3. Metallic Nanoparticles

Three main groups of metallic nanoparticles, gold, silver, and magnetic, can be used for the vectorization of antifungal drugs.

Metallic nanoparticles can be synthetized in three different ways: chemically, physically, and biologically. Chemical synthesis has been associated with many side effects related with the absorption of toxic chemical particles on the surface of nanoparticles [10], thereupon the biological synthesis is acquiring some expression [166].

Gold nanoparticles are used in immunochemical studies to identify protein interactions and in DNA fingerprinting to detect DNA in a sample. They are also used to detect aminoglycosides like streptomycin, gentamicin, and neomycin [10].

Silver nanoparticles are the most efficient on account of their antimicrobial efficacy against bacteria, viruses, and other eukaryotic microorganisms. In fact, they are the most used materials, being applied as antimicrobial agents in textile industry, for water treatment, in solar protectors, etc. [10].

Albeit nanostructures of iron, cobalt, and nickel exhibit superparamagnetic properties and high magnetic susceptibility, superparamagnetic iron oxide nanoparticles such as magnetite (Fe_3O_4), hematite (α-Fe_2O_3), and maghemite (γ-Fe_2O_3), are the most studied types of magnetic nanoparticles. This type of nanoparticle has received special attention by virtue of their capacity to be influenced by magnetic fields, therefore being easily directed and released in a specific site of the organism [10,167].

Superparamagnetic iron oxide nanoparticles present other unique properties, for instance: low toxicity, biocompatibility, potent magnetic targeting capacity, and chemical inertia, thus, they have many biomedical applications, for example in the cancer research field, steam cells, tissue repair, drug release, genetic therapy, DNA analysis, and clinical diagnosis through magnetic resonance [10,167].

Nowadays, nanoparticles of superparamagnetic iron oxide are the ones that answer more efficiently to an external magnetic field, being the ones with more potential to become drug carriers [5]. In order to bypass cytotoxic effects, these Fe_3O_4 magnetic nanoparticles need to be coated, usually with DMSA (meso-2,3-dimercaptosuccinic acid); this is a procedure that is important not only to increase cell internalization and biocompatibility, but also to carry active molecules to the nanoparticle's surface, essential to drug delivery [168].

2.4.4. Other Drug Delivery Systems

Niosomes are non-phospholipid vesicles made of non-ionic surfactants that serve as drug depots in the body as they release the drug in a sustained fashion through its bilayers. They are also able to improve oral bioavailability of poorly soluble drugs, enhance the skin permeability of topical drugs, protect the enclosed active substance from deleterious factors, and increase the stability of the entrapped drug [169].

Nistatin was successfully encapsulated in niosomes and a safe and effective formula for parenteral administration was obtained. This formulation provided reduced nephrotoxicity and hepatoxicity in female Wistar rats and showed pronounced efficacy against *Candida albicans* with a higher level of drug in vital organs [99]. The encapsulation of ciclopirox in niosomes increased the half-life, promoted a prolonged drug release, and minimized the side effects [103]. Given the poor water solubility of griseofulvin and its slow absorption from oral route, a niosome was produced in order to enhance bioavailability of this active substance, to accelerate its absorption and to obtain a sustained release, acting as a depot inside the body [100].

Ketoconazole niosomal gel showed more prolonged action than conventional ketoconazole formulations, hence it can be developed in order to improve the antifungal activity [38].

Spanlastics are termed as modified niosomes which present better permeability because they have edge activators in their composition, like transfersomes and transethosomes [134,145].

These systems show great flexibility allowing them to pass through fenestrations smaller than their own radius in order to enter the cell, simultaneously minimizing the possibility of damaging the vesicles while squashing [138].

Firstly, there were ketoconazole-loaded spanlastics for ocular drug delivery [40] and then spanlastics were loaded with terbinafine hydrochloride for treatment of onychomycosis [79].

Microemulsions are colloidal carriers that consist of a liquid dispersion of oil and water stabilized by an interfacial film of surfactant. Due to this, they are able to incorporate drugs of different lipophilicity [170]. They are promising colloidal carriers because of their transparency, ease of preparation, and long-term stability [171].

When it comes to drug delivery through stratum corneum, microemulsions are very resourceful considering the ability of the oils and surfactants included in their composition to act as skin penetration enhancers [170,172]. Furthermore, they are also good candidates for oral delivery of poorly water-soluble drugs as they can improve their solubilization.

Terbinafine hydrochloride is an example of a slightly water-soluble drug, which presented higher solubility, an increase in the dissolution rate, and better efficacy when incorporated within a microemulsion [170,171]. Likewise, a microemulsion system of voriconazole also showed a significant increase in the antifungal activity against *Candida albicans*, along with better drug skin penetration [173].

Nanoemulsions are thermodynamically and kinetically more stable than emulsions, so they have been evaluated as colloidal carriers to improve the efficacy and tolerability of some antifungal drugs. The capacity of nanoemulsions to dissolve large quantities of drugs with low solubility, their compatibility, their ability to protect drugs from enzymatic degradation and hydrolysis as well as their capacity to penetrate the deeper skin layers, turns them into ideal drug delivery vectors [143,174].

A nystatin nanoemulsion for topical application was developed and was found to have a higher antifungal effect than nystatin itself, representing a therapeutic improvement [97].

Silicon dioxide nanoparticles have been studied as drug carriers to enhance the antimicrobial activity of some drugs, because of their biodegradability, low toxicity, capacity to stimulate macrophages, and the ease by which they are synthetized and modified. The foremost advantage of these nanoparticles is that they can be loaded with large amounts of drug [95,175].

There are four main types of silica nanoparticles, but their antifungal potential is yet to be studied in some cases:

- Nitric oxide-silica nanoparticles with proven anti-biofilm activity [108];
- Metal modified silica nanoparticles, which can include silver or copper, metals that have a very well documented antimicrobial effect, derived from the cell membrane and DNA damages, interaction with enzymes from thiol groups or are associated with generating hydrogen peroxide [176];
- Surface-modified silica nanoparticles by quaternary ammonium compounds loaded with antifungal agents [177,178];
- Bioglasses and bioceramics [179].

Amongst them, mesoporous silica nanoparticles are the ones who have become the most promising candidates for many biomedical applications, specifically for antifungal therapy, because of their uniformed mesoporous tunnels and narrow pore size distribution. Besides that, they present outstanding biocompatibility and chemical stability and can be degraded and metabolized over a relatively short term. These aspects allow high drug loading and reduce the probability of particle-induced toxicity [95,180].

In a study, one group of mice with candidiasis induced by *Candida albicans* was treated with silica nanoparticles functionalized with amphotericin B and the other group was treated with officinal amphotericin B. It was possible to observe that the first group showed a significant increase in survival rates [95]. This confirms the fact that silica nanoparticles coated with quaternary ammonium surfactants have higher fungicidal and fungistatic effect against *Candida albicans* than colloidal silver [177,178].

In order to increase the oral bioavailability of itraconazole, a poorly water-soluble antifungal drug, mesoporous silica particles formulation was developed. It was concluded that ordered mesoporous silica can, in fact, be considered a promising carrier seeing that it enhances the oral bioavailability of extremely low water-soluble drugs [60].

It has been demonstrated that metals can easily accumulate in soil and then enter the food chain, thus the combination of Ag+ ions with silica prevents the formation of these ions and reduces its toxicity [176]. That is the reason why silica nanoparticles have also been studied for agricultural purposes as safe and effective alternative fungicides, for example to manage tomato early blight [180].

3. Hidden Potential and Challenges of Natural Antifungal Compounds

From 1981 to 2014, 32 new chemical entities were placed on the market to treat fungal infections: one from a biological source (interferon gamma-n1), that is a peptide produced by a biotechnological procedure; three derived from a natural product that suffered a semisynthetic modification (anidulafungin, caspofungin, micafungin); 25 totally synthetic discovered by random screening or through the modification of an existing agent (fluconazole, itraconazole, ketoconazole, amorolfine, ciclopirox; three synthetically synthesized with the molecule or the pharmacophore mimicking a natural product (butenafine, liranaftate, terbinafine) [181].

In fact, almost 90% of the antifungal agents approved within this period were from a synthetic origin. This paucity of natural products in modern treatments remains a reality and 1950s agents like amphotericin and griseofulvin are still widely used [181].

One good example of an efficient employment of natural products to nanoparticle synthesis happened with *Mentha pulegium* L., commonly known as pennyroyal, a flowering herb with antitussive, carminative, and antiseptic effects. This herb was successfully used to synthesize stable colloidal silver nanoparticles with promising antifungal effects against *Candida albicans* [182].

On the other hand, the marine environment represents a valuable and unexplored platform to the discovery of new compounds [183]. In Table 4, there is an overview of the natural products that have shown in vitro or in vivo potential as antifungal agents isolated from diverse marine organisms: microorganisms (bacteria and fungi), invertebrates (sponges, corals and sea cucumbers), and marine algae are presented.

Table 4. Overview of antifungal natural compounds produced by marine organisms [183,184].

Marine Organism	Source Organism	Type of Compound	Compound Name	Spectrum of Activity
Bacteria (30% of total)	*Bacillus licheniformis*	Glycolipid	Ledoglucomide C, Iedoglycolipid	*Aspergillus niger, Rhizoctonia solani, Botrytis cinerea, and Colletotrichum acutatum, Candida albicans*
	Bacillus subtilis	Lipopeptide	Gageopeptides A-D	*R. solani, P. capsici, B. cinerea, C. acutatum*
	Actinoalloteichus sp. NPS702	Macrolide	Neomaclafungins A-I	*Trichophyton mentagrophytes*
	Streptomyces sp.	Peptide	Mohangamide A	*C. albicans*
	Bacillus marinus	Macrolide	Macrolactins T and B	*Pyricularia oryzae, A. solani*
	Tolypothrix	Lipopeptide	Hassallidin A	*A. fumigatus and C. albicans*
	Chondromyces pediculatus	Peptide	Pedein A	*Rhodotorula glutinis*
Fungi (15% of total)	*Stagonosporopsis cucurbitacearum*	Alkaloid	Didymellamide A	*C. neoformans, C. albicans, C. glabrata*
	Aspergillus sclerotiorum	Peptide	Sclerotide B	*C. albicans*
	Penicillium bilaiae MA-267	Sesquiterpene	Penicibilaenes A and B	*C. gloeosporioides*

Table 4. *Cont.*

Marine Organism	Source Organism	Type of Compound	Compound Name	Spectrum of Activity
Sponge (35%)	*Theonella swinhoei*	Peptide	Theonegramide, Theonellamide G, Cyclolithistide A	*C. albicans*
	Halichondria cylindrata	Peptide	Halicylindramide D and E	*Mortierella ramanniana*
	Siliquariaspongia mirabilis, Theonella swinhoei	Peptide	Theopapuamide A; B and C	*C. albicans*
	Jaspis johnstoni	Peptide	Jasplakinolide	*C. albicans, C. pseidrotropicalis, C. parapsilosis*
	Monanchora arbuscular	Alkaloid	Batzelladine L	*A. flavus*
	Xestospongia muta	Furan	Mutafuran D	*Cryptococcus neoformans var.grubii*
Corals (5%)	*Clavelina oblonga*	Alkanol	(2S,3R)-2-aminododecan-3-ol	*C. albicans ATCC 10231, C. glabrata*
Sea cucumbers (6%)	*Stichopus variegates*	Triterpene glycoside	Variegatuside D	*C. albicans, C. pseudo- tropicalis, C. parapsilosis, and M. gypseum*
Algae (9%)	*Caulerpa racemos*	Xylene	Caulerprenylol B	*T. rubrum*

Sponges have always interested pharmacologists, chemists, and biologists as a rich source of antimicrobial compounds with peculiar activities. These colonial organisms have a sessile nature, hence the necessity of producing compounds as a way of protecting themselves, communicating, or modulating their cellular functions [184].

Peptides have high relevance as potential drugs, given their large spectrum of bioactivity. Sponges that belong to the Theonella gender are a recognized source of uncommon peptides with antibacterial, antifungal, and anti-HIV properties. The antifungal activity of some of these peptides is even surplus to other commercial formulations, as seen through their diffusion zone in the agar diffusion method [184].

Although some formulations containing marine compounds are already being subjected to clinical trials, none of them target fungal infections [183].

Theopapuamide A is a cyclic depsipeptide (a peptide in which one or more amides were replaced by an ester group) being firstly isolated from the sponge *Theonella swinhoei* from Papua New Guinea [183]. Its isolation, structural elucidation, and stereochemical analysis are well described in literature [185]. It is capable of inhibiting the growth of *Candida albicans* wild strains and also strains resistant to amphotericin B [186]. In addition, it presents anti-HIV activity, thanks to the 3,4-dimethyl-L-glutamine residue in its chemical structure [183,184].

Besides the marine environment, a considerable number of studies have been conducted on medicinal plants and alternative compounds, such as secondary metabolites, phenolic compounds, essential oils, and extracts. Some plant extracts (*Curcuma zedoaria, Psidium guajava, Plectranthus amboinicus, Lippia alba*) have shown activity against *Candida* spp. and others (*Asteraceae, Euphorbiaceae, Rubiaceae,* and *Solanaceae*) against filamentous fungi. Despite the streamline nature of the discovery process, the biological activity found during the screening of plant extracts, may not be experimentally reproducible. This can be due to many reasons: the chemical constituents in the crude extracts may be different, the solvent used to extract may destroy some compounds and chemical composition may vary according to the growth stage or geographic origin. Some components of essential oils, mainly terpenes or terpenoids, such as eugenol, camphor, curcumin, geraniol, and linalol show activity against a wide variety of Candida species and others like clemateol or citral are active against *Trichophyton* spp. or *Malassezia* spp. respectively. Propolis, which represents the resinous substances collected from plants by bees, demonstrated activity against *Candida* spp., some dermatophytes, and onychomycosis. Ajoene, a compound derived from garlic, has shown effectiveness in the treatment of paracoccidioidomycosis and *Fusarium* spp. infections. Other compounds such as saponins, alkaloids, flavonoids, coumarins, xanthones, lignans, and tannins also presented antifungal activity [187].

There is, in fact, a growing awareness of the limited structural diversity in existing compound libraries and that there are many benefits in exploiting the huge chemical diversity and high biological activity of natural compounds. Furthermore, it is possible to use these natural compounds as platforms to discover drug-like characteristics and produce new substances [188]. Therefore, natural compounds with antifungal properties represent a valuable alternative to current antifungals and their incorporation in nanocarriers is a significant step ahead in nanoformulation, besides being a more sustainable option, because it employs marine resources [183].

Since the discovery of penicillin, the pharmaceutical industry has extensively relied on natural products as sources of structural templates for drug discovery and development [188,189].

Regardless of this fact, the discovery and development of natural-derived medicines has been on a steady decline over the last years, possibly due to high throughput screening. This tool has changed the paradigm of drug discovery in the pharmaceutical industry since it allows the automatic screening of thousands to millions of drug candidates within vast libraries. There is every likelihood that these libraries contain a significant representation of all existing compounds, complicating the discovery of a new natural chemical entity itself [190].

Although a valuable and precious resource, natural products brought about their fair share of challenges in a wide variety of features, compromising their inclusion in the clinical pipeline.

The main issue lies in the fact that natural substances are not always abundant and they generally require laborious extraction and purification steps through complex, expensive, and time-consuming processes, often to obtain just few quantities of extract [190]. Moreover, there are no standard protocols and research groups modify the existing procedures, making the studies not reproducible and not comparable [187].

In addition, environmental aspects pose significant hurdles for drug discovery and development because the substance may come from an endangered species and its overexploitation can lead to habitat destruction [188].

The regulatory requirements for substances containing natural substances (medicines, nutraceuticals, and cosmeceuticals) range from rather strict to non-existent and vary between regions, being under the surveillance of different authorities [188].

4. Ongoing Clinical Trials on Myconanotechnology

Several pharmaceutical industries and authors have been performing clinical trials on antifungal nanomedicines. Despite the growing improvement on applying nanotechnology for drug development, just a few of those nanomedicines have been approved for their clinical applications. The major issues with clinical trials are their time-consuming process and the difficulty while accessing and researching information on previous nanomedicine trends. In the mycology field, amphotericin-B is the active substance that represents the majority of the nanomedicines already available in the market: Amphotec® (Three Rivers Pharmaceuticals, approved in 1992), Abelcet® (Sigma-Tau, approved in 1995) and Ambisome® (Gilead Sciences, approved in 1997), all lipid-based formulations [191,192]. An econazole liposomal formulation (Pevaryllipogel®) is also available on the market [193]. In Table 5 some examples of recent clinical trials are presented.

Table 5. Some examples of ongoing clinical trials on myconanotechnology [194].

Trade Name/Sponsor	ClinicalTrials.gov Identifier	Antifungal	Nanoformulation	Clinical Phase	Disease
Sara Botros, Minia University	NCT04110834	Itraconazole	Nanoemulsion gel	II	*Tinea versicolor*
Sara Botros, Minia University	NCT04110860	Voriconazol	Nanoemulsion gel	II	*Tinea versicolor*
Matinas BioPharma	NCT02971007	Amphotericin B	Cochleate lipid-crystal nanoparticle	II	Vulvovaginal candidiasis
Matinas BioPharma	NCT02629419	Amphotericin B	Cochleate lipid-crystal nanoparticle	II	Mucocutaneous candidiasis

Table 5. *Cont.*

Trade Name/Sponsor	ClinicalTrials.gov Identifier	Antifungal	Nanoformulation	Clinical Phase	Disease
Ahmed Abdellatif, Al-Azhar University	NCT03752424	-	Silver nanoparticle gel	I	Mycosis
Mona Badran, Cairo University	NCT03666195	-	Titanium dioxide nanoparticles	Recruiting	Candidiasis
Rasha Hamed, Assiut University	NCT04431804	-	Silver nanoparticle	Recruiting	Invasive aspergillosis
Celtic Pharma Development Services	NCT01145807	Terbinafine (TDT067)	Transfersome	III	Onychomycosis

5. Conclusions

The present pace of antifungal drug development is highly unlikely to keep up with the clinical needs, especially with the uprising of resistance to current agents. Therefore, more therapeutic answers to fungal illnesses are urgently needed.

The subject of sustainability and environmental impact has gained considerable relevance in today's societies and scientific research, motivating a heated debate on whether there should be an active research for new natural compounds with biological activity or if the pillar of today's research for new compounds should be high throughput screening. The fact is that two out of the three major classes of antifungal drugs (polyenes and echinocandins) were screened from natural products. The utilization of natural compounds, such as chitosan is, irrefutably, a more sustainable option and brings both environmental and pharmacokinetic advantages to nanotechnological approaches. Compounds from a marine origin exhibit an undeniable potential, but their activity and toxicity mechanisms are yet to be clarified.

Nanoparticles have been presented as promising solutions, mainly due to their ability to target specific sites where fungi are harbored, their capacity to enhance the pharmacological effect of drugs, optimizing their physiochemical characteristics, thereby allowing an administration through a more comfortable route. All these features can enable lower dosing, more comfortable regimens, increased bioavailability, and less serious adverse effects.

Special attention has been given to certain kinds of nanoparticles nowadays mainly because of the outstanding features they exhibit: (a) magnetic nanoparticles and their capacity to directly restrict fungal growth, (b) ultradeformable vesicles (transethosomes) and their ease on scaling up, (c) mesoporous silica nanoparticles and their high drug loading, (d) polymersomes and their ability to carry both hydrophobic and hydrophilic substances and to respond to external stimuli, (e) PAMAM dendrimers and their versatile and biocompatible structure. We speculate that future antifungal therapies will mostly lie in these five types of nanoparticles and will take advantage of the current knowledge of using them for other purposes (for instance, as anticancer agents).

These new nanotechnological systems should be able to surpass the issues already mentioned and should also mean a significant upgrade when comparing to the conventional treatments, fighting antifungal resistance, presenting a broad spectrum of activity, with an emphasis on potency increase and little host toxicity, thus having the potential to be industrially produced.

Interdisciplinary cooperation may be the key to a striving success of nanomedicine and nanotechnology, not to mention a proper exploitation of natural medicinal products. Physicists, health-care researchers, and clinical researchers have complementary knowledge that could be put together (for example, innovative screening strategies and novel chemical libraries) so that more effective, practical, and safe nanoparticles are designed. That would increase the chances of an industry funding and, ultimately, a rethinking of current antifungal arsenal, while providing a better quality of life for patients.

Author Contributions: Conceptualization, F.S., P.C. and S.R.; writing—original draft preparation, F.S., S.R.; writing—review and editing, F.S., P.C.; supervision, P.C., D.F. and S.R.; project administration, P.C. All authors have read and agreed to the published version of the manuscript.

References

1. Rai, M.; Ingle, A.P.; Pandit, R.; Paralikar, P.; Gupta, I.; Anasane, N.; Dolenc-Voljč, M. Nanotechnology for the Treatment of Fungal Infections on Human Skin. In *The Microbiology of Skin, Soft Tissue, Bone and Joint Infections*; Academic Press: Cambridge, MA, USA, 2017; pp. 169–184.
2. Pianalto, K.M.; Alspaugh, J.A. New Horizons in Antifungal Therapy. *J. Fungi* **2016**, *2*, 26. [CrossRef]
3. Chang, Y.L.; Yu, S.J.; Heitman, J.; Wellington, M.; Chen, Y.L. New facets of antifungal therapy. *Virulence* **2017**, *8*, 222–236. [CrossRef] [PubMed]
4. Nami, S.; Aghebati-Maleki, A.; Morovati, H.; Aghebati-Maleki, L. Current antifungal drugs and immunotherapeutic approaches as promising strategies to treatment of fungal diseases. *Biomed. Pharm.* **2019**, *110*, 857–868. [CrossRef] [PubMed]
5. Souza, A.C.; Amaral, A.C. Antifungal Therapy for Systemic Mycosis and the Nanobiotechnology Era: Improving Efficacy, Biodistribution and Toxicity. *Front. Microbiol.* **2017**, *8*, 336. [CrossRef] [PubMed]
6. Scorzoni, L.; de Paula e Silva, A.C.A.; Marcos, C.M.; Assato, P.A.; de Melo, W.C.M.A.; de Oliveira, H.C.; Costa-Orlandi, C.B.; Mendes-Giannini, M.J.S.; Fusco-Almeida, A.M. Antifungal Therapy: New Advances in the Understanding and Treatment of Mycosis. *Front. Microbiol.* **2017**, *8*, 36. [CrossRef] [PubMed]
7. Sirish Sadhna Khatry, S.N.; Sadanandan, M. Novel Drug Delivery Systems for Antifungal Therapy. *Int. J. Pharm. Pharm. Sci.* **2010**, *2*, 6–9.
8. Perfect, J.R. Is there an emerging need for new antifungals? *Expert Opin Emerg Drugs* **2016**, *21*, 129–131. [CrossRef] [PubMed]
9. Roli Jain, A.P. A Review of Kinetics of Nanoparticulated Delayed Release Formulations. *J. Nanomed. Nanotechnol.* **2015**, *6*, 2.
10. Hasan, S. A review on Nanoparticles: Their Synthesis and Types. *Res. J. Recent Sci.* **2015**, *4*, 1–3.
11. Nagavarma, B.V.N.; Ayaz, A.H.K.S.Y.; Vasudha, L.S.; Shivahumar, H.G. Different Techniques for Preparation of Polymeric Nanoparticles—A review. *Asian J. Pharm. Clin. Res.* **2012**, *5*, 16–23.
12. Bhatt, P.; Lalani, R.; Vhora, I.; Patil, S.; Amrutiya, J.; Misra, A.; Mashru, R. Liposomes encapsulating native and cyclodextrin enclosed Paclitaxel: Enhanced loading efficiency and its pharmacokinetic evaluation. *Int. J. Pharm.* **2017**, *536*, 95–107. [CrossRef]
13. Jinhyun Hannah Lee, Y.Y. Controlled drug release from pharmaceutical nanocarriers. *Chem. Eng. Sci.* **2015**, *125*, 75–84.
14. D'Souza, S. A Review of In Vitro Drug Release Test Methods for Nano-Sized Dosage Forms. *Adv. Pharm.* **2014**, *2014*, 12.
15. Goyal, R.; Macri, L.K.; Kaplan, H.M.; Kohn, J. Nanoparticles and nanofibers for topical drug delivery. *J. Control Release* **2016**, *240*, 77–92. [CrossRef]
16. Rangari, A.T. Polymeric Nanoparticles Based Topical Drug Delivery: An Overview. *Asian J. Biomed. Pharm. Sci.* **2015**, *5*, 5–12. [CrossRef]
17. Siegel, R.A.; Rathbone, M.J. Chapter 2—Overview of Controlled Release Mechanisms. In *Fundamentals and Applications of Controlled Release Drug Delivery, Advances in Delivery Science and Technology*; Society, C.R., Ed.; Springer: New York, NY, USA, 2012.
18. Firthouse, P.U.M.; Halith, S.M.; Wahab, S.U.; Sirajudeen, M.; Mohideen, S.K. Formulation and Evaluation of Miconazole Niosomes. *Int. J. Pharmtech Res.* **2011**, *3*, 1019–1022.
19. Aljaeid, B.M.; Hosny, K.M. Miconazole-loaded solid lipid nanoparticles: Formulation and evaluation of a novel formula with high bioavailability and antifungal activity. *Int. J. Nanomed.* **2016**, *11*, 441–447. [CrossRef]
20. Bhalekar, M.R.; Pokharkar, V.; Madgulkar, A.; Patil, N.; Patil, N. Preparation and evaluation of miconazole nitrate-loaded solid lipid nanoparticles for topical delivery. *AAPS Pharmscitech* **2009**, *10*, 289–296. [CrossRef]

21. Shahzadi, I.; Masood, M.I.; Chowdhary, F.; Anjum, A.A.; Nawaz, M.A.; Maqsood, I.; Zaman, M.Q. Microemulsion Formulation for Topical Delivery of Miconazole Nitrate. *Int. J. Pharm. Sci. Rev. Res.* **2014**, *24*, 30–36.
22. Elmoslemany, R.M.; Abdallah, O.Y.; El-Khordagui, L.K.; Khalafallah, N.M. Propylene glycol liposomes as a topical delivery system for miconazole nitrate: Comparison with conventional liposomes. *AAPS Pharmscitech* **2012**, *13*, 723–731. [CrossRef]
23. Maha, H.L.; Sinaga, K.R.; Masfria, M. Formulation and evaluation of miconazole nitrate nanoemulsion and cream. *Asian J. Pharm. Clin. Res.* **2018**, *11*, 319–321. [CrossRef]
24. Kumar, P.S.; Hematheerthani, N.; Ratna, J.V.; Saikishore, V. Design and characterization of miconazole nitrate loaded nanosponges containing vaginal gels. *Int. J. Pharm. Anal. Res.* **2016**, *5*, 410–417.
25. Qushawy, M.; Nasr, A.; Abd-Alhaseeb, M.; Swidan, S. Design, Optimization and Characterization of a Transfersomal Gel Using Miconazole Nitrate for the Treatment of Candida Skin Infections. *Pharmaceutics* **2018**, *10*, 26. [CrossRef]
26. Ge, S.; Lin, Y.; Lu, H.; Li, Q.; He, J.; Chen, B.; Wu, C.; Xu, Y. Percutaneous delivery of econazole using microemulsion as vehicle: Formulation, evaluation and vesicle-skin interaction. *Int. J. Pharm.* **2014**, *465*, 120–131. [CrossRef] [PubMed]
27. Evelyn, D.; Wooi, C.C.; Kumar, J.R.; Muralidharan, S.; Dhanaraj, S.A. Development and evaluation of microemulsion based gel (MBGs) containing econazole nitrate for nail fungal infection. *J. Pharm. Res.* **2012**, *5*, 2385–2390.
28. Sanna, V.; Gavini, E.; Cossu, M.; Rassu, G.; Giunchedi, P. Solid lipid nanoparticles (SLN) as carriers for the topical delivery of econazole nitrate: In-vitro characterization, ex-vivo and in-vivo studies. *J. Pharm. Pharm.* **2007**, *59*, 1057–1064. [CrossRef]
29. Keshri, L.; Pathak, K. Development of thermodynamically stable nanostructured lipid carrier system using central composite design for zero order permeation of econazole nitrate through epidermis. *Pharm. Dev. Technol.* **2013**, *18*, 634–644. [CrossRef]
30. Xianrong, Q.; Liu, M.H.; Liu, H.Y.; Maitani, Y.; Nagai, T. Topical econazole delivery using liposomal gel. *S.T.P. Pharma Sci.* **2003**, *13*, 241–245.
31. Verma, P.; Pathak, K. Nanosized ethanolic vesicles loaded with econazole nitrate for the treatment of deep fungal infections through topical gel formulation. *Nanomedicine* **2012**, *8*, 489–496. [CrossRef]
32. Verma, S.; Utreja, P. Transethosomes of Econazole Nitrate for Transdermal Delivery: Development, In-vitro Characterization, and Ex-vivo Assessment. *Pharm. Nanotechnol.* **2018**, *6*, 171–179. [CrossRef]
33. Sharma, R.; Walker, R.B.; Pathak, K. Evaluation of the Kinetics and Mechanism of Drug Release from Econazole nitrate Nanosponge Loaded Carbapol Hydrogel. *Indian J. Pharm. Educ. Res.* **2011**, *45*, 25–31.
34. Kumar, Y.P.; Kumar, K.V.; Shekar, R.R.; Ravi, M.; Kishore, V.S. Formulation and Evaluation of Econazole Niosomes. *Sch. Acad. J. Pharm.* **2013**, *2*, 315–318.
35. Bachhav, Y.G.; Mondon, K.; Kalia, Y.N.; Gurny, R.; Möller, M. Novel micelle formulations to increase cutaneous bioavailability of azole antifungals. *J. Control. Release* **2011**, *153*, 126–132. [CrossRef] [PubMed]
36. Youenang Piemi, M.P.; Korner, D.; Benita, S.; Jean-Paul, M. Positively and negatively charged submicron emulsions for enhanced topical delivery of antifungal drugs. *J. Control. Release* **1999**, *58*, 177–187. [CrossRef]
37. Souto, E.B.; Muller, R.H. SLN and NLC for topical delivery of ketoconazole. *J. Microencapsul.* **2005**, *22*, 501–510. [CrossRef]
38. Shirsand, S.; Para, M.; Nagendrakumar, D.; Kanani, K.; Keerthy, D. Formulation and evaluation of Ketoconazole niosomal gel drug delivery system. *Int. J. Pharm. Investig.* **2012**, *2*, 201–207. [CrossRef]
39. Tiwari, N.; Sivakumar, A.; Mukherjee, A.; Chandrasekaran, N. Enhanced antifungal activity of Ketoconazole using rose oil based novel microemulsion formulation. *J. Drug Deliv. Sci. Technol.* **2018**, *47*, 434–444. [CrossRef]
40. Kakkar, S.; Kaur, I.P. Spanlastics—A novel nanovesicular carrier system for ocular delivery. *Int. J. Pharm.* **2011**, *413*, 202–210. [CrossRef]
41. Winnicka, K.; Wroblewska, M.; Wieczorek, P.; Sacha, P.T.; Tryniszewska, E. Hydrogel of ketoconazole and PAMAM dendrimers: Formulation and antifungal activity. *Molecules* **2012**, *17*, 4612–4624. [CrossRef]
42. Ashe, S.; Nayak, D.; Tiwari, G.; Rauta, P.R.; Nayak, B. Development of liposome-encapsulated ketoconazole: Formulation, characterisation and evaluation of pharmacological therapeutic efficacy. *Micro. Nano Lett.* **2015**, *10*, 126–129. [CrossRef]

43. Ning, M.; Guo, Y.; Pan, H.; Chen, X.; Gu, Z. Preparation, in vitro and in vivo evaluation of liposomal/niosomal gel delivery systems for clotrimazole. *Drug Dev. Ind. Pharm.* **2005**, *31*, 375–383. [CrossRef] [PubMed]
44. Kumar, A.S.; Sheri, P.S.; Kuriachan, M.A. Formulation and Evaluation of Antifungal Nanosponge Loaded Hydrogel for Topical Delivery. *Int. J. Pharm. Pharm. Res.* **2018**, *13*, 362–379.
45. Akhtar, N.; Pathak, K. Cavamax W7 Composite Ethosomal Gel of Clotrimazole for Improved Topical Delivery: Development and Comparison with Ethosomal Gel. *Am. Assoc. Pharm. Sci.* **2012**, *13*, 344–355. [CrossRef] [PubMed]
46. Shirsand, S.; Kumar, R.; Keshavshetti, G.; Bushetti, S.S.; Padivala, V.S. Formulation and Evaluation of Clotrimazole Niosomal Gel for Topical Application. *Rajiv Gandhi Univ. Health Sci. J. Pharm. Sci.* **2015**, *5*, 32–38. [CrossRef]
47. Yassin, G.E. Formulation and Evaluation of Optimized Clotrimazole Emulgel Formulations. *Br. J. Pharm. Res.* **2014**, *4*, 1014–1030. [CrossRef]
48. Souto, E.B.; Wissing, S.A.; Barbosa, C.M.; Müller, R.H. Development of a controlled release formulation based on SLN and NLC for topical clotrimazole delivery. *Int. J. Pharm.* **2004**, *278*, 71–77. [CrossRef]
49. Kaewbanjong, J.; Heng, P.W.S.; Boonme, P. Clotrimazole microemulsion and microemulsion-based gel: Evaluation of buccal drug delivery and irritancy using chick chorioallantoic membrane as the model. *J. Pharm. Pharm.* **2017**, *69*, 1716–1723. [CrossRef]
50. Bachhav, Y.G.; Patravale, V.B. Microemulsion-based vaginal gel of clotrimazole: Formulation, in vitro evaluation, and stability studies. *AAPS Pharmscitech* **2009**, *10*, 476–481. [CrossRef]
51. Maheshwari, R.G.S.; Tekade, R.K.; Sharma, P.A.; Darwhekar, G.; Tyagi, A.; Patel, R.P.; Jain, D.K. Ethosomes and ultradeformable liposomes for transdermal delivery of clotrimazole: A comparative assessment. *Saudi Pharm. J. Spj. Off. Publ. Saudi Pharm. Soc.* **2012**, *20*, 161–170. [CrossRef]
52. Zheng, W.S.; Fang, X.Q.; Wang, L.L.; Zhang, Y.J. Preparation and quality assessment of itraconazole transfersomes. *Int. J. Pharm.* **2012**, *436*, 291–298. [CrossRef]
53. Mohanty, B.; Majumdar, D.K.; Mishra, S.K.; Panda, A.K.; Patnaik, S. Development and characterization of itraconazole-loaded solid lipid nanoparticles for ocular delivery. *Pharm. Dev. Technol.* **2015**, *20*, 458–464. [CrossRef] [PubMed]
54. Pardeike, J.; Weber, S.; Haber, T.; Wagner, J.; Zarfl, H.P.; Plank, H.; Zimmer, A. Development of an itraconazole-loaded nanostructured lipid carrier (NLC) formulation for pulmonary application. *Int. J. Pharm.* **2011**, *419*, 329–338. [CrossRef] [PubMed]
55. Wagh, V.D.; Deshmukh, O.J. Itraconazole Niosomes Drug Delivery System and Its Antimycotic Activity against Candida albicans. *Isrn. Pharm.* **2012**, *2012*, 653465. [CrossRef] [PubMed]
56. Chudasama, A.; Patel, V.; Nivsarkar, M.; Vasu, K.; Shishoo, C. Investigation of microemulsion system for transdermal delivery of itraconazole. *J. Adv. Pharm. Technol. Res.* **2011**, *2*, 30–38.
57. Leal, A.F.; Leite, M.C.; Medeiros, C.S.; Cavalcanti, I.M.; Wanderley, A.G.; Magalhaes, N.S.; Neves, R.P. Antifungal activity of a liposomal itraconazole formulation in experimental Aspergillus flavus keratitis with endophthalmitis. *Mycopathologia* **2015**, *179*, 225–229. [CrossRef]
58. Leal, A.F.; Leite, M.C.; Medeiros, C.S.; Cavalcanti, I.M.; Wanderley, A.G.; Magalhaes, N.S.; Neves, R.P. Development of an itraconazole encapsulated polymeric nanoparticle platform for effective antifungal therapy. *J. Mater. Chem. B* **2016**, *4*, 1787–1796.
59. ElMeshad, A.N.; Mohsen, A.M. Enhanced corneal permeation and antimycotic activity of itraconazole against Candida albicans via a novel nanosystem vesicle. *Drug Deliv.* **2016**, *23*, 2115–2123. [CrossRef]
60. Mellaerts, R.; Mols, R.; Jammaer, J.A.G.; Aerts, C.A.; Annaert, P.; Van Humbeeck, J.; Van den Mooter, G.; Augustijns, P.; Martens, J.A. Increasing the oral bioavailability of the poorly water soluble drug itraconazole with ordered mesoporous silica. *Eur. J. Pharm. Biopharm.* **2008**, *69*, 223–230. [CrossRef]
61. Bachhav, Y.G.; Patravale, V.B. Microemulsion based vaginal gel of fluconazole: Formulation, in vitro and in vivo evaluation. *Int. J. Pharm.* **2009**, *365*, 175–179. [CrossRef]
62. Soliman, O.A.E.; Mohamed, E.A.; Khatera, N.A.A. Enhanced ocular bioavailability of fluconazole from niosomal gels and microemulsions: Formulation, optimization, and in vitro-in vivo evaluation. *Pharm. Dev. Technol.* **2017**, *24*, 1–52. [CrossRef]
63. Gupta, S.K.; Dhingra, N.; Velpandian, T.; Jaiswal, J. Efficacy of fluconazole and liposome entrapped fluconazole for C. albicans induced experimental mycotic endophthalmitis in rabbit eyes. *Acta Ophthalmol. Scand* **2000**, *78*, 448–450. [CrossRef] [PubMed]

64. El-Housiny, S.; Shams Eldeen, M.A.; El-Attar, Y.A.; Salem, H.A.; Attia, D.; Bendas, E.R.; El-Nabarawi, M.A. Fluconazole-loaded solid lipid nanoparticles topical gel for treatment of pityriasis versicolor: Formulation and clinical study. *Drug Deliv.* **2017**, *25*, 78–90. [CrossRef] [PubMed]
65. Kelidari, H.R.; Moazeni, M.; Babaei, R.; Saeedi, M.; Akbari, J.; Parkoohi, P.I.; Nabili, M.; Morteza-Semnani, A.A.G.K.; Nokhodchi, A. Improved Yeast Delivery of Fluconazole with a Nanostructured Lipid Carrier System. *Biomed. Pharmacother.* **2017**, *89*, 83–88. [CrossRef] [PubMed]
66. Moin, A.; Deb, T.K.; Osmani, R.A.M.; Bhosale, R.R.; Hani, U. Fabrication, characterization, and evaluation of microsponge delivery system for facilitated fungal therapy. *J. Basic Clin. Pharm.* **2016**, *7*, 39–48. [PubMed]
67. Indora, N.; Kaushik, D. Design, development and evaluation of ethosomal gel of fluconazole for topical fungal infection. *Int. J. Eng. Sci. Invent. Res. Dev.* **2015**, *1*, 280–306.
68. Kaur, I.P.; Rana, C.; Singh, M.; Bhushan, S.; Singh, H.; Kakkar, S. Development and evaluation of novel surfactant-based elastic vesicular system for ocular delivery of fluconazole. *J. Ocul. Pharm.* **2012**, *28*, 484–496. [CrossRef]
69. Lalit, S.K.; Panwar, A.S.; Darwhekar, G.; Jain, D.K. Formulation and Evaluation of Fluconazole Amphiphilogel. *Der. Pharm. Lett.* **2011**, *3*, 125–131.
70. Kumar, R.; Sinha, V.R. Preparation and optimization of voriconazole microemulsion for ocular delivery. *Colloids Surf. B Biointerfaces* **2014**, *117*, 82–88. [CrossRef]
71. Basaran, E.; Karaca, H.; Yenilmez, E.; Guven, U. Voriconazole incorporated polymeric nanoparticles for ocular application. *Lat. Am. J. Pharm.* **2017**, *36*, 1983–1994.
72. Das, P.J.; Paul, P.; Mukherjee, B.; Mazumder, B.; Mondal, L.; Baishya, R.; Debnath, M.C.; Dey, K.S. Pulmonary Delivery of Voriconazole Loaded Nanoparticles Providing a Prolonged Drug Level in Lungs: A Promise for Treating Fungal Infection. *Mol. Pharm.* **2015**, *12*, 2651–2664. [CrossRef]
73. Pandurangan, D.K.; Bodagala, P.; Palanirajan, V.K.; Govindaraj, S. Formulation and evaluation of voriconazole ophthalmic solid lipid nanoparticles in situ gel. *Int. J. Pharm. Investig.* **2016**, *6*, 56–62. [CrossRef] [PubMed]
74. Song, C.K.; Balakrishnan, P.; Shim, C.K.; Chung, S.-J.; Chong, S.; Kim, D.-D. A novel vesicular carrier, transethosome, for enhanced skin delivery of voriconazole: Characterization and in vitro/in vivo evaluation. *Colloids Surf. B Biointerfaces* **2011**, *92*, 299–304. [CrossRef] [PubMed]
75. Faisal, W.; Soliman, G.M.; Hamdan, A.M. Enhanced skin deposition and delivery of voriconazole using ethosomal preparations. *J. Liposome. Res.* **2018**, *28*, 14–21. [CrossRef] [PubMed]
76. Tanriverdi, S.T.; Hilmioglu Polat, S.; Yesim Metin, D.; Kandiloglu, G.; Ozer, O. Terbinafine hydrochloride loaded liposome film formulation for treatment of onychomycosis: In vitro and in vivo evaluation. *J. Liposome Res.* **2016**, *26*, 163–173. [CrossRef]
77. Chen, Y.-C.; Liu, D.-Z.; Liu, J.-J.; Chang, T.-W.; Ho, H.-O.; Sheu, M.-T. Development of terbinafine solid lipid nanoparticles as a topical delivery system. *Int. J. Nanomed.* **2012**, *7*, 4409–4418.
78. Ghannoum, M.; Isham, N.; Henry, W.; Kroon, H.A.; Yurdakul, S. Evaluation of the morphological effects of TDT 067 (terbinafine in Transfersome) and conventional terbinafine on dermatophyte hyphae in vitro and in vivo. *Antimicrob. Agents Chemother.* **2012**, *56*, 2530–2534. [CrossRef]
79. Elsherif, N.I.; Shamma, R.N.; Abdelbary, G. Terbinafine Hydrochloride Trans-ungual Delivery via Nanovesicular Systems: In Vitro Characterization and Ex Vivo Evaluation. *Aaps Pharmscitech* **2017**, *18*, 551–562. [CrossRef]
80. Ozcan, I.; Abaci, O.; Uztan, A.H.; Aksu, B.; Boyacioglu, H.; Guneri, T.; Ozer, O. Enhanced topical delivery of terbinafine hydrochloride with chitosan hydrogels. *Aaps Pharmscitech* **2009**, *10*, 1024–1031. [CrossRef]
81. Erdal, M.S.; Ozhan, G.; Mat, M.C.; Ozsoy, Y.; Gungor, S. Colloidal nanocarriers for the enhanced cutaneous delivery of naftifine: Characterization studies and in vitro and in vivo evaluations. *Int. J. Nanomed.* **2016**, *11*, 1027–1037. [CrossRef]
82. Barakat, H.S.; Darwish, I.A.; El-Khordagui, L.K.; Khalafallah, N.M. Development of naftifine hydrochloride alcohol-free niosome gel. *Drug Dev. Ind. Pharm.* **2009**, *35*, 631–637. [CrossRef]
83. Pillai, A.B.; Nair, J.V.; Gupta, N.K.; Gupta, S. Microemulsion-loaded hydrogel formulation of butenafine hydrochloride for improved topical delivery. *Arch Derm. Res.* **2015**, *307*, 625–633. [CrossRef] [PubMed]
84. Hay, R.J. Liposomal amphotericin B, AmBisome. *J. Infect.* **1994**, *28* (Suppl. 1), 35–43. [CrossRef]
85. Jansook, P.; Pichayakorn, W.; Ritthidej, G.C. Amphotericin B-loaded solid lipid nanoparticles (SLNs) and nanostructured lipid carrier (NLCs): Effect of drug loading and biopharmaceutical characterizations. *Drug Dev. Ind. Pharm.* **2018**, *44*, 1693–1700. [CrossRef] [PubMed]

86. Butani, D.; Yewale, C.; Misra, A. Topical Amphotericin B solid lipid nanoparticles: Design and development. *Colloids Surf. B Biointerfaces* **2016**, *139*, 17–24. [CrossRef]
87. Saldanha, C.A.; Garcia, M.P.; Iocca, D.C.; Rebelo, L.G.; Souza, A.C.; Bocca, A.L.; Almeida Santos Mde, F.; Morais, P.C.; Azevedo, R.B. Antifungal Activity of Amphotericin B Conjugated to Nanosized Magnetite in the Treatment of Paracoccidioidomycosis. *PLoS Negl. Trop Dis.* **2016**, *10*, e0004754. [CrossRef]
88. Sosa, L.; Clares, B.; Alvarado, H.L.; Bozal, N.; Domenech, O.; Calpena, A.C. Amphotericin B releasing topical nanoemulsion for the treatment of candidiasis and aspergillosis. *Nanomedicine* **2017**, *13*, 2303–2312. [CrossRef]
89. Souza, A.C.; Nascimento, A.L.; de Vasconcelos, N.M.; Jeronimo, M.S.; Siqueira, I.M.; R-Santos, L.; Cintra, D.O.; Fuscaldi, L.L.; Pires Junior, O.R.; Titze-de-Almeida, R.; et al. Activity and in vivo tracking of Amphotericin B loaded PLGA nanoparticles. *Eur. J. Med. Chem.* **2015**, *95*, 267–276. [CrossRef]
90. Italia, J.L.; Kumar, M.N.; Carter, K.C. Evaluating the potential of polyester nanoparticles for per oral delivery of amphotericin B in treating visceral leishmaniasis. *J. Biomed. Nanotechnol.* **2012**, *8*, 695–702. [CrossRef]
91. Tang, X.; Zhu, H.; Sun, L.; Hou, W.; Cai, S.; Zhang, R.; Liu, F. Enhanced antifungal effects of amphotericin B-TPGS-b-(PCL-ran-PGA) nanoparticles in vitro and in vivo. *Int. J. Nanomed.* **2014**, *9*, 5403–5413.
92. Jay Prakash Jain, N.K. Development of amphotericin B loaded polymersomes based on (PEG)3-PLA co-polymers: Factors affecting size and in vitro evaluation. *Eur. J. Pharm. Sci.* **2010**, *40*, 456–465. [CrossRef]
93. Perez, A.P.; Altube, M.J.; Schilrreff, P.; Apezteguia, G.; Celes, F.S.; Zacchino, S.; de Oliveira, C.I.; Romero, E.L.; Morilla, M.J. Topical amphotericin B in ultradeformable liposomes: Formulation, skin penetration study, antifungal and antileishmanial activity in vitro. *Colloids Surf. B Biointerfaces* **2016**, *139*, 190–198. [CrossRef] [PubMed]
94. Moreno-Rodriguez, A.C.; Torrado-Duran, S.; Molero, G.; Garcia-Rodriguez, J.J.; Torrado-Santiago, S. Efficacy and toxicity evaluation of new amphotericin B micelle systems for brain fungal infections. *Int. J. Pharm.* **2015**, *494*, 17–22. [CrossRef] [PubMed]
95. Lykov, A.; Gaidul, K.; Goldina, I.; Konenkov, V.; Kozlov, V.; Lyakhov, N.; Dushkin, A. Silica Nanoparticles as a Basis for Efficacy of Antimicrobial Drugs. In *Nanostructures for Antimicrobial Therapy*; Elsevier: Amsterdam, The Netherlands, 2017; pp. 551–575.
96. Khalil, R.M.; Rahman, A.A.A.E.; Kassem, M.A.; Ridi, M.S.E.; Samra, M.M.A.; Awad, G.E.A.; Mansy, S.S. Preparation and in vivo Assessment of Nystatin-Loaded Solid Lipid Nanoparticles for Topical Delivery against Cutaneous Candidiasis. *Int. J. Pharmacol. Pharm. Sci.* **2014**, *8*, 401–409.
97. Fernandez-Campos, F.; Clares Naveros, B.; Lopez Serrano, O.; Alonso Merino, C.; Calpena Campmany, A.C. Evaluation of novel nystatin nanoemulsion for skin candidosis infections. *Mycoses* **2013**, *56*, 70–81. [CrossRef] [PubMed]
98. Offner, F.; Krcmery, V.; Boogaerts, M.; Doyen, C.; Engelhard, D.; Ribaud, P.; Cordonnier, C.; de Pauw, B.; Durrant, S.; Marie, J.P.; et al. Liposomal nystatin in patients with invasive aspergillosis refractory to or intolerant of amphotericin B. *Antimicrob. Agents Chemother.* **2004**, *48*, 4808–4812. [CrossRef]
99. El-Ridy, M.S.; Abdelbary, A.; Essam, T.; Abd El-Salam, R.M.; Aly Kassem, A.A. Niosomes as a potential drug delivery system for increasing the efficacy and safety of nystatin. *Drug Dev. Ind. Pharm.* **2011**, *37*, 1491–1508. [CrossRef]
100. Jadon, P.S.; Gajbhiye, V.; Jadon, R.S.; Gajbhiye, K.R.; Ganesh, N. Enhanced oral bioavailability of griseofulvin via niosomes. *Aaps Pharmscitech* **2009**, *10*, 1186–1192. [CrossRef]
101. Shirsand, S.B.; Keshavshetti, G.G. Formulaiton and characterization of drug loaded niosomes for antifungal activity. *Sper. J. Adv. Nov. Drug Deliv.* **2016**, *1*, 12–17.
102. Jaya raja Kumar, S.M.; Subramani, P. Antifugal Agents: New Approach for Novel Delivery Systems. *J. Pharm. Sci. Res.* **2014**, *6*, 229–235.
103. Srinivasan, A.; Lopez-Ribot, J.L.; Ramasubramanian, A.K. Overcoming antifungal resistance. *Drug Discov. Today Technol.* **2014**, *11*, 65–71. [CrossRef]
104. Pelgrift, R.Y.; Friedman, A.J. Nanotechnology as a therapeutic tool to combat microbial resistance. *Adv. Drug Deliv. Rev.* **2013**, *65*, 1803–1815. [CrossRef] [PubMed]
105. Schairer, D.O.; Chouake, J.S.; Nosanchuk, J.D.; Friedman, A.J. The potential of nitric oxide releasing therapies as antimicrobial agents. *Virulence* **2012**, *3*, 271–279. [CrossRef] [PubMed]
106. Blecher, K.; Nasir, A.; Friedman, A. The growing role of nanotechnology in combating infectious disease. *Virulence* **2011**, *2*, 395–401. [CrossRef] [PubMed]

107. Zhang, L.D.P.; Hu, C.-M.J.; Huang, C.-M. Development of Nanoparticles for Antimicrobial Drug Delivery. *Curr. Med. Chem.* **2010**, *17*, 585–594. [CrossRef]
108. Hetrick, E.M.; Shin, J.H.; Paul, H.S.; Schoenfisch, M.H. Anti-biofilm efficacy of nitric oxide-releasing silica nanoparticles. *Biomaterials* **2009**, *30*, 2782–2789. [CrossRef]
109. Hajipour, M.J.; Fromm, K.M.; Akbar Ashkarran, A.; Jimenez de Aberasturi, D.; Larramendi, I.R.d.; Rojo, T.; Serpooshan, V.; Parak, W.J.; Mahmoudi, M. Antibacterial properties of nanoparticles. *Trends Biotechnol.* **2012**, *30*, 499–511. [CrossRef]
110. Mashitah, M.D.; Chan, Y.S.; Jason, J. Antifungal nanomaterials: Syntesis, properties and applications. In *Nanobiomaterials in Antimicrobial Therapy*; William Andrew: San Diego, CA, USA, 2016; pp. 343–383.
111. Mashitah, M.D.; Chan, Y.S.; Jason, J. Antimicrobial properties of nanobiomaterials and the mechanism. In *Nanobiomaterials in Antimicrobial Therapy*; William Andrew: San Diego, CA, USA, 2016; pp. 261–312.
112. Slavin, Y.N.; Asnis, J.; Häfeli, U.O.; Bach, H. Metal nanoparticles: Understanding the mechanisms behind antibacterial activity. *J. Nanobiotechnol.* **2017**, *15*, 65. [CrossRef]
113. Qidway, A.; Pandey, A.; Kumar, R.; Shukla, S.K.; Dikshit, A. Advances in Biogenic Nanoparticles and the Mechanisms of Antimicrobial Effects. *Indian J. Pharm. Sci.* **2018**, *80*, 592–603. [CrossRef]
114. Zhang, X.F.; Liu, Z.G.; Shen, W.; Gurunathan, S. Silver Nanoparticles: Synthesis, Characterization, Properties, Applications, and Therapeutic Approaches. *Int. J. Mol. Sci.* **2016**, *17*, 1534. [CrossRef]
115. Bocate, K.P.; Reis, G.F.; de Souza, P.C.; Oliveira Junior, A.G.; Duran, N.; Nakazato, G.; Furlaneto, M.C.; de Almeida, R.S.; Panagio, L.A. Antifungal activity of silver nanoparticles and simvastatin against toxigenic species of Aspergillus. *Int. J. Food Microbiol.* **2018**, *291*, 79–86. [CrossRef]
116. Calvo, N.L.; Sreekumar, S.; Svetaz, L.A.; Lamas, M.C.; Moerschbacher, B.M.; Leonardi, D. Design and Characterization of Chitosan Nanoformulations for the Delivery of Antifungal Agents. *Int. J. Mol. Sci.* **2019**, *20*, 3686. [CrossRef] [PubMed]
117. Kucharska, M.S.; Sikora, M.; Brzoza-Malczewska, K.; Owczarek, M. Antimicrobial Properties of Chitin and Chitosan. In *Chitin and Chitosan: Properties and Applications*; John Wiley & Sons, Ltd.: West Sussex, UK, 2020.
118. Sun, Q.; Li, J.; Le, T. Zinc Oxide Nanoparticle as a Novel Class of Antifungal Agents: Current Advances and Future Perspectives. *J. Agric. Food Chem.* **2018**, *66*, 11209–11220. [CrossRef] [PubMed]
119. Singh, P.N.; Nanda, A. Antimicrobial and antifungal potential of zinc oxide nanoparticles in comparison to conventional zinc oxide particles. *J. Chem. Pharm. Res.* **2013**, *5*, 457–463.
120. Rai, M.; Yadav, A.; Bridge, P.; Gade, A. Myconanotechnology: A New and Emerging Science. In *Applied Mycology*, 14th ed.; York, C.I.N., Ed.; CABI: Wallingford, UK, 2009.
121. Ingle, A.; Rai, M.; Gade, A.; Bawaskar, M. Fusarium solani: A novel biological agent for the extracellular synthesis of silver nanoparticles. *J. Nanoparticle Res.* **2009**, *11*, 2079–2085. [CrossRef]
122. Korbekandi, H.; Ashari, Z.; Iravani, S.; Abbasi, S. Optimization of Biological Synthesis of Silver Nanoparticles using Fusarium oxysporum. *Iran. J. Pharm. Res. IJPR* **2013**, *12*, 289–298.
123. Kamil, D.; Prameeladevi, T.; Ganesh, S.; Prabhakaran, N.; Nareshkumar, R.; Thomas, S.P. Green synthesis of silver nanoparticles by entomopathogenic fungus Beauveria bassiana and their bioefficacy against mustard aphid (Lipaphis erysimi Kalt.). *Indian J. Exp. Biol.* **2017**, *55*, 555–561.
124. Huang, W.; Fang, X.; Wang, H.; Chen, F.; Duan, H.; Bi, Y.; Yu, H. Biosynthesis of AgNPs by B. maydis and its antifungal effect against Exserohilum turcicum. *IET Nanobiotechnol.* **2018**, *12*, 585–590. [CrossRef]
125. Ogar, A.; Tylko, G.; Turnau, K. Antifungal properties of silver nanoparticles against indoor mould growth. *Sci. Total Environ.* **2015**, *521–522*, 305–314. [CrossRef]
126. Hariharan, H.; Al-Harbi, N.A.; Karuppiah, P.; Rajaram, S.K. Microbial synthesis of Selenium Nanocomposite using Saccharomyces cerevisiae and its antimicrobial activity against pathogens causing nosocomial infection. *Chalcogenide Lett.* **2012**, *9*, 509–515.
127. Muthupandian Saravanan, T.A.; Letemichael, N.; Araya, G.; Arokiyaraj, S.; Vinoth, R.; Karthik, D. Extracellular Biosynthesis and Biomedical Application of Silver Nanoparticles Synthesized from Baker's Yeast. *Int. J. Res. Pharm. Biomed. Sci.* **2013**, *4*, 822–828.
128. Shanbhaga, P.P.; Janib, U. Drug delivery through nails: Present and future. *New Horiz. Transl. Med.* **2017**, *3*, 252–263.
129. Rajendra, V.B.; Baro, A.; Kumari, A.; Dhamecha, D.L.; Lahoti, S.R.; Shelke, S.D. Transungual Drug Delivery: An Overview. *J. Appl. Pharm. Sci.* **2012**, *2*, 203–209.

130. Tiwary, A.K.; Sapra, B. High failure rate of transungal drug delivery: Need for new strategies. *Ther. Deliv.* **2017**, *8*, 239–242. [CrossRef] [PubMed]
131. Beloqui, A.; Solinis, M.A.; Rodriguez-Gascon, A.; Almeida, A.J.; Preat, V. Nanostructured lipid carriers: Promising drug delivery systems for future clinics. *Nanomedicine* **2016**, *12*, 143–161. [CrossRef]
132. Puglia, C.; Blasi, P.; Ostacolo, C.; Sommella, E.; Bucolo, C.; Platania, C.B.M.; Romano, G.L.; Geraci, F.; Drago, F.; Santonocito, D.; et al. Innovative Nanoparticles Enhance N-Palmitoylethanolamide Intraocular Delivery. *Front Pharm.* **2018**, *9*, 285. [CrossRef]
133. Kumar, L.; Verma, S.; Bhardwaj, A.; Vaidya, S.; Vaidya, B. Eradication of superficial fungal infections by conventional and novel approaches: A comprehensive review. *Artif. Cells Nanomed. Biotechnol.* **2014**, *42*, 32–46. [CrossRef]
134. Soliman, G.M. Nanoparticles as safe and effective delivery systems of antifungal agents: Achievements and challenges. *Int. J. Pharm.* **2017**, *523*, 15–32. [CrossRef]
135. Mishra, G.P.; Bagui, M.; Tamboli, V.; Mitra, A.K. Recent applications of liposomes in ophthalmic drug delivery. *J. Drug Deliv.* **2011**, *2011*, 863734. [CrossRef]
136. Habib, F.S.; Fouad, E.A.; Abdel-Rhaman, M.S.; Fathalla, D. Liposomes as an ocular delivery system of fluconazole: In-vitro studies. *Acta Ophthalmol.* **2010**, *88*, 901–904. [CrossRef]
137. Fetih, G. Fluconazole-loaded niosomal gels as a topical ocular drug delivery system for corneal fungal infections. *J. Drug Deliv. Sci. Technol.* **2016**, *35*, 8–15. [CrossRef]
138. Mohanta, P.; Pandey, N.; Kapoor, D.N.; Singh, S.; Sarvi, Y.; Sharma, P. Development of surfactant-based nanocarrier system for delivery of an antifungal drug. *J. Pharm. Res.* **2017**, *11*, 1153–1158.
139. Baishakhi Bhowmik, A.R.A.S.; Gowda, D.V.; Singh, A.; Srivastava, A.; Ali, R.; Osmani, M. Recent trends and advances in fungal drug delivery. *J. Chem. Pharm. Res.* **2016**, *8*, 169–178.
140. Jensen, G.M. The care and feeding of a commercial liposomal product: Liposomal amphotericin B (AmBisome((R))). *J. Liposome Res.* **2017**, *27*, 173–179. [CrossRef]
141. Jung, S.H.; Lim, D.H.; Jung, S.H.; Lee, J.E.; Jeong, K.S.; Seong, H.; Shin, B.C. Amphotericin B-entrapping lipid nanoparticles and their in vitro and in vivo characteristics. *Eur. J. Pharm Sci.* **2009**, *37*, 313–320. [CrossRef] [PubMed]
142. Korting, H.C.; Klövekorn, W.; Klövekorn, G. Comparative Efficacy and Tolerability of Econazole Liposomal Gel 1%, Branded Econazole Conventional Cream 1% and Generic Clotrimazole Cream 1% in Tinea Pedis. *Clin. Drug Investig.* **1997**, *14*, 286–293. [CrossRef]
143. Dhawade Nakusha, K.P.; Pande, V. Emerging Trends in Topical Antifungal Therapy: A Review. *Inventi J.* **2015**, *2015*, 1–5.
144. Ascenso, A.; Raposo, S.; Batista, C.; Cardoso, P.; Mendes, T.; Praca, F.G.; Bentley, M.V.; Simoes, S. Development, characterization, and skin delivery studies of related ultradeformable vesicles: Transfersomes, ethosomes, and transethosomes. *Int. J. Nanomed.* **2015**, *10*, 5837–5851. [CrossRef]
145. Verma, S.; Utreja, P. Vesicular nanocarrier based treatment of skin fungal infections: Potential and emerging trends in nanoscale pharmacotherapy. *Asian J. Pharm. Sci.* **2018**, *14*, 117–129. [CrossRef]
146. Shaji, J.; Bajaj, R. Transethosomes: A new prospect for enhanced transdermal delivery. *Int. J. Pharm. Sci. Res.* **2018**, *9*, 2681–2685.
147. Ramasamy, T.; Khandasami, U.S.; Ruttala, H.; Shanmugam, S. Development of solid lipid nanoparticles enriched hydrogels for topical delivery of anti-fungal agent. *Macromol. Res.* **2012**, *20*, 682–692. [CrossRef]
148. Pardeike, J.; Hommoss, A.; Muller, R.H. Lipid nanoparticles (SLN, NLC) in cosmetic and pharmaceutical dermal products. *Int. J. Pharm.* **2009**, *366*, 170–184. [CrossRef] [PubMed]
149. Jain, S.; Jain, S.; Khare, P.; Gulbake, A.; Bansal, D.; Jain, S.K. Design and development of solid lipid nanoparticles for topical delivery of an anti-fungal agent. *Drug Deliv.* **2010**, *17*, 443–451. [CrossRef] [PubMed]
150. Crucho, C.I.C.; Barros, M.T. Polymeric nanoparticles: A study on the preparation variables and characterization methods. *Mater Sci. Eng. C Mater Biol. Appl.* **2017**, *80*, 771–784. [CrossRef] [PubMed]
151. Patel, E.K.; Oswal, R. Nanosponge and Micro Sponges: A Novel Drug Delivery System. *Int. J. Res. Pharm. Chem.* **2012**, *2*, 2281–2781.
152. Amaral, A.C.; Bocca, A.L.; Ribeiro, A.M.; Nunes, J.; Peixoto, D.L.; Simioni, A.R.; Primo, F.L.; Lacava, Z.G.; Bentes, R.; Titze-de-Almeida, R.; et al. Amphotericin B in poly(lactic-co-glycolic acid) (PLGA) and dimercaptosuccinic acid (DMSA) nanoparticles against paracoccidioidomycosis. *J. Antimicrob. Chemother.* **2009**, *63*, 526–533. [CrossRef]

153. Nazila Kamaly, B.Y.; Wu, J.; Farokhzad, O.C. Degradable Controlled-Release Polymers and Polymeric Nanoparticles: Mechanisms of Controlling Drug Release. *Chem. Rev.* **2016**, *116*, 2602–2663. [CrossRef]
154. Caon, T.; Porto, L.C.; Granada, A.; Tagliari, M.P.; Silva, M.A.; Simoes, C.M.; Borsali, R.; Soldi, V. Chitosan-decorated polystyrene-b-poly(acrylic acid) polymersomes as novel carriers for topical delivery of finasteride. *Eur. J. Pharm. Sci.* **2014**, *52*, 165–172. [CrossRef]
155. Ing, L.Y.; Zin, N.M.; Sarwar, A.; Katas, H. Antifungal activity of chitosan nanoparticles and correlation with their physical properties. *Int. J. Biomater.* **2012**, *2012*, 632698. [CrossRef]
156. Serrano, D.R.; Lalatsa, A.; Dea-Ayuela, M.A.; Bilbao-Ramos, P.E.; Garrett, N.L.; Moger, J.; Guarro, J.; Capilla, J.; Ballesteros, M.P.; Schätzlein, A.G.; et al. Oral Particle Uptake and Organ Targeting Drives the Activity of Amphotericin B Nanoparticles. *Mol. Pharm.* **2015**, *12*, 420–431. [CrossRef]
157. Makhmalzade, B.S.; Chavoshy, F. Polymeric micelles as cutaneous drug delivery system in normal skin and dermatological disorders. *J. Adv. Pharm. Technol. Res.* **2018**, *9*, 2–8.
158. Thambi, T.; Deepagan, V.G.; Ko, H.; Lee, D.S.; Park, J.H. Bioreducible polymersomes for intracellular dual-drug delivery. *J. Mater. Chem.* **2012**, *22*, 22028–22036. [CrossRef]
159. Lee, J.S.; Feijen, J. Polymersomes for drug delivery: Design, formation and characterization. *J. Control. Release* **2012**, *161*, 473–483. [CrossRef] [PubMed]
160. Sun, H.; Meng, F.; Cheng, R.; Deng, C.; Zhong, Z. Reduction and pH dual-bioresponsive crosslinked polymersomes for efficient intracellular delivery of proteins and potent induction of cancer cell apoptosis. *Acta Biomater.* **2014**, *10*, 2159–2168. [CrossRef] [PubMed]
161. Sherje, A.P.; Jadhav, M.; Dravyakar, B.R.; Kadam, D. Dendrimers: A versatile nanocarrier for drug delivery and targeting. *Int. J. Pharm.* **2018**, *548*, 707–720. [CrossRef] [PubMed]
162. Caminade, A.M.; Laurent, R.; Majoral, J.P. Characterization of dendrimers. *Adv. Drug Deliv. Rev.* **2005**, *57*, 2130–2146. [CrossRef] [PubMed]
163. Gupta, U.; Perumal, O. Dendrimers and Its Biomedical Applications. In *Natural and Synthetic Biomedical Polymers*; Elsevier: Amsterdam, The Netherlands, 2014; pp. 243–257.
164. Nimesh, S. Dendrimers. In *Gene therapy: Potential Applications of Nanotechnology*; Woodhead Publishing Limited: Cambridge, UK, 2013; pp. 259–285.
165. Nanjwade, B.K.; Bechra, H.M.; Derkar, G.K.; Manvi, F.V.; Nanjwade, V.K. Dendrimers: Emerging polymers for drug-delivery systems. *Eur. J. Pharm. Sci.* **2009**, *38*, 185–196. [CrossRef] [PubMed]
166. Abbasi, E.; Milani, M.; Fekri Aval, S.; Kouhi, M.; Akbarzadeh, A.; Tayefi Nasrabadi, H.; Nikasa, P.; Joo, S.W.; Hanifehpour, Y.; Nejati-Koshki, K.; et al. Silver nanoparticles: Synthesis methods, bio-applications and properties. *Crit. Rev. Microbiol.* **2016**, *42*, 173–180. [CrossRef]
167. Vallabani, N.V.S.; Singh, S. Recent advances and future prospects of iron oxide nanoparticles in biomedicine and diagnostics. *3 Biotech* **2018**, *8*, 279. [CrossRef]
168. Seabra, A.B.; Pasquoto, T.; Ferrarini, A.C.; Santos Mda, C.; Haddad, P.S.; de Lima, R. Preparation, characterization, cytotoxicity, and genotoxicity evaluations of thiolated- and s-nitrosated superparamagnetic iron oxide nanoparticles: Implications for cancer treatment. *Chem. Res. Toxicol.* **2014**, *27*, 1207–1218. [CrossRef]
169. Sankhyan, A.; Pawar, P. Recent Trends in Niosome as Vesicular Drug Delivery System. *J. Appl. Pharm. Sci.* **2012**, *2*, 20–32.
170. Boonme, P.; Kaewbanjong, J.; Amnuaikit, T.; Andreani, T.; Silva, A.M.; Souto, E.B. Microemulsion and Microemulsion-Based Gels for Topical Antifungal Therapy with Phytochemicals. *Curr. Pharm. Des.* **2016**, *22*, 4257–4263. [CrossRef] [PubMed]
171. Mehta, K.; Bhatt, D. Preparation, Optimization and in vitro Microbiological Efficacy of Antifungal Microemulsion. *Int. J. Pharm. Sci. Res.* **2011**, *2*, 2424–2429.
172. Güngör, S.; Erdal, M.S.; Aksu, B. New Formulation Strategies in Topical Antifungal Therapy. *J. Cosmet. Dermatol. Sci. Appl.* **2013**, *3*, 56–65. [CrossRef]
173. El-Hadidy, G.N.; Ibrahim, H.K.; Mohamed, M.I.; El-Milligi, M.F. Microemulsions as vehicles for topical administration of voriconazole: Formulation and in vitro evaluation. *Drug Dev. Ind. Pharm.* **2012**, *38*, 64–72. [CrossRef]
174. De Souza, M.L.; Oliveira, D.D.; Pereira, N.P.; Soares, D.M. Nanoemulsions and dermatological diseases: Contributions and therapeutic advances. *Int. J. Derm.* **2018**, *57*, 894–900. [CrossRef]

175. Zazo, H.; Colino, C.I.; Lanao, J.M. Current applications of nanoparticles in infectious diseases. *J. Control Release* **2016**, *224*, 86–102. [CrossRef]
176. Peszke, J.; Dulski, M.; Nowak, A.; Balin, K.; Zubko, M.; Sułowicz, S.; Nowak, B.; Piotrowska-Seget, Z.; Talik, E.; Wojtyniak, M.; et al. Unique properties of silver and copper silica-based nanocomposites as antimicrobial agents. *RSC Adv.* **2017**, *7*, 28092–28104. [CrossRef]
177. Botequim, D.; Maia, J.; Lino, M.M.; Lopes, L.M.; Simoes, P.N.; Ilharco, L.M.; Ferreira, L. Nanoparticles and surfaces presenting antifungal, antibacterial and antiviral properties. *Langmuir* **2012**, *28*, 7646–7656. [CrossRef]
178. Cristiana, S.; Vidal, M.; Ferreira, L.S. Antifungal Nanoparticles and Surfaces. *Biomacromolecules* **2010**, *11*, 2810–2817.
179. Camporotondi, D.E.; Foglia, M.L.; Alvarez, G.S.; Mebert, A.; Diaz, L.E.; Coradin, T. Antimicrobial properties of silica modified nanoparticles. In *Microbial Pathogens and Strategies for Combating Them: Science, Technology and Education*; Méndez-Vilas, A., Ed.; Formatex Research Center: Badajoz, Spain, 2013.
180. Derbalah, A.; Shenashen, M.; Hamza, A.; Mohamed, A.; El Safty, S. Antifungal activity of fabricated mesoporous silica nanoparticles against early blight of tomato. *Egypt. J. Basic Appl. Sci.* **2018**, *5*, 145–150. [CrossRef]
181. Newman, D.J.; Cragg, G.M. Natural Products as Sources of New Drugs from 1981 to 2014. *J. Nat. Prod.* **2016**, *79*, 629–661. [CrossRef] [PubMed]
182. Kelkawi, A.H.A.; Kajani, A.A.; Bordbar, A.K. Green synthesis of silver nanoparticles using Mentha pulegium and investigation of their antibacterial, antifungal and anticancer activity. *IET Nanobiotechnol.* **2017**, *11*, 370–376. [CrossRef]
183. El-Hossary, E.M.; Cheng, C.; Hamed, M.M.; El-Sayed Hamed, A.N.; Ohlsen, K.; Hentschel, U.; Abdelmohsen, U.R. Antifungal potential of marine natural products. *Eur. J. Med. Chem.* **2017**, *126*, 631–651. [CrossRef] [PubMed]
184. Vitali, A. Antimicrobial Peptides Derived from Marine Sponges. *Am. J. Clin. Microbiol. Antimicrob.* **2018**, *1*, 1006.
185. Ratnayake, A.S.; Bugni, T.S.; Feng, X.; Harper, M.K.; Skalicky, J.J.; Mohammed, K.A.; Andjelic, C.D.; Barrows, L.R.; Ireland, C.M. Theopapuamide, a Cyclic Depsipeptide from a Papua New Guinea Lithistid Sponge Theonella swinhoei. *J. Nat. Prod.* **2006**, *69*, 1582–1586. [CrossRef] [PubMed]
186. Alberto Plaza, G.B.; Jessica, L.K.; John, R.L.; Heather, L.B.; Carole, A.B. Celebesides A-C and Theopapuamides B-D, Depsipeptides from an Indonesian Sponge that Inhibit HIV-1 Entry. *J. Org. Chem.* **2010**, *74*, 504–512. [CrossRef]
187. Negri, M.; Salci, T.P.; Shinobu-Mesquita, C.S.; Capoci, I.R.G.; Svidzinski, T.I.E.; Kioshima, E.S. Early state research on antifungal natural products. *Molecules* **2014**, *19*, 2925–2956. [CrossRef] [PubMed]
188. Krause, J.; Tobi, G. Discovery, Development, and Regulation of Natural Products. In *Using Old Solutions to New Problems—Natural Drug Discovery in the 21st Century*; BoD–Books on Demand: Norderstedt, Germany, 2013.
189. Roemer, T.; Xu, D.; Singh, S.B.; Parish, C.A.; Harris, G.; Wang, H.; Davies, J.E.; Bills, G.F. Confronting the Challenges of Natural Product-Based Antifungal Discovery. *Chem. Biol.* **2011**, *18*, 148–164. [CrossRef]
190. Wright, G.D. Unlocking the potential of natural products in drug discovery. *Microb. Biotechnol.* **2018**, *12*, 55–57. [CrossRef]
191. Gupta, N.; Rai, D.B.; Jangid, A.K.; Kulhari, H. Use of nanotechnology in antimicrobial therapy. In *Nanotechnology*; Academic Press: Cambridge, MA, USA, 2019; pp. 143–172.
192. Pooja, D.; Kadari, A.; Kulhari, H.; Sistla, R. Lipid-based nanomedicines. In *Lipid Nanocarriers for Drug Targeting*; William Andrew: San Diego, CA, USA, 2018; pp. 509–528.
193. Koppa Raghu, P.; Bansal, K.K.; Thakor, P.; Bhavana, V.; Madan, J.; Rosenholm, J.M.; Mehra, N.K. Evolution of Nanotechnology in Delivering Drugs to Eyes, Skin and Wounds via Topical Route. *Pharmaceuticals* **2020**, *13*, 167. [CrossRef]
194. NIH. *ClinicalTrials*. Available online: https://clinicaltrials.gov/ct2/home (accessed on 10 September 2020).

2

Antimicrobial Peptides in Reptiles

Monique L. van Hoek

National Center for Biodefense and Infectious Diseases, and School of Systems Biology, George Mason University, MS1H8, 10910 University Blvd, Manassas, VA 20110, USA; mvanhoek@gmu.edu;

Abstract: Reptiles are among the oldest known amniotes and are highly diverse in their morphology and ecological niches. These animals have an evolutionarily ancient innate-immune system that is of great interest to scientists trying to identify new and useful antimicrobial peptides. Significant work in the last decade in the fields of biochemistry, proteomics and genomics has begun to reveal the complexity of reptilian antimicrobial peptides. Here, the current knowledge about antimicrobial peptides in reptiles is reviewed, with specific examples in each of the four orders: Testudines (turtles and tortosises), Sphenodontia (tuataras), Squamata (snakes and lizards), and Crocodilia (crocodilans). Examples are presented of the major classes of antimicrobial peptides expressed by reptiles including defensins, cathelicidins, liver-expressed peptides (hepcidin and LEAP-2), lysozyme, crotamine, and others. Some of these peptides have been identified and tested for their antibacterial or antiviral activity; others are only predicted as possible genes from genomic sequencing. Bioinformatic analysis of the reptile genomes is presented, revealing many predicted candidate antimicrobial peptides genes across this diverse class. The study of how these ancient creatures use antimicrobial peptides within their innate immune systems may reveal new understandings of our mammalian innate immune system and may also provide new and powerful antimicrobial peptides as scaffolds for potential therapeutic development.

Keywords: antimicrobial peptides; antibacterial; reptile; biofilm; broad-spectrum; Gram-positive; Gram-negative

---

1. Introduction

Reptiles are among the oldest amniotes. They are cold-blooded (ectothermic) vertebrates with dry and scaly skin that usually lay soft-shelled eggs with amniotic membranes. They thrive in diverse environments, ranging as far north as Hudson's Bay in Canada, and as far south as Cape Horn, Chile. They range from very small geckos to enormous crocodiles and have survived millennia of evolution. They are highly adapted to their environment, including their innate immune systems, allowing them to be such successful animals. Antimicrobial peptides are part of the innate immune system, and may contribute to the survival of these animals in microbe-filled, challenging environment. This paper will review the known and predicted antimicrobial peptides of reptiles. A set of known host defense antimicrobial peptides is collected in the Antimicrobial Peptide Database [1,2] and the examples from reptiles have been annotated (Table 1). Recently, many reptilian genomes have been sequenced. From these genomes, potential antimicrobial peptide genes have been predicted here by bioinformatics analysis (Tables 2–8), which should be synthesized and tested for activity in future work. Overall, the Reptile class thrives in diverse and challenging environments, partly due to their robust innate immune system, and our hypothesis is that antimicrobial peptides contribute to the evolutionary success of reptiles as they do in mammals and other species.

Table 1. Known reptile antimicrobial peptides identified in the Antimicrobial Peptide Database (APD2) [2].

Peptide name	Sequence	APD Identified	Source Organism	Comment Reference	Activity (*)
		Cathelicidin			
OH-CATH	KRFKKFFKKLKNSVKK RAKKFFKKPRVIGVSIPF	AP00895	*O. Hannah* (Snake)	Derivatives: OH-CATH30; OH-CM6 [3,4]	G+, G−
Derivative OH-CATH30	KFFKKLKNSVKKRA KKFFKKPRVIGVSIPF			[5,6]	G+, G−
Derivative OH-CM6	KFFKKLKKAVKKGFKKFAKV			[3,4]	G+, G−
BF-CATH	KRFKKFFKKLKKSVKK RAKKFFKKPRVIGVSIPF	AP00896	*Bungarus fasciatus* (Snake)	[7]	G+, G−, F, Cancer cells
Derivative BF-30	KFFRKLKKSVKKRAK EFFKKPRVIGVSIPF	AP01239	*B. fasciatus*	[8–10]	G+, G−
Derivative BF-15	KFFRKLKKSVVKRFK		*B. fasciatus*	[8]	G+, G−
NA-CATH	KRFKKFFKKLKNSVKKRA KKFFKKPKVIGVTFPF	AP00897	*N. atra* (Snake)	[3]	G+, G−
		Waprin			
Omwaprin	KDRPKKPGLCPPRPQKPCVK ECKNDDSCPGQQKCCN YGCKDECRDPIFVG	AP01589	*Oxyuranus microlepidotus* (Snake)	4S = S [11,12]	G+
		Proline Rich			
Lethal peptide I/Waglerin	GGKPDLRPCHPP CHYIPRPKPR	AP00238	*Trimeresurus wagleri*, Wagler's pit viper (Snake)	P24335, [13]	Tx
		β-Defensin or defensin-like			
TBD-1 (Turtle β-defensin 1)	YDLSKNCRLRGGICYIGK CPRRFFRSGSCSRGNVCCLRFG	AP01380	Turtle	3S = S [14]	G+, G−, F
Pelovaterin	DDTPSSRCGSGGWGPCLPI VDLLCIVHVTVGCSGGFGCCRIG	AP01381	Turtle	2JR3 BBBh2o [15,16]	G−
TEWP (turtle egg-white protein)	EKKCPGRCTLKCGKHER PTLPYNCGKYICCVPVKVK	AP01382	Turtle	2B5B XXQ [17–19]	G-, V
		Crotamine defensin-like toxin			
Crotamine	YKQCHKKGGHCFPKEKICLPP SSDFGKMDCRWRWKCCKKGSG	AP01650	Snake Venom	1Z99, 3S = S ZZP [20,21]	G+, G−, F, P, Mammalian and Cancer cells

(*) Activity abbreviations: G+, G−, inhibiting both G+ and G− bacteria; G+, Gram-positive bacteria only, G−, Gram-negative bacteria only; V, antiviral; F, antifungal; P: antiparasitic, Tx: Toxin activity to mammals.

2. Four Orders of Reptiles

The structural and sequence diversity of antimicrobial peptides is impressive (see below), but it is useful to first review the phylogenetic and physiological diversity of the Reptilia class in order to appreciate all the ecosystems and environments that they live in and the prey that they eat.

All living reptiles fall within the kingdom Animalia, the phylum Chordata, the class Reptilia, and the clade Sauropsida [22]. There are four orders within the class Reptilia: turtles and tortoises (Testudines), tuataras (Sphenodontia), snakes and lizards (Squamata), and crocodilans (Crocodilia). Each order will be briefly introduced below. Many reptile species are endangered, including the painted turtle, and the Siamese crocodile. Although considered by phylogenetic analysis to be "monophyletic" with avians (Sauropsida; See Cladogram, Figure 1), reptiles are still generally considered to be separate from birds. Some researchers use the term avian reptile and non-avian reptile to distinguish the two groups [23]. Within the non-avian reptilians, the crocodilians are considered to be the most closely related to the avian branch. Interestingly, this evolutionary connection is reflected in the antimicrobial profile in that neither avians nor reptilians encode α-defensin antimicrobial peptides, for example, which are a critical part of mammalian innate immunity. In contrast, avians do not appear to express hepcidin peptides, while reptiles do, highlighting a potential difference.

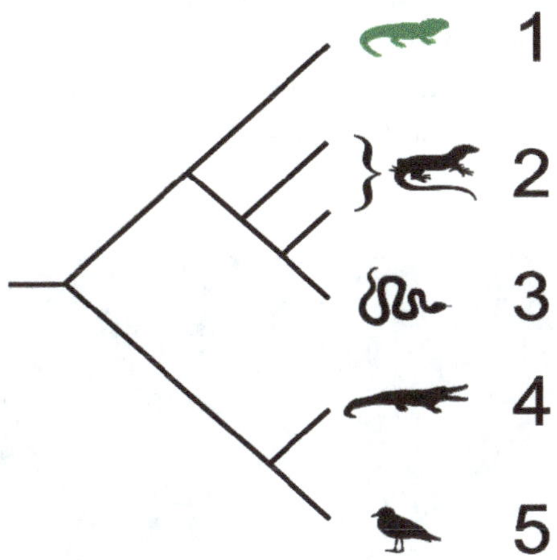

Figure 1. Cladogram showing the relationships of extant members of the Sauria (Sauropsida) which includes birds and reptiles. Branch lengths are not representative of divergence time. 1. Tuataras; 2. Lizards; 3. Snakes; 4. Crocodiles; 5. Birds. Cladogram by Benchill, licensed under the Creative Commons Attribution 3.0 Unported license [24].

2.1. Testudines (Turtles and Tortises)

The testudine order includes the turtles and tortosises. The western painted turtle (*Chrysemys picta bellii*) is a small turtle of North America, commonly found in ponds and other slow-moving fresh water [25].

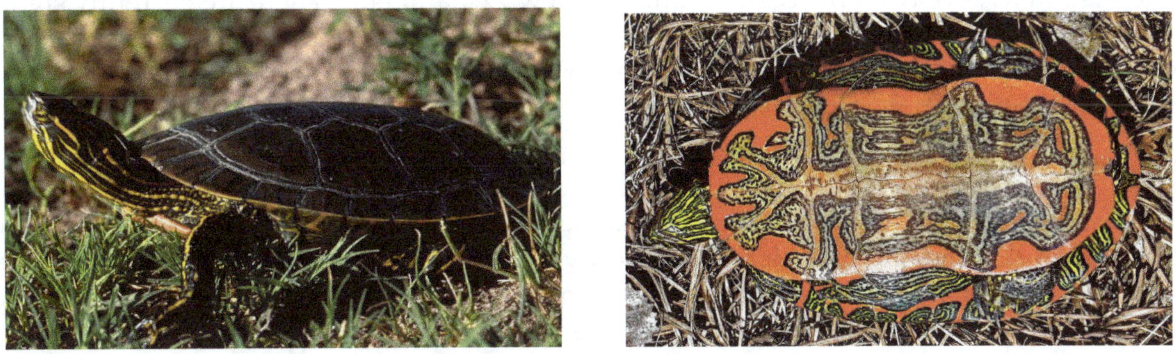

(a) **(b)**

Figure 2. Western Painted Turtle *Chrysemys picta bellii*. (**a**) Western painted turtle. Photo by Gary M. Stolz, U.S. Fish and Wildlife Service in the Public domain [26]. (**b**) Underside of a Western Painted Turtle. Photo by Matt Young [27].

This intensely colorful turtle (Figure 2) has existed for approximately 15 million years, according to the fossil record [25]. The genomes of three turtles have recently been sequenced, including the green sea turtle (*Chelonia mydas*) and the Chinese softshell turtle *Pelodiscus sinensis* [28], as well as the western painted turtle, *Chrysemys picta bellii* [29,30]. Interestingly, these papers place the turtles as a sister group to crocodiles and birds, which is different than their prior morphological classification [31]. The precise evolutionary relationship of the testudine class with other reptiles is a matter of current debate [32–36]. Their genomes appear to encode cathelicidin antimicrobial peptides that are "snake-like" but encode defensin type peptides (gallinacin-like) that may be more similar to "avian" antimicrobial peptides.

2.2. Sphenodontia (Tuataras)

The family Sphenodontidae (within Lepidosauromorpha) contains the genus of Sphenodon, which has one species, *S. puctatus* (previously thought to have three species including *S. guntheri*, and *S. diversum*, now considered sub-species) all commonly referred to as tuatara lizards [37,38], although they are not classified as lizards. The tuatara (Figure 3) is the farthest removed from the avian lineage in terms of evolution and is considered to be the most "ancient" extant reptile, in existence in its current form for 100 million years.

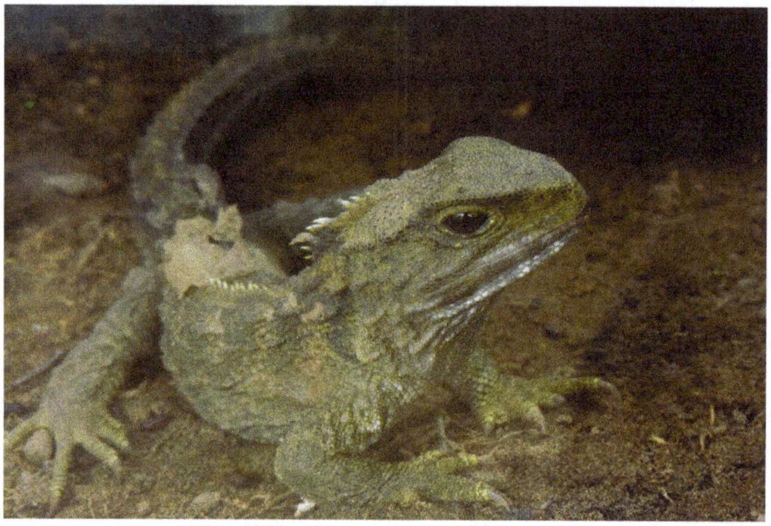

Figure 3. *Sphenodon punctatus*, Tuatara, Nga Manu, Waikanae, New Zealand. Photo by PhillipC [39].

The tuatara lives only on the costal islands of New Zealand [40]. There are currently significant efforts underway to sequence the tuatara genome [41]. However, until the genomes and transcriptomes can be analyzed for antimicrobial peptides and verified from tuatara samples, there are no known antimicrobial peptides from the tuatara.

2.3. Squamata (Snakes and Lizards)

The Squamata order of Lepidosauromorpha includes lizards and snakes. In the group of snakes which although limbless are considered tetrapod vertebrates and are descended from four legged ancestors, we will consider elapid snakes and pythons. Elapid snakes are venomous, fanged snakes commonly found in warm climates. Pythons are nonvenomous snakes that are found in Africa, Asia and Australia. The King cobra (*Ophiophagus (O.) hannah*) is one of the longest venomous snakes [42], with lengths up to 18 ft (Figure 4a). The genus *Naja* is a group of venomous elapid snakes in southern Africa and South Asia, including the species *Naja (N.) atra*, the Chinese King cobra (Figure 4b). The Banded Krait (*Bungarus (B.) fasciatus*) is commonly found in Southeast Asia and India and has distinctive banding markings (Figure 4c). The Burmese python (*Python bivittatus*) is typically found in tropical areas including Southeast Asia and is one of the largest snakes, typically reaching 12 ft long. This snake is also found as an invasive species in the Florida Everglades in the Southeast United States [43]. Snakes encode well-studied cathelicidin peptides that appear to be generally similar throughout the reptiles, despite the well-known sequence diversity of cathelicidin antimicrobial peptides in general.

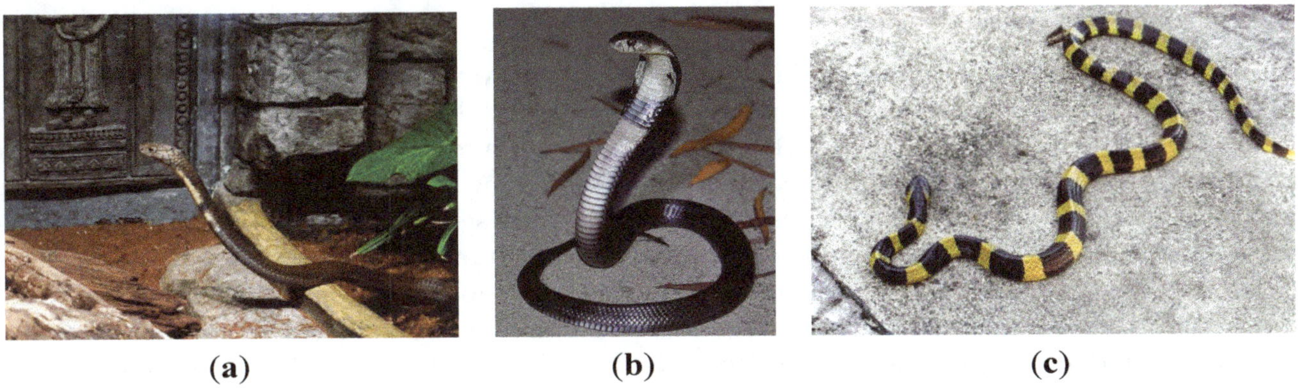

Figure 4. Elapid snakes (a) The King cobra (*O. hannah*) [44] (b) A juvenile Chinese cobra *(N. atra)* [45] (c) Banded Krait *(B. fasciatus)* [46].

The Squamata order also includes the lizards. Unlike snakes, lizards have four legs and external ears. There are more than 6,000 species of lizards, making it the largest group of reptiles. Lizards inhabit a wide range of ecological niches, from hot, dry desserts to cool, moist forests. The main groups of lizards include Gekkota, Iguania, Scincomorpha and Platynota (Varanoidea). Although the tuatara looks much like a lizard, it is excluded from the lizard group. The Gekkota suborder includes geckos, while skinks fall into the suborder Scincomorpha. Monitor lizards, Komodo dragons and Gila monsters are classified as Platynota (Varanoidea). The suborder Iguania includes chameleons, anoles and iguanas. The Carolina green anole lizard (*Anolis carolinensis)* is a small tree-living lizard, often green or brown, commonly found in the southeastern United States. It has intense green, blue and white coloring, especially evident on the male, and has a pink dewlap on its throat (Figure 5). The Anole lizard genome encodes for many β-defensin antimicrobial peptide genes and lysozyme genes.

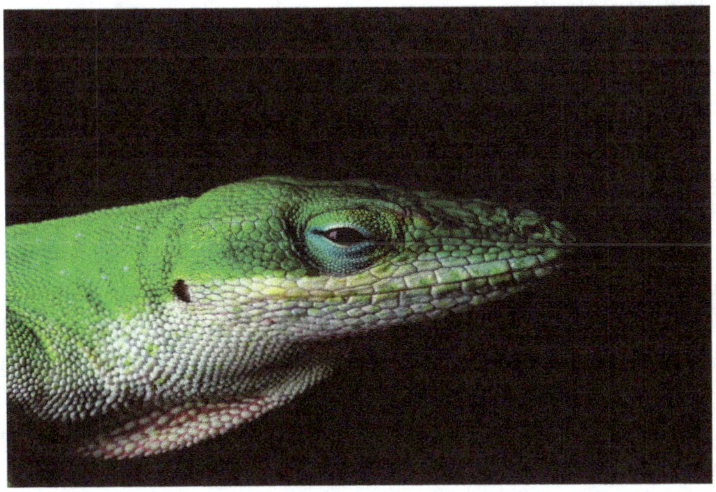

Figure 5. Male Carolina Anole with partially expanded dewlap [47].

The genomes of several members of the Squamata have recently been sequenced including the anole lizard [23], the elapid snakes *O. hannah* [15], *B. fasciatus*, and *N. atra* [30]. High-throughput sequencing and mass-spectrometry proteomics has been recently performed on snake venom, which should provide a deep view of proteins and peptides produced in the venom [48]. Antimicrobial peptides have been identified in the anole (defensins) [49], as well as cathelicidins in all three species of elapid snakes (see below) [3]. Very recently, the python genome has been sequenced [30]. Genome projects are also underway for other reptiles, such as the common garter snake (*Thamnophis sirtalis*) [23].

2.4. Crocodilia (Crocodilians)

The order of crocodilians (Crocodilia) within the group Archosauromorpha includes alligators and caimans (family Alligatoridae), crocodiles (family Crocodylidae), and gharials (gavials, family Gavialidae) (Figure 6). Most species live in fresh-water, but a few have also adapted to salt-water conditions. These animals are evolutionarily ancient, and along with birds, are considered the only surviving relatives of dinosaurs (Archosauria). Within their semi-aquatic ecosystems, these large animals are the apex predators, using their powerful jaws to capture large and small prey [50]. They are cold-blooded and egg-laying. They can be found around the world, in the Americas, in Asia, South America, and Africa [51]. The ancestors of alligators and crocodiles first emerged in the Late Cretaceous era, and the modern alligators and crocodiles are estimated to be as much as 83 million years old.

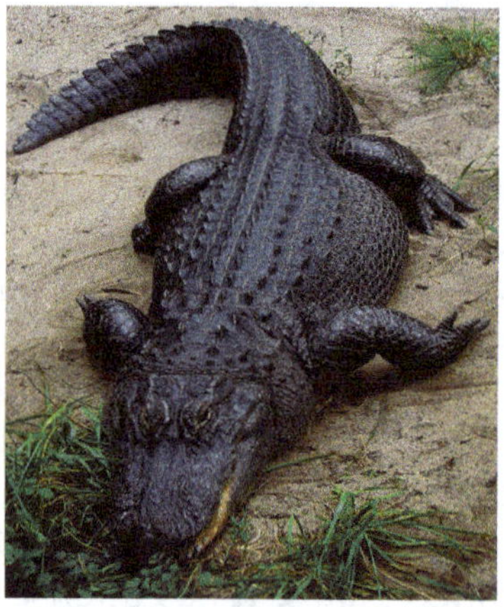

(a)

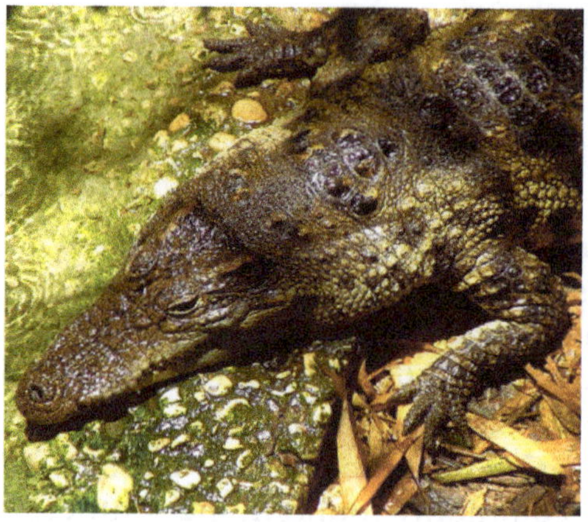

(b)

Figure 6. Crocodilians. (**a**) The American alligator, *Alligator mississippiensis* [52]. (**b**) The Siamese crocodile, *Crocodylus siamesnsis* [53].

Today, the American alligator is commonly found all around the Gulf of Mexico and Southeastern United States, having made a comeback from near extinction due to overhunting. The meat and skins of farmed alligators are now harvested for consumption and use. This large animal is typically 8–11 ft long and 200–500 lbs depending on gender and age [54]. The alligator has a broad snout and the top teeth come down over the bottom lips, unlike the crocodile. Alligators inhabit swamps such as the Great Dismal Swamp, rivers and streams, ponds and lakes, with a preference for fresh water over brackish water, and intolerance for salt water. Alligators can be infected by *Mycoplasma alligatoris* [55] as well as other bacterial pathogens. In terms of temperature preference, alligators are more cold tolerant than most other crocodilian species, accounting for their location as far north as South Carolina in the United States [54].

The Siamese crocodile (*Crocodylus siamensis*) [56,57] is a critically endangered freshwater crocodilian found in Southeast Asia (Cambodia, Vietnam, Thailand, Indonesia and Burma for example). Like most crocodiles, it is a tropical animal with low tolerance for the cold [3]. This animal is smaller than the alligator, typically about 7 ft long and 80–150 lbs when fully grown, although larger specimens have been recorded [4]. These animals are being intensively studied as part of their conservation, and are bred in captivity, and thus are accessible to researchers for DNA or blood samples [58–60].

Crocodilians such as alligators can carry a high burden of fecal coliforms from their aquatic environment [61], yet despite their potentially near-constant exposure to potential pathogens, alligators and other crocodilians do not seem to be susceptible to infection by these organisms, either systemically or on their skin, via wounds or lesions. This has led to the idea that these animals may have highly potent antimicrobial components to their immune systems [57,62–67]. Several crocodilian genomes have been published [68] or are underway [69]. The peptides that have been discovered in crocodilians are outlined in the sections below and include lysozyme, defensin, hepcidin, hemocidin and other antimicrobial peptides. Several important crocodilian genomes have been sequenced, including the Chinese alligator (*Alligator sinensis*), the American alligator (*Alligator mississippiensis*), the saltwater crocodile (*Crocodylus porosus*) and the Indian gharial (*Gavialis gangeticus*) [69,70]. It will be very interesting to compare freshwater species to saltwater species in terms of their innate immune response profiles, as the environmental organisms will be significantly different between the two types of water.

3. Antimicrobial Peptides of Reptiles

Reptiles are highly adapted to their environments, which often include many bacteria, allowing them to be such successful animals. Antimicrobial peptides are part of the innate immune system, and may contribute to the survival of reptiles. However, to date there has been no direct data in reptiles such as gene knock-out experiments to demonstrate their importance to overall survival, development and resistance to infection, as has been done in mice [71]. There has been some suggestion that β-defensin peptides are associated with fur color in dogs [72,73], but again no studies of this kind have yet been done on reptiles. This area of research presents many opportunities for scientists to explore the role of antimicrobial peptides in these animals. This paper will review the known (Table 1) and predicted antimicrobial peptides of reptiles. Recently, new reptilian genomes have been sequenced. From these genomes, additional antimicrobial peptide genes have been predicted here by bioinformatics analysis (Tables 2–8), which should be synthesized and tested for activity.

Antimicrobial peptides are well-characterized peptides, and exhibit significant structure-function specificity. Following the identification of magainin peptides in amphibians in 1987 [74], scientists have been exploring the diversity of peptides expressed in different animals, looking for new structures and new functions of antimicrobial peptides. The structure and function of each of the major classes of antimicrobial peptides is described below, in addition to the data pertaining to its known or predicted expression in reptiles.

3.1. Defensin Peptides in Reptiles

Defensins are one of the major classes of antimicrobial peptides in higher vertebrates. These 3–4 kDa cationic peptides are characterized by having six cysteines arranged in three disulfide bonds, with the characteristic pairing of the bonds highly characteristic for each type of defensin. Defensins have predominantly β-sheet characteristic with some α-helices. Defensins are encoded in the genome and are processed from a pro-defensin molecule by proteases [75].

3.1.1. Three Sub-Classes of Defensins

Defensins are known to be critical components of innate immunity in many animals [76]. The three main sub-classes of defensins are α, β- and θ-defensins. In humans, α-defensins are commonly found in neutrophils and other leukocytes (for example, Human Neutrophil peptide HNP-1 = α-defensin 1), and are important in the ability of white blood cells to deal with pathogens [77]. The β-defensins are defined as having a Cys1-Cys5, Cys2-Cys4, and Cys3-Cys6 bonding pattern of cysteines. In humans, β-defensins are commonly expressed in epithelial cells, and are widely expressed in the body [78]. The expression of these cationic antimicrobial peptides are often induced following bacterial or viral infection as part of the innate immune response, except for hBD1 which appears to be constitutively expressed in humans. The third class of defensins is the θ-defensins. θ-Defensins are not known outside of primates, and are not expressed in humans [21] but are very active antiviral peptides [76].

Within the reptiles, there are no known genes for α-defensins, and only the β-defensins appear to be expressed, similar to what is found in avians. Within some species of reptiles, β-defensin genes and peptides have been identified, for example in the red-eared slider turtle [79]. Lizards are known to be highly resistant to infection, and recently genes encoding up to 32 different β-defensin-like peptides were identified in the *Anole carolinensis* genome [49]. Indeed, using an antibody that reacts to AcBD15 (one of those β-defensin-like peptides in anole), staining was observed in some (but not all) of the granules of heterophilic and basophilic granulocytes in lizards, a snake, a turtle and the tuatara, but not alligator nor chicken granulocytes. Cells from other tissues such as epidermis were negative for staining. Alibardi *et al.* describe that not all the granules within a granulocyte stained with the antibody, suggesting that there may be different types of granules as is seen in mammalian neutrophils [22].

Similarly, turtle leukocytes were found to contain TBD-1, the first β-defensin identified in reptile leukocytes [14]. In the turtle system, TBD-1 was also identified in other tissues, such as the skin [18,80, 81]. These fascinating and unique results suggest that further study of the antimicrobial peptidome of reptilian granulocytes should be performed.

3.1.2. Inducible Expression of β-Defensins in Wounded Lizards

The first extensive report of an *in vivo* role for β-defensin peptide expression was in the anole lizard (Table 2). It has long been known that lizards can lose their tails as a method of predator escape, and that these tail then regenerate from the wound site. In this process, a wound is formed, which does not typically get infected. β-Defensin peptides are found to be expressed both within the azurophilic granulocytes in the wound-bed as well as in the associated epithelium [82,83], and are observed in phagosomes containing degraded bacteria. While there is a distinct lack of inflammation in the wound, which is associated with regeneration, there is a high level of expression of AcBD15 and AcBD27 (two of the most highly expressed β-defensins in that tissue) [84,85]. Overall, there appears to be a fascinating role of AcBD15 and AcBD27 in the wound healing and regeneration in the anole lizard.

Table 2. Predicted defensin-like protein genes in multiple reptilian species.

Organism	Peptide annotation	aa	Locus- Accession #
Alligator mississippiensis	Gallinacin-14-like	58	XP_006270781.1
Alligator sinensis	Gallinacin-14-like	58	XP_006033878.1
Anolis carolinensis	β-Defensin-like protein 5	62	CBY85058.1
Anolis carolinensis	β-Defensin-like protein 8	65	CBY85059.1
Anolis carolinensis	β-Defensin-like protein 9	66	CBY85060.1
Anolis carolinensis	β-Defensin-like protein 10	67	CBY85061.1
Anolis carolinensis	β-Defensin-like protein 15	63	CCA62931.1
Anolis carolinensis	β-Defensin-like protein 21	89	CBY85062.1
Anolis carolinensis	β-Defensin-like protein 22	95	CBY85063.1
Anolis carolinensis	β-Defensin-like protein 27	81	CBY85064.1
Anolis carolinensis	Gallinacin-10-like	68	XP_003225602.1
Anolis carolinensis	Gallinacin-13-like	60	XP_003225598.1
Anolis carolinensis	Hypothetical protein LOC100555370		XP_003227809.1
Anolis carolinensis	Hypothetical protein LOC100555565		XP_003227810.1
Anolis carolinensis	Hypothetical protein LOC100555756		XP_003227811.1
Anolis carolinensis	Hypothetical protein LOC100562305		XP_003225604.1
Anolis carolinensis	Hypothetical protein LOC100562502	65	XP_003225605.1
Anolis carolinensis	Hypothetical protein LOC100562898		XP_003225607.1
Anolis carolinensis	Hypothetical protein LOC100563098		XP_003225608.1
Chrysemys picta bellii	β-Defensin 1-like	80	XP_005308390.1
Chrysemys picta bellii	Gallinacin-5-like		XP_005290738.1
Chrysemys picta bellii	Gallinacin-5-like, partial		XP_005314963.1
Chrysemys picta bellii	Gallinacin-14-like	58	XP_005308403.1
Pelodiscus sinensis	Gallinacin-1 α-like		XP_006137072.1
Pelodiscus sinensis	Lingual antimicrobial peptide-like isoform X2		XP_006127561.1
Bothrops neuwiedi	β-Defensin-like protein		AGF25392.1
Bothrops jararacussu	β-Defensin-like protein		AGF25388.1
Bothrops leucurus	β-Defensin-like protein		AGF25389.1
Bothrops matogrossensis	β-Defensin-like protein		AGF25391.1, AGF25390.1
Bothrops diporus	β-Defensin-like protein		AGF25384.1
Bothrops pauloensis	β-Defensin-like protein		AGF25393.1
Bothrops jararaca	β-Defensin-like protein		AGF25386.1, AGF25387.1
Bothrops atrox	β-Defensin-like protein		AGF25383.1
Bothrops erythromelas	β-defensin-like protein		AGF25385.1

3.1.3. Expression of β-Defensins in Reptile Eggs

Reptile eggs are a good biological sample for the purification of peptides and proteins, since there is so much material within each egg. Recently, it was found that while the β-defensin-like peptide pelovaterin (Table 1) identified in the eggshell of the Chinese soft-shelled turtle does indeed have antimicrobial activity, these peptides may also play an additional role in the formation of the eggshell, through aggregation [15]. This is similar to the role of the gallin defensin-like peptide in avian eggs [86–90].

3.2. Cathelicidin Peptides in Reptiles

Cathelicidins are a second major class of antimicrobial peptides in higher eukaryotes. They are characterized as being antimicrobial peptides derived by proteolytic cleavage from a pre-propeptide that includes the cathelin domain in mammals and less-well conserved cathelin domain in other eukaryotes [91,92]. In humans, cathelicidins are stored in the azurophilic granules of neutrophils as the inactive prepropeptide, and are processed by enzymes (neutrophil elastase [93] or a serine protease [19]) to the mature active peptide [94]. In humans and higher vertebrates, the active cathelicidin peptide is always encoded on Exon 4 of the cathelicidin encoding gene [91,95,96]. Four cathelicidin-like peptides have been identified in the chicken (*Gallus gallus domesticus*) [97], including fowlicidin-1, -2 and -3 (also known as chCATH-1, chCATH-2/CMAP27, chCATH-3) [98], and chCATH-B1/chCATH-4 [99]. In humans, the hCAP18 cathelicidin is processed by proteinase 3 inside the granule [19] or neutrophil elastase in the extracellular space [4] to its active form. In the case of chicken cathelicidin, the pre-pro-cathelin domain peptide is cleaved by a serine protease to release the mature peptide following stimulation of heterophils with LPS [100].

3.3. Cathelicidin Peptides in Snakes

Cathelicidin peptides have been identified and characterized in the snake family (Table 1) [1,2], although there may be similar genes in other reptiles by genomic analysis (see below). Highly related cathelicidins were identified in *B. fasciatus*, *O. hannah* and *N. atra* [3] (Table 3). We identified additional genes for antimicrobial peptides by BLAST searching the genomes of the pit vipers (*Bothrops atrox*, *Trimeresurus wagler* and *Crotalus durissus*) [13] and the Eastern brown snake (*Pseudonaja textilis*) (Table 3). The genes of these cathelicidins have the general structure of the cathelicidin genes, including a poorly conserved cathelin domain and the c-terminal active peptide. The snake cathelicidins have been well studied. The functional cathelicidin peptide of the snake family is highly divergent from the functional cathelicidin peptide of humans, for example, confirming the "general rule" of cathelicidins, which is that the active peptides are highly divergent, but the pre-pro-regions in the gene and the peptide are more highly conserved [101].

3.3.1. King Cobra (*Ophiophagus (O.) Hannah*)

Zhao *et al.* determined the hemolytic and antimicrobial activity of the predicted *O. hannah* cathelicidin, OH-CATH [3] (Table 1). The OH-CATH peptide proved to be an excellent inhibitor of bacterial growth and demonstrated broad-spectrum activity against bacterial isolates including multi-drug resistant strains. The OH-CATH peptide displayed greater potency than the human cathelicidin LL-37 against a variety of known human bacterial pathogens and the antimicrobial potency of OH-CATH was not significantly impacted by the concentration of salt in the media. They demonstrated that OH-CATH showed no hemolytic activity against erythrocytes, even at a concentration of 200 μg/mL, suggesting low cytotoxicity of the peptide to eukaryotic cells [3]. Additional studies with smaller fragments of OH-CATH (Table 1) have also been tested and found to be active both *in vitro* and *in vivo*, even against antibiotic resistant bacteria [4,6]. Their strong antimicrobial activity and lack of hemolytic activity make the reptile cathelicidins strong candidates for development into new therapeutics.

Table 3. Known and predicted cathelicidin open reading frames in multiple snake species. The active antimicrobial peptides NA-CATH, BF-CATH and OH-CATH are highlighted.

Protein name [Organism]	Accession		Sequence
Cathelicidin-NA antimicrobial peptide [Naja atra]	B6S2X0.1	1 81 157	MEGFFWKTLLVVGALTISGTSSFPHKPLTYEEAVDLAVSVYN SKSGEDSLYRLLEAVPALKWDALSESNQELNFSVKETV 80 CQMAEERSLEECDFQEAGAVMGCTGYYFFGESPPVLVLTCK SVGNE-EEQKQEEGNEEEKEVEKEEKEEDQKDQPKR 156 VKRFKKFFKKLKNSVKKRAKKFFKKPKVIGVTFPF191
Cathelicidin-BF antimicrobial peptide [Bungarus fasciatus]	B6D434.1	1 81 157	MEGFFWKTLLVVGALAIAGTSSLPHKPLIYEEAVDLAVSIYN SKSGEDSLYRLLEAVSPPKWDPLSESNQELNFTMKETV 80 CLVAEERSLEECDFQEDGAIMGCTGYYFFGESPPVLVLTCK PVGEE-EEQKQEEGNEEEKEVEKEEKEEDEKDQPRR 156 VKRFKKFFRKLKKSVKKRAKEFFKKPRVIGVSIPF 191
Cathelicidin-OH antimicrobial peptide [Ophiophagus hannah]	B6S2X2.1	1 81 157	MEGFFWKTLLVVGALAIGGTSSLPHKPLTYEEAVDLAVSIYNS KSGEDSLYRLLEAVPPPEWDPLSESNQELNFTIKETV 80 CLVAEERSLEECDFQEDGVVMGCTGYYFFGESPPVVVLTCKP VGEE-GEQKQEEGNEEEKEVEEEEQEEDEKDQPRR 156 VKRFKKFFKKLKNSVKKRAKKFFKKPRVIGVSIPF 191
cathelicidin-like peptide precursor [Bothrops atrox]	AGS36140.1	1 79 155	MQGFFWKTWLVVALC–GTSSSLAHRPLSYGEALELALSIYNSK AGEESLFRLLEAVPQPEWDPLSEGSQQLNFTIKETV 78 CQVEEERPLEECGFQEDGVVLECTGYYFFGETPPVVVLTCVPV GGV-EEEEEDE-EEQKAEVEKDEKEDEEKDRPKR 154 VKRFKKFFKKLKNSVKKRVKKFFRKPRVIGVTFPF 189
cathelicidin-related antimicrobial peptide isoform precursor [Pseudonaja textilis]	AGS36144.1	1 81 150	MEGFFWKTWLVVAAFAIGGTSSLPHKPLTYEEAVDLAVSTYN GKSGEESLYRLLEAVPPPKWDPLSESNQELNLTIKETV 80 CLVAEERSLEECDFQDDGAVMGCTGYFFFGESPPVLVLTCEPL GED-EEQNQEEE——-EEEEKEEDEKDQPRR 149 VKRFKKFFMKLKKSVKKRVMKFFKKPMVIGVTFPF 184
cathelicidin-related antimicrobial peptide precursor [Pseudonaja textilis]	AGS36143.1	1 81 150	MDGFFWKTWLVVAALAIGGTSSLPHKPLTYEEAVDLAVSTYN GKSGEESLYRLLEAVPPPKWDPLSESNQELNLTIKETV 80 CLVAEERSLEECDFQDDGAVMGCTGYFFFGESPPVLVLTCEP LGED-EEQNQEEE——-EEEEKEEDEKDQPRR 149 VKRFKKFFRKLKKSVKKRVKKFFKKPRVIGVTIPF 184
cathelicidin-like peptide precursor [Bothrops lutzi]	AGS36141.1	1 79 155	MQGFFWKTLLVVALC—GTSSSLAHRPLSYGEALELALSVYNS KAGEESLFRLLEAVPQPEWDPLSEGSQQLNFTIKETV 78 CQVEEERPLEECGFQEDGVVLECTGYYFFGETPPVVVLTCVP VGGV-EEEEEDE-EEQKAEVEKDEKEDEEKDRPKR 154 VKRFKKFFKKLKNNVKKRVKKFFRKPRVIGVTIPF 189
cathelicidin-like peptide precursor [Lachesis muta rhombeata]	AGS36142.1	1 79 160	MQGFFWKTWLVLAVC–GTPASLAHRPLSYGEALELAVSVYN GKAGEASLYRLLEAVPQPEWDPSSEGSQQLNFTLKETA 78 CQVEEERSLEECGFQEDGVVLECTGYYFFGETPPVVVLSCVP VGGVeEEEEEEE-EEQKAEAENDEKEDEEKDQPKR 159 160 VKRFKKFFKKVKKSVKKRLKKIFKKPMVIGVTFPF 194
cathelicidin-like peptide precursor [Crotalus durissus terrificus]	AGS36138.1	1 79 160	MQGFFWKTWLVLAVC—GTPASLAHRPLSYGEALELAVSVYN GKAGEASLYRLLEAVPQPEWDPSSEGSQQLNFTLKETA 78 CQVEEERSLEECGFQEDGVVLECTGYYFFGETPPVVVLSCVP VGGVeEEEEEEE-EEQKAEAENDEKGDEEKDQPKR 159 VKRFKKFFKKVKKSVKKRLKKIFKKPMVIGVTIPF 194

3.3.2. Chinese King Cobra *(Naja (N.) Atra)*

The genus *Naja* is a group of venomous elapid snakes in the southern Africa and South Asia, including the species *N. atra*, the Chinese King cobra. The cathelicidin peptide from the Chinese King cobra, *N. atra* (NA-CATH) (Table 1), has been well studied. The full-length NA-CATH peptide was synthesized and was found to be antimicrobial against a wide variety of bacteria [102–105]. Smaller fragments of this peptide have been identified and found to be effective [102–105].

Interestingly, while the human cathelicidin peptide (LL-37) was found to exert antibiofilm activity against bacterial pathogens such as *Pseudomonas* [103] and *Staphylococcus* [105], NA-CATH did not exhibit antibiofilm effect against *Pseudomonas*, despite similar overall biophysical properties (length, size, charge) to LL-37.

The smallest identified fragment of NA-CATH is an 11-amino acid peptide, called ATRA, which imperfectly repeats in the NA-CATH sequence (Figure 7a) [102]. Variants of the ATRA peptide have been found to be very informative regarding the role of charged residues and proline residues in the activity of small antimicrobial peptides [102]. The peptide ATRA-1 is almost identical to the ATRA-2 peptide, with the exception of the 3d (A/F) and 10th (L/P) residues. Variants of these peptides were made to switch out the 3rd and 10th position amino acids, such that ATRA-1A contains alanine at position 3 rather than phenylalanine (F). Another variant was ATRA-1P, which contains proline at position 10 rather than leucine (L). All the peptides were the same length, similar molecular weight, and the same net charge. It was found for multiple gram-negative bacteria that ATRA-1P was almost as ineffective as ATRA-2, while ATRA-1A was as effective as ATRA-1 [102]. These results suggested that the introduction of a proline in ATRA-1P may have affected the charge distribution on that peptide, which then may disrupt the antibacterial activity of the peptide (Figure 7b,c).

Further studies have examined the D-amino acid enantiomer of the ATRA peptides [106], and found that D-ATRA-1A is as effective as ATRA-1A, and as it is protease resistant, potentially has a longer half-life. The ATRA peptides have also been demonstrated to be highly antimicrobial both *in vitro* and *in vivo* against both gram-negative bacteria such as *Escherichia coli* K12 strain and *Aggregatibacter actinomycetemcomitans*-Y4 [102], *Pseudomonas aeruginosa* [103] and *Francisella novicida* [104]. ATRA peptides are also antimicrobial against the gram-positive bacteria *Staphylococcus aureus* [105].

3.3.3. Banded Krait *(B. fasciatus)*

The cathelicidin peptide from *B. fasciatus* (BF-CATH, Table 1, Table 3) is also very well studied. The full-length BF-CATH peptide has been shown to have antimicrobial activity against a variety of bacteria including antibiotic resistant bacteria [7,107]. Smaller fragments of BF-CATH have also been expressed and studied [10,108] (Table 1). For example, BF-30 showed significant activity against drug-resistant *E. coli* and *S. aureus* both *in vitro* and *in vivo* [109]. BF-15 is a shorter version of BF-CATH with lower hemolytic activity, and broad-spectrum antimicrobial activity even against antibiotic-resistant bacteria [8].

Peptide Description	Peptide Sequence
NA-CATH Active Peptide	**KRFKKFFKKLK**NSVK**KRAKKFFKKPK**VIGVTFPF
ATRA-1	**KRFKKFFKKLK**
ATRA-2	------------------------------ **KRAKKFFKKPK**
ATRA-1A	**KAFKKFFKKLK**
ATRA-1P	**KRFKKFFKKPK**

(a) Sequence of the Chinese King Cobra *Naja atra* cathelicidin and ATRA derivatives.

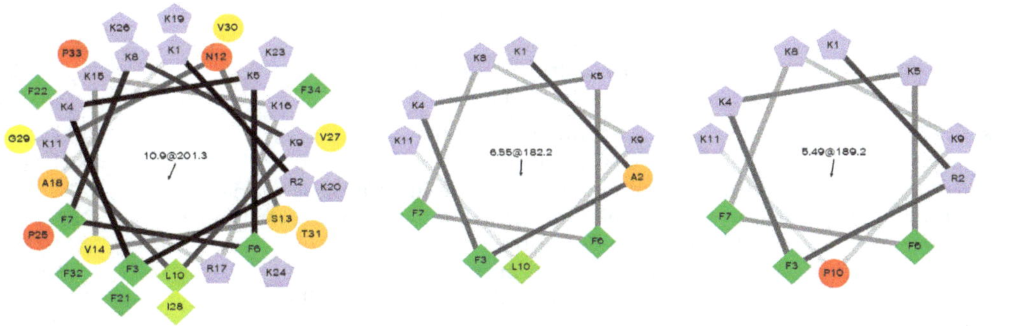

(b) **(c)** **(d)**

Figure 7. *Naja atra* cathelicidin peptide analysis. (**a**) Sequences of the NA-CATH active peptide and derivatives [102–105]. (**b**) Helical wheel projection of NA-CATH. (**c**) Analysis of the active ATRA-1A peptide (**d**) Analysis of the inactive ATRA-1P peptide. From Rzlab.ucr.edu/scripts/wheel/wheel.cgi: "The hydrophilic residues are presented as circles, hydrophobic residues as diamonds, potentially negatively charged as triangles, and potentially positively charged as pentagons. Hydrophobicity is color coded as well: the most hydrophobic residue is green, and the amount of green is decreasing proportionally to the hydrophobicity, with zero hydrophobicitycoded as yellow. Hydrophilic residues are coded red with pure red being the most hydrophilic (uncharged) residue, and the amount of red decreasing proportionally to the hydrophilicity. The potentially charged residues are light blue."

3.3.4. Predicted Cathelicidins in Other Snake Species

By performing BLAST analysis with the elapid snake cathelicidins against other snake sequences in the database, we identified cathelicidin-like gene sequences in the venomous pit viper, *Bothrops atrox*, and the Eastern brown snake, *Pseudonaja textilis* (Table 3). These genes should be further studied to verify that cathelicidin-like peptides are produced and to determine the activity of these peptides.

3.4. Cathelicidin Peptides in Lizards

Cathelicidin-like peptides Ac-CATH-1, Ac-CATH-2a, Ac-CATH -2b, and Ac-CATH -3 have been reported in the genome of the Carolina anole lizard (*Anolis carolinensis*) [110] (Table 4). In addition, cathelicidin 1 and 2 antibody reactive peptides have been identified by immunocytochemistry staining within granules of heterophilic and basophilic granulocytes [111]. This study also identified cathelicidin-antibody staining material in wound epidermis and associated with bacteria within wounds [111].

Table 4. Predicted active cathelicidin peptides in the anole lizard [91,92].

Organism	Peptide annotation
Anolis carolinensis	Ac-CATH-1 MGRITRSRWGRFWRGAKRFVKKHGVSIALAGLRFG (+10)
Anolis carolinensis	Ac-CATH-2a/b DPQMTRFRGLGHFFKGFGRGFIWGLNH (+3)
Anolis carolinensis	Ac-CATH-3—no active peptide encoded.

3.5. Cathelicidin Peptides in Turtles

Analysis of the recently published genomes revealed that there are many cathelicin-like genes in turtles. While no active cathelicidin peptides have been demonstrated yet in the turtle (Table 1), there are at many predicted cathelicidin-like peptide genes (Table 5). Many of these are annotated as being similar to the snake cathelicidins (eg OH-CATH).

Table 5. Predicted cathelicidin pre-pro-protein genes in multiple turtle species.

Organism	Peptide annotation	Locus- Accession #
Chrysemys picta bellii	Cathelicidin-OH antimicrobial peptide-like	XM_005295113.1
Chrysemys picta bellii	Cathelicidin-OH antimicrobial peptide-like	XP_005295170.1
Chrysemys picta bellii	Cathelicidin-2-like	XP_005295171.1
Chrysemys picta bellii	Uncharacterized LOC101951069	XR_255838.1
Chrysemys picta bellii	Uncharacterized LOC101951243	XR_255839.1
Pelodiscus sinensis	Cathelicidin-2-like	XM_006114422.1
Pelodiscus sinensis	Cathelicidin-2-like	XM_006114419.1
Pelodiscus sinensis	Cathelicidin-OH antimicrobial peptide-like transcript variant X1	XM_006129620.1
Pelodiscus sinensis	Cathelicidin-OH antimicrobial peptide-like transcript variant X2	XM_006129621.1
Pelodiscus sinensis	Cathelicidin-OH antimicrobial peptide-like	XM_006129625.1
Pelodiscus sinensis	Cathelicidin-BF antimicrobial peptide-like	XP_006114480.1
Pelodiscus sinensis	Cathelicidin-BF antimicrobial peptide-like	XM_006114418.1
Pelodiscus sinensi	Cathelicidin-2-like	XP_006114484.
Pelodiscus sinensis	Cathelicidin-2-like	XP_006114481.1
Pelodiscus sinensis	Cathelicidin-OH antimicrobial peptide-like isoform X1	XP_006129682.1
Pelodiscus sinensis	Cathelicidin-OH antimicrobial peptide-like isoform X2	XP_006129683.1
Pelodiscus sinensis	Cathelicidin-OH antimicrobial peptide-like	XP_006129687.1
Chelonia mydas	Hypothetical protein UY3_13361	EMP29519.1
Chelonia mydas	Hypothetical protein UY3_13360	EMP29518.1

3.6. Cathelicidin Peptides in Crocodilians

Analysis of the databases revealed that there are many cathelicidin-like genes in alligators. While no active cathelicidin peptides have been demonstrated yet in the alligator (Table 1), there are at many predicted cathelicidin-like peptide genes (Table 6). Many of these genes are annotated as being similar to the snake cathelicidins (e.g., OH-CATH).

Table 6. Predicted cathelicidin pre-pro-protein genes in Alligator species.

Organism	Peptide annotation	Locus- Accession #
Alligator mississippiensis	Cathelicidin-2-like	XM_006262429.1
Alligator mississippiensis	Cathelicidin-2-like	XP_006262491.1
Alligator mississippiensis	Cathelicidin-OH antimicrobial peptide-like	XM_006262431.1
Alligator mississippiensis	Cathelicidin-OH antimicrobial peptide-like	XM_006262430.1
Alligator mississippiensis	Cathelicidin-OH antimicrobial peptide-like	XP_006262492.1
Alligator mississippiensis	Cathelicidin-OH antimicrobial peptide-like	XP_006262493.1
Alligator sinensis	Cathelicidin-2-like	XM_006026412.1
Alligator sinensis	Cathelicidin-2-like	XP_006026474.1
Alligator sinensis	Cathelicidin-2-like	XP_006026475.1
Alligator sinensis	Cathelicidin-3-like	XM_006026409.1
Alligator sinensis	Cathelicidin-3-like	XP_006026471.1
Alligator sinensis	Cathelicidin-OH antimicrobial peptide-like	XM_006037224.1
Alligator sinensis	Cathelicidin-OH antimicrobial peptide-like	XM_006026410.1
Alligator sinensis	Cathelicidin-OH antimicrobial peptide-like	XM_006026411.1
Alligator sinensis	Cathelicidin-OH antimicrobial peptide-like	XM_006037211.1
Alligator sinensis	Cathelicidin-OH antimicrobial peptide-like	XP_006037286.1
Alligator sinensis	Cathelicidin-OH antimicrobial peptide-like	XP_006026472.1
Alligator sinensis	Cathelicidin-OH antimicrobial peptide-like	XP_006037273.1
Alligator sinensis	Cathelicidin-OH antimicrobial peptide-like	XP_006026487.1

3.7. *Liver-Derived Peptides in Reptiles*

3.7.1. Hepcidin (HAMP1)

Hepcidin antimicrobial peptides are liver-expressed peptides containing eight cysteines (four disulfide bonds) that are broadly antimicrobial, binds iron and is involved in ferroportin binding [112, 113]. A gene encoding a hepcidin-like peptide (E8ZAD0_CROSI) was recently proposed to be encoded by the Siamese crocodile (*Crocodylus siamensis*). A 26 aa peptide (Cshepc), representing the predicted active peptide (FNSHFPICSYCCNCCRNKGCGLCCRT), was expressed in yeast, and the unpurified product was found to have antimicrobial activity against both Gram-positive bacteria such as *S. aureus* and *Bacillus subtilis*, as well as Gram-negative bacteria *Escherichia coli* and *Aeromonas sobria* [114]. Hepcidin-like sequences were also identified in the anole lizard, although interestingly hepcidins appear to be missing in most avians [115].

3.7.2. LEAP-2, Liver Expressed Antimicrobial Peptide-2

Another liver-expressed peptide, LEAP-2, is expressed in many different organisms, has broad-spectrum antibacterial and antifungal activity, and can be induced following bacterial challenge [116–118]. This 40 aa, 4-cysteine, cationic peptide differs significantly from hepcidin in sequence and predicted structure [119], but is also predominantly expressed in the liver.

The Leap-2 gene is annotated in many of the sequenced reptiles (Table 7), including *Pelodiscus sinensis, Chrysemys picta bellii, Alligator sinensis, Alligator mississippiensis*, as identified by a BLAST analysis we performed with the LEAP-2 from *Anolis carolinensis*. The antimicrobial activity or biological role of this peptide in reptiles has not been studied.

Table 7. Predicted LEAP-2 pre-propeptide amino-acid sequences identified in reptiles.

Species	Predicted LEAP-2 full sequence	Accession Number
Anolis carolinensis	MTPLKITAVILICSALLFQTQGASLYPPNSQLVRQR RMTPFWRGISRPIGASCRDNSECSTRLCRSKHCSLRTSQE	XP_003217432.1
Alligator sinensis	MHWLKVIAVMLLFALHLFQIHCASLHQPNSQPKRQRRM TPFWRGVSSLRPIGASCRDDIECVTMLCRKSHCSLRTSRE	XP_006023615.1
Alligator mississippiensis	MHWLKVIAVMLLFALHLFQIHCASLHQPNSQPKRQRRM TPFWRGVSSLRPIGASCKDDGECITMRCRKSHCSLRTSRE	XP_006263463.1
Pelodiscus sinensis	MQCLKVIALLLFCAALLTQTHCASLHHSSSQLTRQRRMTP FWRGISLRPIGALCRHDNECISMLCRKNRCSLRISCE	XP_006128591.1
Chrysemys picta belli	MQYLKVIAVLLLCAALLSQIHSASLHRPSSHLTRQRRMTPF WRGISLRPIGAICRDDSECVSRLCRKNHCSIRISRA	XP_005302895.1

3.8. Lysozyme in Reptiles

Lysozyme is a very important part of innate immunity in most animals. In humans, it is packaged into neutrophil granules, released in tears and other secretions, and is very effective against a broad spectrum of bacteria. Not surprisingly, reptiles have also been found to use lysozyme as part of their innate immune response. In the crocodilians, a lysozyme-like enzyme was identified with broad-spectrum antibacterial activity [67]. Lysozyme proteins very similar to chicken lysozymes (~130 aa) have been identified from some species of turtles, including the soft shelled turtle (*Trionyx sinensis*), the Asiatic soft shelled turtle (*Amyda cartilagenea*) and the green sea turtle (*Chelonia mydas*) [17,19,120–122], although the antimicrobial activity of these molecules has not yet been proven. Lysozyme peptide has also been identified from *Crocodylus siamensis* [67]. Lysozyme-like genes were identified by analysis of reptile genomes (Table 8).

3.9. Crotamine Peptides in Reptiles

Defensins are one example of cysteine-stabilized polypeptides with antimicrobial function. A similar family of peptides is the crotamine toxin family isolated from rattlesnakes with a similar gamma-core motif to defensins [123,124], which is considered a cell-penetrating peptide The sequence of crotamine is YKQ**C**HKKGGH**C**FPKEKI**C**LPPSSDFGKMD**C**RWRWK**CC**KKGSG (+8) [2]. This cationic peptide contains nine lysines (underlined), three disulfide bonds (6 cysteines, shown in bold) and has a defensin-like fold (Figure 8).

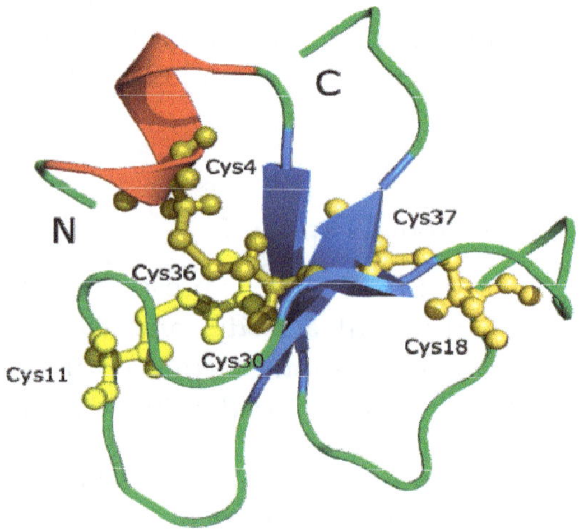

Figure 8. The crotamine chemical structure. Crotamine, a Na+ channel-affecting toxin from *Crotalus durissus terrificus* venom (PDB 1H5O) [125].

Table 8. Selected predicted lysozyme genes identified in reptiles.

Reptile name	Enzyme Name	Accession Number
Softshell turtle lysozyme C(SSTL)	Lysozyme C (1,4-β-N-acetylmuramidase C)	Q7LZQ1.3
Asiatic softshell turtle lysozyme C (ASTL)	Lysozyme C	P85345.1
Pelodiscus sinensis	Lysozyme	ADR51676.1
Pelodiscus sinensis	PREDICTED: lysozyme g-like isoform X2	XP_006113603.1
Pelodiscus sinensis	PREDICTED: lysozyme g-like isoform X1	XP_006113602.1
Pelodiscus sinensis	PREDICTED: lysozyme g-like	XP_006113601.1
Chelonia mydas	Lysozyme C	EMP38935.1
Chelonia mydas	Lysozyme G	EMP27176.1
Chrysemys picta bellii	PREDICTED: lysozyme C-like	XP_005314893.1
Chrysemys picta bellii	PREDICTED: lysozyme C-like	XP_005312037.1
Chrysemys picta bellii	PREDICTED: lysozyme g-like protein 2	XP_005283410.1
Chrysemys picta bellii	PREDICTED: lysozyme G-like	XP_005283294.1
Ophiophagus hannah	Lysozyme C, partial	ETE58503.1
Anolis carolinensis	Lysozyme C, milk isozyme-like	XP_003225844.1, XP_003216710.1, XP_003216704.1
Anolis carolinensis	Lysozyme C II-like	XP_003224512.1
Anolis carolinensis	Lysozyme g-like	XP_003227178.1
Alligator sinensis	Lysozyme C-like	XP_006027022.1, XP_006027021.1
Alligator sinensis	Lysozyme G-like	XP_006026406.1, XP_006026397.1, XP_006026395.1, XP_006026396.1

Some reptiles are known to express crotamine-like peptides, and The X-ray structure of crotamine, from the Brazilian snake *Crotalus durissus terrificus*, was recently solved (PDB 4GV5_A) [126]. We found that some species of reptiles have genes that are annotated as crotamine-like (Table 9).

Table 9. Crotamine-like peptide genes in reptiles.

Reptile	AA	Name	Accession numbers
Uromastyx aegyptia	67	crotamine-Uro-1	AGI97143.1
Crotalus durissus terrificus	65	crotamine	AAF34911.1, AAF34910.1, AAC02995.1, AAC06241.1
Crotalus durissus	34	crotamine	ACA63453.1, ACA63452.1, ACA63451.1, ACA63450.1, ACA63449.1, ACA63448.1, ACA63447.1, ACA63446.1
Crotalus oreganus helleri	65	crotamine 7	AEU60015.1
Crotalus oreganus helleri	65	crotamine 6	AEU60014.1
Crotalus oreganus helleri	65	crotamine 5	AEU60013.1
Crotalus oreganus helleri	70	crotamine 4	AEU60012.1
Crotalus oreganus helleri	70	crotamine 3	AEU60011.1
Crotalus oreganus helleri	83	crotamine 2	AEU60010.1
Crotalus oreganus helleri	70	crotamine 1	AEU60009.1
Pogona barbata	102	CLP-POGL1	AAZ75614.1
Pogona barbata	67	CLP-POGL2	AAZ75615.1
Pogona barbata	61	CLP-POGU3	AAZ75613.1
Pogona barbata	98	CLP-POGU2	AAZ75612.1
Pogona barbata	76	CLP-POGU1	AAZ75611.1
Varanus tristis	83	crotamine-Var-5	AGI97148.1
Varanus glauerti	83	crotamine-Var-4	AGI97147.1
Varanus glauerti	83	crotamine-Var-3	AGI97146.1
Varanus glauerti	83	crotamine-Var-2	AGI97145.1
Varanus glauerti	83	crotamine-Var-1	AGI97144.1

It has been a matter of some debate whether crotamine peptides are antimicrobial or if they just contain a similar cysteine-stabilized core structure. Recently, it was demonstrated that crotamine toxin is expressed similarly on epithelial or mucosal surfaces, and displays some antimicrobial activity against *Bacillus subtilis*, and was able to permeabilize *Staphylococcus aureus* cells, for example [20]. In addition, crotamine has been shown to be antifungal [127]. Thus, it seems that crotamine should be considered as an antimicrobial peptide of reptiles.

3.10. Other Peptides in Reptiles

3.10.1. Leucrocin

There are a handful of peptides identified in reptiles that were not easily classified in the categories above. One interesting example is the peptide leucrocin, an antibacterial compound from white blood cells of the Siamese crocodile (*Crocodylus siamensis*). Unlike Crocosin [65], which does not appear to be peptide based, leucrocins are very small peptides with antibacterial activity. The amino acid sequence of Leucrocin I is NGVQPKY, and of Leucrocin II is NAGSLLSGWG [66]. No known genes encode for these peptides, so their source is unclear. Recently, a synthetic peptide based on the Leucrocin sequence was found to have broad-spectrum antibacterial activity [128].

3.10.2. Omwaprin

Another example of an unusual antimicrobial peptide in reptiles is omwaprin, which is a member of the waprin family of venom proteins (Sequence shown in Table 1) [11,12], and was isolated from the Australian inland taipan (*Oxyuranus microlepidotus*), considered the most venomous snake (a member of the Elapid family of snakes). This 50 aa peptide has relatively salt-tolerant antibacterial activity against gram-positive bacteria and was found to be non-toxic to mice upon injection. Its activity was found to be highly dependent upon the four disulfide-bonds, similar to the hepcidins and defensins [11]. Thus, except for its large size, this peptide appears to have many favorable properties as a potential therapeutic candidate.

3.10.3. Hemocidin

Fragments of hemoglobin have been found to have some antimicrobial activity, and have been referred to as hemocidins [129–131]. In the study of the Siamese crocodile, 13 fragments of crocodile hemoglobin were found to have antimicrobial activity, including peptides similar to hemoglobin β subunit [59,60]. Recently, the hemoglobin α- and β-chains of crocodilian species (*Crocodylus siamensis*, *Alligator mississippiensis*, *Crocodylus niloticus* and *Caiman crocodilus*) have been reported [132]. The *in vivo* relevance of these peptides in the crocodile remains to be determined, but it represents a potential other class of antimicrobial peptides from reptiles that should be investigated.

3.10.4. Other Peptides

Other peptides have been identified in reptiles that do not fall into the various classes of antimicrobial peptides described above. These include a short, synthetic tryptophan-rich cationic antimicrobial peptide, pEM-2 (KKWRWWLKALAKK) that was shown to have broad-spectrum bactericidal activities, and was identified as a fragment of myotoxin II, a snake venom Lys49 phospholipase A2 [133,134]. Synthetic variants of this peptide were shown to have improved antimicrobial activity, salt resistance and reduced hemolytic activity [135,136]. These peptides have led to other advances in rational design of synthetic peptides, including peptides with exclusively arginine and tryptophan residues [137].

Gomes et al isolated, but did not sequence, a small 1370 Da peptide from the venom of a pit viper (*Borthrops jaracaca*), which showed very good activity against different fungi and yeast [138].

Another group identified an antimicrobial peptide derived from *N. atra* venom, the vgf-1 peptide, and found that this peptide had significant antimicrobial activity against drug-resistant clinical strains of *Mycobacterium tuberculosis* [139].

4. Conclusions

Reptiles are evolutionarily ancient, found in diverse and microbially challenging environments and appear to have robust immune systems. Some reptiles, especially lizards, have unique properties such as tail regeneration. All of these features suggest that reptiles may express many interesting antimicrobial peptides. A few reptilian antimicrobial peptides have been isolated and studied which demonstrate broad-spectrum antimicrobial and antifungal activity. These include members of the cathelicidin and defensin and lysozyme class.

Antimicrobial peptides are known in three of the four orders of reptiles: the testudines, crocodilians, and the squamata. No peptides are known from the sphenodontia (tuataras), as this organism has just been sequenced [41]. Reptile neutrophils appear to have granules that contain both cathelicidin-like peptides as well as β-defensin peptides, although unlike mammals, there are no genes encoding α-defensins. β-defensin-like peptides and lysozyme are also found in reptile eggs. These peptides are expressed in wounds, such as when lizards lose their tails. Detailed study of the Chinese cobra Naja atra cathelicidin peptides has revealed smaller peptides that could be useful for therapeutic applications.

Overall, reptiles reflect the diversity of antimicrobial peptides within higher organisms. They appear to express cathelicidins and β-defensins, and express hepcidins unlike avians. Additional classes of antimicrobial peptides such as lysozyme, LEAP-2 and crotamine also appear to be highly expressed in reptiles. With the advent of high-throughput genomics, new reptilian genomes have been sequenced and their transcriptomes determined. Analysis of these sequences has revealed that there are additional genes that may encode AMPs in reptiles. Future studies may reveal the in vivo role of antimicrobial peptides in reptiles. In the face of the emerging challenges due to antibiotic resistant bacteria, new and useful molecules that could be developed into future antibiotics may potentially be found in the reptilian AMPs.

Acknowledgments: MVH was partially supported by HDTRA1-12-C-0039, Translational Peptides for Personnel Protection.

References

1. Wang, G. Antimicrobial Peptide Database. Available online: http://aps.unmc.edu/AP (accessed on 9 May 2014).
2. Wang, G.; Li, X.; Wang, Z. APD2: The updated antimicrobial peptide database and its application in peptide design. *Nucleic Acids Res.* **2009**, *37*, D933–D937. [CrossRef]
3. Zhao, H.; Gan, T.X.; Liu, X.D.; Jin, Y.; Lee, W.H.; Shen, J.H.; Zhang, Y. Identification and characterization of novel reptile cathelicidins from elapid snakes. *Peptides* **2008**, *29*, 1685–1691. [CrossRef]
4. Li, S.A.; Lee, W.H.; Zhang, Y. Efficacy of OH-CATH30 and its analogs against drug-resistant bacteria *in vitro* and in mouse models. *Antimicrob. Agents Chemother.* **2012**, *56*, 3309–3317. [CrossRef]
5. Zhang, B.Y.; Li, S.M.; Gao, Z.H.; Shen, J.H. Protective effects of snake venom antimicrobial peptide OH-CATH on *E. coli* induced rabbit urinary tract infection models. *Dong Wu Xue Yan Jiu* **2013**, *34*, 27–32.
6. Zhang, Y.; Zhao, H.; Yu, G.Y.; Liu, X.D.; Shen, J.H.; Lee, W.H.; Zhang, Y. Structure-function relationship of king cobra cathelicidin. *Peptides* **2010**, *31*, 1488–1493. [CrossRef]
7. Wang, Y.; Hong, J.; Liu, X.; Yang, H.; Liu, R.; Wu, J.; Wang, A.; Lin, D.; Lai, R. Snake cathelicidin from Bungarus fasciatus is a potent peptide antibiotics. *PloS One* **2008**, *3*, e3217.
8. Chen, W.; Yang, B.; Zhou, H.; Sun, L.; Dou, J.; Qian, H.; Huang, W.; Mei, Y.; Han, J. Structure-activity relationships of a snake cathelicidin-related peptide, BF-15. *Peptides* **2011**, *32*, 2497–2503. [CrossRef]

9. Wang, H.; Ke, M.; Tian, Y.; Wang, J.; Li, B.; Wang, Y.; Dou, J.; Zhou, C. BF-30 selectively inhibits melanoma cell proliferation via cytoplasmic membrane permeabilization and DNA-binding *in vitro* and in B16F10-bearing mice. *Eur. J. Pharmacol.* **2013**, *707*, 1–10.
10. Zhou, H.; Dou, J.; Wang, J.; Chen, L.; Wang, H.; Zhou, W.; Li, Y.; Zhou, C. The antibacterial activity of BF-30 *in vitro* and in infected burned rats is through interference with cytoplasmic membrane integrity. *Peptides* **2011**, *32*, 1131–1138. [CrossRef]
11. Nair, D.G.; Fry, B.G.; Alewood, P.; Kumar, P.P.; Kini, R.M. Antimicrobial activity of omwaprin, a new member of the waprin family of snake venom proteins. *Biochem. J.* **2007**, *402*, 93–104. [CrossRef]
12. Banigan, J.R.; Mandal, K.; Sawaya, M.R.; Thammavongsa, V.; Hendrickx, A.P.; Schneewind, O.; Yeates, T.O.; Kent, S.B. Determination of the X-ray structure of the snake venom protein omwaprin by total chemical synthesis and racemic protein crystallography. *Protein Sci.* **2010**, *19*, 1840–1849. [CrossRef]
13. Schmidt, J.J.; Weinstein, S.A.; Smith, L.A. Molecular properties and structure-function relationships of lethal peptides from venom of Wagler's pit viper, *Trimeresurus wagleri*. *Toxicon* **1992**, *30*, 1027–1036. [CrossRef]
14. Stegemann, C.; Kolobov, A., Jr.; Leonova, Y.F.; Knappe, D.; Shamova, O.; Ovchinnikova, T.V.; Kokryakov, V.N.; Hoffmann, R. Isolation, purification and de novo sequencing of TBD-1, the first beta-defensin from leukocytes of reptiles. *Proteomics* **2009**, *9*, 1364–1373. [CrossRef]
15. Lakshminarayanan, R.; Vivekanandan, S.; Samy, R.P.; Banerjee, Y.; Chi-Jin, E.O.; Teo, K.W.; Jois, S.D.; Kini, R.M.; Valiyaveettil, S. Structure, self-assembly, and dual role of a beta-defensin-like peptide from the Chinese soft-shelled turtle eggshell matrix. *J. Am. Chem. Soc.* **2008**, *130*, 4660–4668. [CrossRef]
16. Lakshminarayanan, R.; Chi-Jin, E.O.; Loh, X.J.; Kini, R.M.; Valiyaveettil, S. Purification and characterization of a vaterite-inducing peptide, pelovaterin, from the eggshells of Pelodiscus sinensis (Chinese soft-shelled turtle). *Biomacromolecules* **2005**, *6*, 1429–1437. [CrossRef]
17. Thammasirirak, S.; Ponkham, P.; Preecharram, S.; Khanchanuan, R.; Phonyothee, P.; Daduang, S.; Srisomsap, C.; Araki, T.; Svasti, J. Purification, characterization and comparison of reptile lysozymes. *Comp. biochem. Phys. Toxicol. Pharmacol.* **2006**, *143*, 209–217.
18. Chattopadhyay, S.; Sinha, N.K.; Banerjee, S.; Roy, D.; Chattopadhyay, D.; Roy, S. Small cationic protein from a marine turtle has beta-defensin-like fold and antibacterial and antiviral activity. *Proteins* **2006**, *64*, 524–531. [CrossRef]
19. Ponkham, P.; Daduang, S.; Kitimasak, W.; Krittanai, C.; Chokchaichamnankit, D.; Srisomsap, C.; Svasti, J.; Kawamura, S.; Araki, T.; Thammasirirak, S. Complete amino acid sequence of three reptile lysozymes. *Comp. Biochem. Phys. Toxicol. Pharmacol.* **2010**, *151*, 75–83. [CrossRef]
20. Yount, N.Y.; Kupferwasser, D.; Spisni, A.; Dutz, S.M.; Ramjan, Z.H.; Sharma, S.; Waring, A.J.; Yeaman, M.R. Selective reciprocity in antimicrobial activity *versus* cytotoxicity of hBD-2 and crotamine. *Proc. Natl. Acad. Sci. USA* **2009**, *106*, 14972–14977. [CrossRef]
21. Coronado, M.A.; Georgieva, D.; Buck, F.; Gabdoulkhakov, A.H.; Ullah, A.; Spencer, P.J.; Arni, R.K.; Betzel, C. Purification, crystallization and preliminary X-ray diffraction analysis of crotamine, a myotoxic polypeptide from the Brazilian snake Crotalus durissus terrificus. *Acta Crystallogr. F* **2012**, *68*, 1052–1054. [CrossRef]
22. Modesto, S.P.; Anderson, J.S. The phylogenetic definition of reptilia. *Syst. Biol.* **2004**, *53*, 815–821. [CrossRef]
23. Alfoldi, J.; Di Palma, F.; Grabherr, M.; Williams, C.; Kong, L.; Mauceli, E.; Russell, P.; Lowe, C.B.; Glor, R.E.; Jaffe, J.D.; *et al.* The genome of the green anole lizard and a comparative analysis with birds and mammals. *Nature* **2011**, *477*, 587–591. [CrossRef]
24. Cladogram by Benchill, licensed under the Creative Commons Attribution 3.0 Unported license. Available online: http://en.wikipedia.org/wiki/File:Tuatara_cladogram.svg (accessed on 9 May 2014).
25. Ernst, C.H.; Lovich, J.E. *Turtles of the United States and Canada*, 2nd ed.; Johns Hopkins University Press: Baltimore, MD, USA, 2009; pp. 185–259.
26. Photo from Oregon Department of Fish & Wildlife, licensed under the Creative Commons Attribution-Share Alike 2.0 Generic license. Photo by Gary M. Stolz/U. S. Fish and Wildlife Service in the Public domain. Available online: http://en.wikipedia.org/wiki/FileA4_Western_painted_turtle.jpg (accessed on 9 May 2014).
27. Underside of a Western Painted Turtle. Photo by Matt Young, l.u.t.C.C.A.-S.A.G.l. Available online: http://en.wikipedia.org/wiki/File:B4_Western_painted_turtle_underside.jpg (accessed on 9 May 2014).
28. Wang, Z.; Pascual-Anaya, J.; Zadissa, A.; Li, W.; Niimura, Y.; Huang, Z.; Li, C.; White, S.; Xiong, Z.; Fang, D.; *et al.* The draft genomes of soft-shell turtle and green sea turtle yield insights into the development and evolution of the turtle-specific body plan. *Nat. Genet.* **2013**, *45*, 701–706. [CrossRef]

29. Jiang, J.J.; Xia, E.H.; Gao, C.W.; Gao, L.Z. The complete mitochondrial genome of western painted turtle, *Chrysemys picta bellii* (Chrysemys, Emydidae). *Mitochondrial DNA* **2014**. [CrossRef]
30. Shaffer, H.B.; Minx, P.; Warren, D.E.; Shedlock, A.M.; Thomson, R.C.; Valenzuela, N.; Abramyan, J.; Amemiya, C.T.; Badenhorst, D.; Biggar, K.K.; *et al.* The western painted turtle genome, a model for the evolution of extreme physiological adaptations in a slowly evolving lineage. *Genome Biol.* **2013**, *14*, R28. [CrossRef]
31. Gilbert, S.F.; Corfe, I. Turtle origins: Picking up speed. *Dev. Cell* **2013**, *25*, 326–328. [CrossRef]
32. Zardoya, R.; Meyer, A. Complete mitochondrial genome suggests diapsid affinities of turtles. *Proc. Natl. Acad. Sci. USA* **1998**, *95*, 14226–14231. [CrossRef]
33. Iwabe, N.; Hara, Y.; Kumazawa, Y.; Shibamoto, K.; Saito, Y.; Miyata, T.; Katoh, K. Sister group relationship of turtles to the bird-crocodilian clade revealed by nuclear DNA-coded proteins. *Mol. Biol. Evol.* **2005**, *22*, 810–813. [CrossRef]
34. Roos, J.; Aggarwal, R.K.; Janke, A. Extended mitogenomic phylogenetic analyses yield new insight into crocodylian evolution and their survival of the Cretaceous-Tertiary boundary. *Mol. Phylogenet. Evol.* **2007**, *45*, 663–673. [CrossRef]
35. Katsu, Y.; Matsubara, K.; Kohno, S.; Matsuda, Y.; Toriba, M.; Oka, K.; Guillette, L.J., Jr.; Ohta, Y.; Iguchi, T. Molecular cloning, characterization, and chromosome mapping of reptilian estrogen receptors. *Endocrinology* **2010**, *151*, 5710–5720.
36. Lyson, T.R.; Sperling, E.A.; Heimberg, A.M.; Gauthier, J.A.; King, B.L.; Peterson, K.J. MicroRNAs support a turtle + lizard clade. *Biol. Lett.* **2012**, *8*, 104–107. [CrossRef]
37. Jones, M.E.; Cree, A. Tuatara. *Curr. Biol.* **2012**, *22*, R986–R987. [CrossRef]
38. Hay, J.M.; Sarre, S.D.; Lambert, D.M.; Allendorf, F.W.; Daugherty, C.H. Genetic diversity and taxonomy: A reassessment of species designation in tuatara (Sphenodon: Reptilia). *Conserv. Genet.* **2010**, *11*, 1063–1081.
39. Photo by PhillipC, licensed under the Creative Commons Attribution 2.0 Generic license. Available online: http://en.wikipedia.org/wiki/File:Sphenodon_punctatus_in_Waikanae,_New_Zealand.jpg (accessed on 9 May 2014).
40. Ramstad, K.M.; Nelson, N.J.; Paine, G.; Beech, D.; Paul, A.; Paul, P.; Allendorf, F.W.; Daugherty, C.H. Species and cultural conservation in New Zealand: maori traditional ecological knowledge of tuatara. *Conserv. Biol.* **2007**, *21*, 455–464. [CrossRef]
41. Miller, H.C.; Biggs, P.J.; Voelckel, C.; Nelson, N.J. De novo sequence assembly and characterisation of a partial transcriptome for an evolutionarily distinct reptile, the tuatara (*Sphenodon punctatus*). *BMC Genomics* **2012**, *13*, 439. [CrossRef]
42. Vonk, F.J.; Casewell, N.R.; Henkel, C.V.; Heimberg, A.M.; Jansen, H.J.; McCleary, R.J.; Kerkkamp, H.M.; Vos, R.A.; Guerreiro, I.; Calvete, J.J.; *et al.* The king cobra genome reveals dynamic gene evolution and adaptation in the snake venom system. *Proc. Natl. Acad. Sci. US A* **2013**, *110*, 20651–20656. [CrossRef]
43. Pyron, R.A.; Burbrink, F.T.; Guiher, T.J. Claims of potential expansion throughout the U.S. by invasive python species are contradicted by ecological niche models. *PloS One* **2008**, *3*, e2931. [CrossRef]
44. Photo by Greg Hume, licensed under the Creative Commons Attribution 2.0 Generic license. Available online: http://en.wikipedia.org/wiki/File:King_Cobra_25.jpg (accessed on 9 May 2014).
45. Found inside a water catchment on Lantau. 2011, Photo by: Thomas Brown. This file is licensed under the Creative Commons Attribution 2.0 Generic license. Available online: http://en.wikipedia.org/wiki/File: Naja_atra_juvenile.jpg (accessed on 9 May 2014).
46. Photo by AshLin. Photo of Banded Krait captured in Binnaguri, N.B., India on 19 Sep 2006. This file is licensed under the Creative Commons Attribution-Share Alike 2.5 Generic license. Available online: http://en.wikipedia.org/wiki/File:AB_054_Banded_Krait.JPG (accessed on 9 May 2014).
47. Photo by PiccoloNamek at en.wikipedia, licensed under the Creative Commons Attribution-Share Alike 3.0 Unported license. Available online: http://en.wikipedia.org/wiki/File:Anolis_carolinensis.jpg (accessed on 9 May 2014).
48. Aird, S.D.; Watanabe, Y.; Villar-Briones, A.; Roy, M.C.; Terada, K.; Mikheyev, A.S. Quantitative high-throughput profiling of snake venom gland transcriptomes and proteomes (*Ovophis okinavensis* and *Protobothrops flavoviridis*). *BMC Genomics* **2013**, *14*, 790. [CrossRef]

49. Dalla Valle, L.; Benato, F.; Maistro, S.; Quinzani, S.; Alibardi, L. Bioinformatic and molecular characterization of beta-defensins-like peptides isolated from the green lizard Anolis carolinensis. *Dev. Comp. Immunol.* **2012**, *36*, 222–229. [CrossRef]
50. Erickson, G.M.; Gignac, P.M.; Steppan, S.J.; Lappin, A.K.; Vliet, K.A.; Brueggen, J.D.; Inouye, B.D.; Kledzik, D.; Webb, G.J. Insights into the ecology and evolutionary success of crocodilians revealed through bite-force and tooth-pressure experimentation. *PloS One* **2012**, *7*, e31781. [CrossRef]
51. Shirley, M.H.; Vliet, K.A.; Carr, A.N.; Austin, J.D. Rigorous approaches to species delimitation have significant implications for African crocodilian systematics and conservation. *Proc. Biol. Sci.* **2014**, *281*, 20132483.
52. An American Alligator (One of two) in captivity at the Columbus Zoo, Powell, Ohio. This file is licensed under the Creative Commons Attribution-Share Alike 3.0 Unported license. Available online: http://en.wikipedia.org/wiki/File:American_Alligator.jpg (accessed on 9 May 2014).
53. A Siamese Crocodile (Crocodylus siamensis) at the Jerusalem Biblical Zoo. This file is licensed under the Creative Commons Attribution-Share Alike 3.0 Unported license. Available online: http://commons.wikimedia.org/wiki/File:Siamese_Crocodile-Biblical_Zoo.JPG (accessed on 9 May 2014).
54. Lance, V.A. Alligator physiology and life history: The importance of temperature. *Exp. Gerontol.* **2003**, *38*, 801–805. [CrossRef]
55. Brown, D.R.; Schumacher, I.M.; Nogueira, M.F.; Richey, L.J.; Zacher, L.A.; Schoeb, T.R.; Vliet, K.A.; Bennett, R.A.; Jacobson, E.R.; Brown, M.B. Detection of antibodies to a pathogenic mycoplasma in American alligators (*Alligator mississippiensis*), broad-nosed Caimans (*Caiman latirostris*), and Siamese crocodiles (*Crocodylus siamensis*). *J. Clin. Microbiol.* **2001**, *39*, 285–292. [CrossRef]
56. Meganathan, P.R.; Dubey, B.; Batzer, M.A.; Ray, D.A.; Haque, I. Molecular phylogenetic analyses of genus Crocodylus (Eusuchia, Crocodylia, Crocodylidae) and the taxonomic position of *Crocodylus porosus*. *Mol. Phylogenet. Evol.* **2010**, *57*, 393–402. [CrossRef]
57. Kommanee, J.; Preecharram, S.; Daduang, S.; Temsiripong, Y.; Dhiravisit, A.; Yamada, Y.; Thammasirirak, S. Antibacterial activity of plasma from crocodile (*Crocodylus siamensis*) against pathogenic bacteria. *Ann. Clin. Microbiol. Antimicrob.* **2012**, *11*, 22. [CrossRef]
58. Theansungnoen, T.; Yaraksa, N.; Daduang, S.; Dhiravisit, A.; Thammasirirak, S. Purification and Characterization of Antioxidant Peptides from Leukocyte Extract of *Crocodylus siamensis*. *Protein J.* **2014**, *33*, 24–31.
59. Srihongthong, S.; Pakdeesuwan, A.; Daduang, S.; Araki, T.; Dhiravisit, A.; Thammasirirak, S. Complete amino acid sequence of globin chains and biological activity of fragmented crocodile hemoglobin (*Crocodylus siamensis*). *Protein J.* **2012**, *31*, 466–476.
60. Jandaruang, J.; Siritapetawee, J.; Thumanu, K.; Songsiriritthigul, C.; Krittanai, C.; Daduang, S.; Dhiravisit, A.; Thammasirirak, S. The effects of temperature and pH on secondary structure and antioxidant activity of *Crocodylus siamensis* hemoglobin. *Protein J.* **2012**, *31*, 43–50.
61. Johnston, M.A.; Porter, D.E.; Scott, G.I.; Rhodes, W.E.; Webster, L.F. Isolation of faecal coliform bacteria from the American alligator (*Alligator mississippiensis*). *J. Appl. Microbiol.* **2010**, *108*, 965–973. [CrossRef]
62. Merchant, M.E.; Mills, K.; Leger, N.; Jerkins, E.; Vliet, K.A.; McDaniel, N. Comparisons of innate immune activity of all known living crocodylian species. *Com. Biochem. Physiol. Part B* **2006**, *143*, 133–137.
63. Merchant, M.E.; Leger, N.; Jerkins, E.; Mills, K.; Pallansch, M.B.; Paulman, R.L.; Ptak, R.G. Broad spectrum antimicrobial activity of leukocyte extracts from the American alligator (*Alligator mississippiensis*). *Vet. Immunol. Immunopathol.* **2006**, *110*, 221–228. [CrossRef]
64. Merchant, M.E.; Roche, C.; Elsey, R.M.; Prudhomme, J. Antibacterial properties of serum from the American alligator (*Alligator mississippiensis*). *Comp. biochem. Physiol. Part B* **2003**, *136*, 505–513. [CrossRef]
65. Preecharram, S.; Jearranaiprepame, P.; Daduang, S.; Temsiripong, Y.; Somdee, T.; Fukamizo, T.; Svasti, J.; Araki, T.; Thammasirirak, S. Isolation and characterisation of crocosin, an antibacterial compound from crocodile (*Crocodylus siamensis*) plasma. *Nihon chikusan Gakkaiho* **2010**, *81*, 393–401.
66. Pata, S.; Yaraksa, N.; Daduang, S.; Temsiripong, Y.; Svasti, J.; Araki, T.; Thammasirirak, S. Characterization of the novel antibacterial peptide Leucrocin from crocodile (*Crocodylus siamensis*) white blood cell extracts. *Dev. Comp. Immunol.* **2011**, *35*, 545–553.
67. Pata, S.; Daduang, S.; Svasti, J.; Thammasirirak, S. Isolation of Lysozyme like protein from crocodile leukocyte extract (*Crocodylus siamensis*). *KMITL Sci. Technol. J.* **2007**, *7*, 70–85.
68. Castoe, T.A.; Pollock, D.D. Chinese alligator genome illustrates molecular adaptations. *Cell res.* **2013**, *23*, 1254–1255. [CrossRef]

69. St John, J.A.; Braun, E.L.; Isberg, S.R.; Miles, L.G.; Chong, A.Y.; Gongora, J.; Dalzell, P.; Moran, C.; Bed'hom, B.; Abzhanov, A.; *et al.* Sequencing three crocodilian genomes to illuminate the evolution of archosaurs and amniotes. *Genome Biol.* **2012**, *13*, 415. [CrossRef]
70. Wan, Q.H.; Pan, S.K.; Hu, L.; Zhu, Y.; Xu, P.W.; Xia, J.Q.; Chen, H.; He, G.Y.; He, J.; Ni, X.W.; *et al.* Genome analysis and signature discovery for diving and sensory properties of the endangered Chinese alligator. *Cell Res.* **2013**, *23*, 1091–1105. [CrossRef]
71. Chromek, M.; Arvidsson, I.; Karpman, D. The antimicrobial peptide cathelicidin protects mice from Escherichia coli O157:H7-mediated disease. *PloS One* **2012**, *7*, e46476. [CrossRef]
72. Oguro-Okano, M.; Honda, M.; Yamazaki, K.; Okano, K. Mutations in the melanocortin 1 receptor, beta-defensin103 and agouti signaling protein genes, and their association with coat color phenotypes in Akita-inu dogs. *J. Vet. Med. Sci.* **2011**, *73*, 853–858. [CrossRef]
73. Schmutz, S.M.; Berryere, T.G. Genes affecting coat colour and pattern in domestic dogs: A review. *Anim. Genet.* **2007**, *38*, 539–549. [CrossRef]
74. Zasloff, M. Magainins, a class of antimicrobial peptides from Xenopus skin: isolation, characterization of two active forms, and partial cDNA sequence of a precursor. *Proc. Natl. Acad. Sci. USA* **1987**, *84*, 5449–5453. [CrossRef]
75. Wilson, C.L.; Schmidt, A.P.; Pirila, E.; Valore, E.V.; Ferri, N.; Sorsa, T.; Ganz, T.; Parks, W.C. Differential Processing of {alpha}- and {beta}-Defensin Precursors by Matrix Metalloproteinase-7 (MMP-7). *J. Biol. Chem.* **2009**, *284*, 8301–8311.
76. Zhao, L.; Lu, W. Defensins in innate immunity. *Curr. Opin. Hematol.* **2014**, *21*, 37–42. [CrossRef]
77. Lehrer, R.I.; Lu, W. alpha-Defensins in human innate immunity. *Immunol. Rev.* **2012**, *245*, 84–112. [CrossRef]
78. Garcia, J.R.; Jaumann, F.; Schulz, S.; Krause, A.; Rodriguez-Jimenez, J.; Forssmann, U.; Adermann, K.; Kluver, E.; Vogelmeier, C.; Becker, D.; *et al.* Identification of a novel, multifunctional beta-defensin (human beta-defensin 3) with specific antimicrobial activity. Its interaction with plasma membranes of Xenopus oocytes and the induction of macrophage chemoattraction. *Cell Tissue Res.* **2001**, *306*, 257–264. [CrossRef]
79. Kaplinsky, N.J.; Gilbert, S.F.; Cebra-Thomas, J.; Lillevali, K.; Saare, M.; Chang, E.Y.; Edelman, H.E.; Frick, M.A.; Guan, Y.; Hammond, R.M.; *et al.* The Embryonic Transcriptome of the Red-Eared Slider Turtle. *PloS one* **2013**, *8*, e66357.
80. Lorenzo, A. Immunolocalization of a beta-defensin (Tu-BD-1) in the skin and subdermal granulocytes of turtles indicate the presence of an antimicrobial skin barrier. *Ann. Anat.* **2013**, *195*, 554–561. [CrossRef]
81. Benato, F.; Dalla Valle, L.; Skobo, T.; Alibardi, L. Biomolecular identification of beta-defensin-like peptides from the skin of the soft-shelled turtle Apalone spinifera. *J. Exp. Zool. Part B* **2013**, *320*, 210–217. [CrossRef]
82. Alibardi, L. Ultrastructural immunolocalization of beta-defensin-27 in granulocytes of the dermis and wound epidermis of lizard suggests they contribute to the anti-microbial skin barrier. *Anat. Cell Biol.* **2013**, *46*, 246–253. [CrossRef]
83. Alibardi, L. Histochemical, Biochemical and Cell Biological aspects of tail regeneration in lizard, an amniote model for studies on tissue regeneration. *Prog. Histochem. Cytochem.* **2014**, *48*, 143–244. [CrossRef]
84. Alibardi, L. Granulocytes of reptilian sauropsids contain beta-defensin-like peptides: a comparative ultrastructural survey. *J. Morphol.* **2013**, *274*, 877–886. [CrossRef]
85. Alibardi, L.; Celeghin, A.; Dalla Valle, L. Wounding in lizards results in the release of beta-defensins at the wound site and formation of an antimicrobial barrier. *Dev. Comp. Immunol.* **2012**, *36*, 557–565. [CrossRef]
86. Abdel Mageed, A.M.; Isobe, N.; Yoshimura, Y. Immunolocalization of avian beta-defensins in the hen oviduct and their changes in the uterus during eggshell formation. *Reproduction* **2009**, *138*, 971–978. [CrossRef]
87. Gong, D.; Wilson, P.W.; Bain, M.M.; McDade, K.; Kalina, J.; Herve-Grepinet, V.; Nys, Y.; Dunn, I.C. Gallin; an antimicrobial peptide member of a new avian defensin family, the ovodefensins, has been subject to recent gene duplication. *BMC Immunol.* **2010**, *11*, 12.
88. Herve, V.; Meudal, H.; Labas, V.; Rehault Godbert, S.; Gautron, J.; Berges, M.; Guyot, N.; Delmas, A.F.; Nys, Y.; Landon, C. 3D NMR structure of hen egg gallin (chicken ovo-defensin) reveals a new variation of the beta-defensin fold. *J. Biol. Chem.* 2014.
89. Herve-Grepinet, V.; Rehault-Godbert, S.; Labas, V.; Magallon, T.; Derache, C.; Lavergne, M.; Gautron, J.; Lalmanach, A.C.; Nys, Y. Purification and characterization of avian beta-defensin 11, an antimicrobial peptide of the hen egg. *Antimicrob. Agents Chemother.* **2010**, *54*, 4401–4409. [CrossRef]

90. Mine, Y.; Oberle, C.; Kassaify, Z. Eggshell matrix proteins as defense mechanism of avian eggs. *J. Agric. Food Chem.* **2003**, *51*, 249–253. [CrossRef]
91. Kosciuczuk, E.M.; Lisowski, P.; Jarczak, J.; Strzalkowska, N.; Jozwik, A.; Horbanczuk, J.; Krzyzewski, J.; Zwierzchowski, L.; Bagnicka, E. Cathelicidins: family of antimicrobial peptides. A review. *Mol. Biol. Reports* **2012**, *39*, 10957–10970. [CrossRef]
92. Lehrer, R.I.; Ganz, T. Cathelicidins: A family of endogenous antimicrobial peptides. *Curr. Opin. Hematol.* **2002**, *9*, 18–22. [CrossRef]
93. Cole, A.M.; Shi, J.; Ceccarelli, A.; Kim, Y.H.; Park, A.; Ganz, T. Inhibition of neutrophil elastase prevents cathelicidin activation and impairs clearance of bacteria from wounds. *Blood* **2001**, *97*, 297–304. [CrossRef]
94. Tongaonkar, P.; Golji, A.E.; Tran, P.; Ouellette, A.J.; Selsted, M.E. High fidelity processing and activation of the human alpha-defensin HNP1 precursor by neutrophil elastase and proteinase 3. *PloS One* **2012**, *7*, e32469.
95. Nizet, V.; Gallo, R.L. Cathelicidins and innate defense against invasive bacterial infection. *Scand. J. Infect. Dis.* **2003**, *35*, 670–676. [CrossRef]
96. Zanetti, M.; Gennaro, R.; Scocchi, M.; Skerlavaj, B. Structure and biology of cathelicidins. *Adv. Exp. Med. Biol.* **2000**, *479*, 203–218.
97. van Dijk, A.; Molhoek, E.M.; Bikker, F.J.; Yu, P.L.; Veldhuizen, E.J.; Haagsman, H.P. Avian cathelicidins: Paradigms for the development of anti-infectives. *Vet. Microbiol.* **2011**, *153*, 27–36. [CrossRef]
98. Van Dijk, A.; Veldhuizen, E.J.; van Asten, A.J.; Haagsman, H.P. CMAP27, a novel chicken cathelicidin-like antimicrobial protein. *Vet. Immunol. Immunopathol.* **2005**, *106*, 321–327. [CrossRef]
99. Xiao, Y.; Cai, Y.; Bommineni, Y.R.; Fernando, S.C.; Prakash, O.; Gilliland, S.E.; Zhang, G. Identification and functional characterization of three chicken cathelicidins with potent antimicrobial activity. *J. Biol. Chem.* **2006**, *281*, 2858–2867.
100. Van Dijk, A.; Tersteeg-Zijderveld, M.H.; Tjeerdsma-van Bokhoven, J.L.; Jansman, A.J.; Veldhuizen, E.J.; Haagsman, H.P. Chicken heterophils are recruited to the site of Salmonella infection and release antibacterial mature Cathelicidin-2 upon stimulation with LPS. *Mol. Immunol.* **2009**, *46*, 1517–1526. [CrossRef]
101. Sorensen, O.E.; Borregaard, N. Cathelicidins–nature's attempt at combinatorial chemistry. *Comb. Chem. High Throughput Screen.* **2005**, *8*, 273–280. [CrossRef]
102. De Latour, F.A.; Amer, L.S.; Papanstasiou, E.A.; Bishop, B.M.; van Hoek, M.L. Antimicrobial activity of the Naja atra cathelicidin and related small peptides. *Biochem. Biophys. Res. Commun.* **2010**, *396*, 825–830. [CrossRef]
103. Dean, S.N.; Bishop, B.M.; van Hoek, M.L. Susceptibility of Pseudomonas aeruginosa Biofilm to Alpha-Helical Peptides: D-enantiomer of LL-37. *Front. Microbiol.* **2011**, *2*, 128.
104. Amer, L.S.; Bishop, B.M.; van Hoek, M.L. Antimicrobial and antibiofilm activity of cathelicidins and short, synthetic peptides against Francisella. *Biochem. Biophys. Res. Commun.* **2010**, *396*, 246–251. [CrossRef]
105. Dean, S.N.; Bishop, B.M.; van Hoek, M.L. Natural and synthetic cathelicidin peptides with anti-microbial and anti-biofilm activity against *Staphylococcus aureus*. *BMC Microbiol.* **2011**, *11*, 114. [CrossRef]
106. Juba, M.; Porter, D.; Dean, S.; Gillmor, S.; Bishop, B. Characterization and performance of short cationic antimicrobial peptide isomers. *Biopolymers* **2013**, *100*, 387–401. [CrossRef]
107. Wang, Y.; Zhang, Z.; Chen, L.; Guang, H.; Li, Z.; Yang, H.; Li, J.; You, D.; Yu, H.; Lai, R. Cathelicidin-BF, a snake cathelicidin-derived antimicrobial peptide, could be an excellent therapeutic agent for acne vulgaris. *PloS One* **2011**, *6*, e22120.
108. Hao, Q.; Wang, H.; Wang, J.; Dou, J.; Zhang, M.; Zhou, W.; Zhou, C. Effective antimicrobial activity of Cbf-K16 and Cbf-A7 A13 against NDM-1-carrying Escherichia coli by DNA binding after penetrating the cytoplasmic membrane *in vitro*. *J. Pept. Sci.* **2013**, *19*, 173–180. [CrossRef]
109. Wang, J.; Li, B.; Li, Y.; Dou, J.; Hao, Q.; Tian, Y.; Wang, H.; Zhou, C. BF-30 effectively inhibits ciprofloxacin-resistant bacteria *in vitro* and in a rat model of vaginosis. *Arch. Pharm. Res.* **2013**. [CrossRef]
110. Dalla Valle, L.; Benato, F.; Paccanaro, M.C.; Alibardi, L. Bioinformatic and molecular characterization of cathelicidin-like peptides isolated from the green lizard Anolis carolinensis (Reptilia: Lepidosauria: Iguanidae). *Ital. J. Zool.* **2013**, *80*, 177–186. [CrossRef]
111. Alibardi, L. Ultrastructural immunolocalization of chatelicidin-like peptides in granulocytes of normal and regenerating lizard tissues. *Acta Histochem.* 2013.
112. Park, C.H.; Valore, E.V.; Waring, A.J.; Ganz, T. Hepcidin, a urinary antimicrobial peptide synthesized in the liver. *J. Biol. Chem.* **2001**, *276*, 7806–7810.

113. Rodriguez, R.; Jung, C.L.; Gabayan, V.; Deng, J.C.; Ganz, T.; Nemeth, E.; Bulut, Y. Hepcidin induction by pathogens and pathogen-derived molecules is strongly dependent on interleukin-6. *Infect. Immun.* **2014**, *82*, 745–752. [CrossRef]
114. Hao, J.; Li, Y.W.; Xie, M.Q.; Li, A.X. Molecular cloning, recombinant expression and antibacterial activity analysis of hepcidin from Simensis crocodile (*Crocodylus siamensis*). *Comp. Biochem. Phys. Part B* **2012**, *163*, 309–315. [CrossRef]
115. Hilton, K.B.; Lambert, L.A. Molecular evolution and characterization of hepcidin gene products in vertebrates. *Gene* **2008**, *415*, 40–48.
116. Sang, Y.; Ramanathan, B.; Minton, J.E.; Ross, C.R.; Blecha, F. Porcine liver-expressed antimicrobial peptides, hepcidin and LEAP-2: cloning and induction by bacterial infection. *Dev. Comp. Immunol.* **2006**, *30*, 357–366. [CrossRef]
117. Hocquellet, A.; Odaert, B.; Cabanne, C.; Noubhani, A.; Dieryck, W.; Joucla, G.; le Senechal, C.; Milenkov, M.; Chaignepain, S.; Schmitter, J.M.; *et al.* Structure-activity relationship of human liver-expressed antimicrobial peptide 2. *Peptides* **2010**, *31*, 58–66. [CrossRef]
118. Henriques, S.T.; Tan, C.C.; Craik, D.J.; Clark, R.J. Structural and functional analysis of human liver-expressed antimicrobial peptide 2. *Chembiochem* **2010**, *11*, 2148–2157. [CrossRef]
119. Krause, A.; Sillard, R.; Kleemeier, B.; Kluver, E.; Maronde, E.; Conejo-Garcia, J.R.; Forssmann, W.G.; Schulz-Knappe, P.; Nehls, M.C.; Wattler, F.; *et al.* Isolation and biochemical characterization of LEAP-2, a novel blood peptide expressed in the liver. *Protein Sci.* **2003**, *12*, 143–152. [CrossRef]
120. Araki, T.; Yamamoto, T.; Torikata, T. Reptile lysozyme: the complete amino acid sequence of soft-shelled turtle lysozyme and its activity. *Biosci. Biotechnol. Biochem.* **1998**, *62*, 316–324. [CrossRef]
121. Chijiiwa, Y.; Kawamura, S.; Torikata, T.; Araki, T. Amino acid sequence and activity of green turtle (*Chelonia mydas*) lysozyme. *Protein J.* **2006**, *25*, 336–344. [CrossRef]
122. Prajanban, B.O.; Shawsuan, L.; Daduang, S.; Kommanee, J.; Roytrakul, S.; Dhiravisit, A.; Thammasirirak, S. Identification of five reptile egg whites protein using MALDI-TOF mass spectrometry and LC/MS-MS analysis. *J. Proteomics* **2012**, *75*, 1940–1959. [CrossRef]
123. Radis-Baptista, G.; Kerkis, I. Crotamine, a small basic polypeptide myotoxin from rattlesnake venom with cell-penetrating properties. *Curr. Pharm. Design* **2011**, *17*, 4351–4361. [CrossRef]
124. Kerkis, I.; Silva Fde, S.; Pereira, A.; Kerkis, A.; Radis-Baptista, G. Biological versatility of crotamine—A cationic peptide from the venom of a South American rattlesnake. *Expert Opin. Investig. Drugs* **2010**, *19*, 1515–1525. [CrossRef]
125. Structure of crotamine, a Na+ channel affecting toxin from Crotalus durissus terrificus venom (PDB 1H5O). This image is licensed under the Creative Commons Attribution-Share Alike 3.0 Unported license. Available online: http://en.wikipedia.org/wiki/File:Crotamin_1H5O.png (accessed on 9 May 2014).
126. Radis-Baptista, G.; Kubo, T.; Oguiura, N.; Prieto da Silva, A.R.; Hayashi, M.A.; Oliveira, E.B.; Yamane, T. Identification of crotasin, a crotamine-related gene of Crotalus durissus terrificus. *Toxicon* **2004**, *43*, 751–759. [CrossRef]
127. Yamane, E.S.; Bizerra, F.C.; Oliveira, E.B.; Moreira, J.T.; Rajabi, M.; Nunes, G.L.; de Souza, A.O.; da Silva, I.D.; Yamane, T.; Karpel, R.L.; *et al.* Unraveling the antifungal activity of a South American rattlesnake toxin crotamine. *Biochimie* **2013**, *95*, 231–240.
128. Yaraksa, N.; Anunthawan, T.; Theansungnoen, T.; Daduang, S.; Araki, T.; Dhiravisit, A.; Thammasirirak, S. Design and synthesis of cationic antibacterial peptide based on Leucrocin I sequence, antibacterial peptide from crocodile (*Crocodylus siamensis*) white blood cell extracts. *J. Antibiot.* **2013**, *67*, 205–212.
129. Mak, P. Hemocidins in a functional and structural context of human antimicrobial peptides. *Front. Biosci.* **2008**, *13*, 6859–6871.
130. Sheshadri, P.; Abraham, J. Antimicrobial properties of hemoglobin. *Immunopharm. Immunotoxicol.* **2012**, *34*, 896–900. [CrossRef]
131. Parish, C.A.; Jiang, H.; Tokiwa, Y.; Berova, N.; Nakanishi, K.; McCabe, D.; Zuckerman, W.; Xia, M.M.; Gabay, J.E. Broad-spectrum antimicrobial activity of hemoglobin. *Bioorg. Med. Chem.* **2001**, *9*, 377–382.
132. Anwised, P.; Kabbua, T.; Temsiripong, T.; Dhiravisit, A.; Jitrapakdee, S.; Araki, T.; Yoneda, K.; Thammasirirak, S. Molecular cloning and expression of alpha-globin and beta-globin genes from crocodile (*Crocodylus siamensis*). *Protein J.* **2013**, *32*, 172–182.

133. Santamaria, C.; Larios, S.; Quiros, S.; Pizarro-Cerda, J.; Gorvel, J.P.; Lomonte, B.; Moreno, E. Bactericidal and antiendotoxic properties of short cationic peptides derived from a snake venom Lys49 phospholipase A2. *Antimicrob. Agents Chemother.* **2005**, *49*, 1340–1345. [CrossRef]
134. Santamaria, C.; Larios, S.; Angulo, Y.; Pizarro-Cerda, J.; Gorvel, J.P.; Moreno, E.; Lomonte, B. Antimicrobial activity of myotoxic phospholipases A2 from crotalid snake venoms and synthetic peptide variants derived from their C-terminal region. *Toxicon* **2005**, *45*, 807–815. [CrossRef]
135. Yu, H.Y.; Huang, K.C.; Yip, B.S.; Tu, C.H.; Chen, H.L.; Cheng, H.T.; Cheng, J.W. Rational design of tryptophan-rich antimicrobial peptides with enhanced antimicrobial activities and specificities. *Chembiochem* **2010**, *11*, 2273–2282. [CrossRef]
136. Chu, H.L.; Yu, H.Y.; Yip, B.S.; Chih, Y.H.; Liang, C.W.; Cheng, H.T.; Cheng, J.W. Boosting salt resistance of short antimicrobial peptides. *Antimicrob. Agents Chemother.* **2013**, *57*, 4050–4052. [CrossRef]
137. Deslouches, B.; Steckbeck, J.D.; Craigo, J.K.; Doi, Y.; Mietzner, T.A.; Montelaro, R.C. Rational design of engineered cationic antimicrobial peptides consisting exclusively of arginine and tryptophan, and their activity against multidrug-resistant pathogens. *Antimicrob. Agents Chemother.* **2013**, *57*, 2511–2521. [CrossRef]
138. Gomes, V.M.; Carvalho, A.O.; Da Cunha, M.; Keller, M.N.; Bloch, C., Jr.; Deolindo, P.; Alves, E.W. Purification and characterization of a novel peptide with antifungal activity from Bothrops jararaca venom. *Toxicon* **2005**, *45*, 817–827. [CrossRef]
139. Xie, J.P.; Yue, J.; Xiong, Y.L.; Wang, W.Y.; Yu, S.Q.; Wang, H.H. In vitro activities of small peptides from snake venom against clinical isolates of drug-resistant Mycobacterium tuberculosis. *Int. J. Antimicrob. Agents* **2003**, *22*, 172–174. [CrossRef]

3

Thermoreversible Gel-Loaded Amphotericin B for the Treatment of Dermal and Vaginal Candidiasis

Lilian Sosa [1], Ana Cristina Calpena [1,2], Marcelle Silva-Abreu [1,2,*], Lupe Carolina Espinoza [1,3], María Rincón [1], Nuria Bozal [4], Oscar Domenech [1], María José Rodríguez-Lagunas [5,6] and Beatriz Clares [2,7]

1 Department of Pharmacy and Pharmaceutical Technology and Physical Chemistry, School of Pharmacy and Food Sciences, University of Barcelona, 08028 Barcelona, Spain
2 Institute de Nanoscience and Nanotechnology (IN2UB), University of Barcelona, 08028 Barcelona, Spain
3 Departamento de Química y Ciencias Exactas, Universidad Técnica Particular de Loja, Loja 1101608, Ecuador
4 Department of Biology, Healthcare and the Environment, School of Pharmacy and Food Sciences, University of Barcelona, 08028 Barcelona, Spain
5 Department of Biochemistry and Physiology, Faculty of Pharmacy and Food Sciences, University of Barcelona, 08028 Barcelona, Spain
6 Institut de Recerca en Nutrició i Seguretat Alimentària (INSA), Universitat de Barcelona, 08921 Barcelona, Spain
7 Department of Pharmacy and Pharmaceutical Technology, School of Pharmacy, University of Granada, 18071 Granada, Spain
* Correspondence: marcellesabreu@gmail.com

Abstract: The present study was designed to develop a thermoreversible gel of Pluronic (P407) loaded amphotericin B (AmB-gel) for the dermal and vaginal treatment of candidiasis. P407 was used as a copolymer to exploit potential advantages related to increasing drug concentration in the tissue layer in order to provide a local effect. Parameters including internal structure, swelling, porosity, and short-term stability were determined. In addition, drug release profile and ex vivo skin and vaginal permeation studies were carried out. Antifungal efficacy was evaluated against strains of *Candida* spp. and atomic force microscopy (AFM) supported the results. The tolerance of AmB-gel was studied by evaluating biomechanical properties of skin and determining the irritation level in scarified rabbit skin supported by histological analysis. Results confirmed the development of a thermoreversible AmB-gel with high porosity exhibiting Newtonian behavior at 4 °C and pseudoplasticity at 32 °C as well as optimal stability for at least 90 days. The Amb-gel provided a sustained drug release following a Boltzmann sigmoidal model. Non permeation was observed in skin and vaginal mucosa, showing a high retained amount of AmB of 960.0 and 737.3 μg/g/cm^2, respectively. In vitro antifungal efficacy showed that AmB-gel was more effective than Free-AmB in inhibiting strains of *Candida* spp. and these results were corroborated by AFM. Finally, tolerance studies showed that its application did not induce skin irritation nor alter its biophysical properties. Together, these results confirmed that AmB-gel could be proposed as a promising candidate for the clinical status in the treatment of skin and vaginal candidiasis.

Keywords: thermoreversible gel; poloxamer 407; candidiasis; amphotericin B; skin and vaginal mucosa

1. Introduction

Cutaneous fungal infections are a significant cause of morbidity and constitute a critical health issue on a global scale. The most identified fungal pathogenesis that affects people worldwide is based on superficial skin, vaginal and nail infections, with approximately 1.7 billion individuals affected. This has led to an increase of superficial mycoses higher than 20% in recent decades, especially in patients who are immunocompromised or hospitalized [1,2] as well as in cases of topical burn wound infections [3]. Among these fungal infections, various species of Candida cause superficial complications known as candidiasis [4]. Categorically, *Candida albicans* is reported to be the fourth most frequent cause of infection [5].

The first-line drugs used for the treatment of these mycoses are the Azoles antifungal compounds such as fluconazole, ketoconazole, voriconazole, itraconazole, clotrimazole, among others [6,7]. However, mechanisms of resistance to these antifungals have been detected [8,9]. The appearance of these resistance mechanisms leads to the use of other antifungals such as amphotericin B (AmB), especially in immunosuppressed patients [10,11].

AmB is a polyene macrolide of a broad-spectrum with high activity against the most frequently occurring fungi involved in cutaneous mycoses, including Candida [12]. It is considered the gold standard in the treatment of fungal infections and has been found to be effective against azole-resistant fungi due to the creation of transmembrane channels by complexation with the membrane sterols which results in fungal cell death. However, it is not without side effects in systemic administration due to the self-assembly process into higher-order molecular forms [13]. From a physicochemical point of view, AmB is a poorly hydrosoluble, amphoteric, amphiphilic molecule and is difficult to solubilize in organic solvents. These properties block an optimal permeation of the drug through the stratum corneum (SC), which is the major barrier that limits permeation of external substances. For this reason, there is no topical formulation of AmB commercially available at the moment [14]. This fact evidences the need to develop new formulations using excipients with permeation-enhancing properties in order to facilitate the penetration of drug into SC and its distribution from SC to epidermis and dermis. Therefore, the research of new therapeutic approaches for the treatment of superficial mycoses, including dermal and vaginal administration from galenical perspective, is a challenging yet necessary undertaking.

The topical administration of antimicrobials for superficial mycoses offers several advantages, particularly for direct application at the site of infection. Among these are the prevention of systemic toxicity of the drug, effectiveness at an eminently local level and insurance that a sufficient amount of drug is retained in the skin [15].

With the aim of achieving an improved release of AmB, this drug was incorporated to Poloxamer 407 (P407), which is a copolymer of amphiphilic nature consisting of a central hydrophobic block of polypropylene oxide (PPO) flanked by hydrophilic polyethylene (PEG) blocks (PEG–PPO–PEG). The P407 prepared above >18% shows an aqueous solution (4–5 °C) that turns into a gel ~32 °C, making it an ideal candidate for thermoreversible delivery [16]. P407 is a low toxicity excipient approved by the Food and Drug Administration (FDA) [17]. Moreover, it has beneficial properties that help to promote and improve drug permeation through the skin and mucosa [18].

Therefore, an approach to deliver AmB formulated into P407 gel form specifically developed for skin and vaginal treatment against *Candida* spp. was developed. This work has accomplished detailed research of (i) development and physicochemical characterization of AmB-gel for topical administration, (ii) biopharmaceutical studies (release profile) and ex vivo permeation studies, (iii) in vitro antifungal activity and its effect on yeast cells by atomic force microscopy (AFM), and (iv) biomechanical properties and tolerance assay complemented with histological studies.

2. Materials and Methods

2.1. Materials

AmB was obtained from Acofarma (Barcelona, Spain). Pluronic®® F127 (P407) was obtained from Fagron (Barcelona, Spain). Dimethyl sulfoxide (DMSO), methanol, castor oil and *N,N*-dimethylformamide were obtained from Sigma-Aldrich (Darmstadt, Germany). Transcutol®® P and Propylene glycol were kindly provided by Gattefossé (Barcelona, Spain). The water used in all experiments was obtained from a Milli-Q®® Plus System (Millipore Co., Burlington, MA, USA). All the chemicals and reagents were of analytical grade.

2.2. *Preparation of AmB-Gel*

Firstly, a selection of solvents was tested to determine the solubility of AmB. Transcutol®® P, Propylene glycol, *N,N*-dimethyformamide, Castor oil and DMSO were analyzed. The DMSO was selected as the best solubilizing component of AmB. Shortly afterwards 25 g of P407 were dispersed on ultrapure water at 4 °C up to 100 mL. Subsequently, 60 mg of AmB were dissolved in 10 mL of DMSO, of which 1 mL was slowly added under stirring to 20 mL of P407 solution at 4 °C. The resulting solution was adjusted to pH 6.5 with NaOH 2N solution, thus obtaining an AmB-gel at a final concentration of 0.03%.

2.3. *Physiochemical Characterization*

To analyze the morphology, the AmB-gel was dried over a period of 8 days using a desiccator with provision for a vacuum. Once it was dried, a small quantity was coated with carbon as a conductor agent. The internal structure of the gel was examined by scanning electron microscopy (SEM) using a JEOL J-7100F (Peabody, Massachusetts, MA, USA).

2.3.1. Swelling and Degradation Tests

The swelling ratio (SR) and degradation as percentage of weight loss (WL) were accomplished by a gravimetric method. Half a gram of dried AmB-gel or fresh AmB-gel was used to carry out swelling and degradation tests, respectively. In both experiments the sample was incubated in PBS (pH = 5.5) at 32 °C for 30 min. Samples (n = 3) were removed and weighed after blotting the surface water at predetermined time intervals of 5 min. The PBS uptake was carried out in triplicate.

The SR ratio was calculated using the following equation and expressed by kinetic modeling:

$$\mathrm{SR} = \frac{W_s - W_d}{W_d} \tag{1}$$

where W_s is the weight of the swollen AmB-gel at 5 min intervals and W_d is the weight of dried gel.

WL was calculated following the equation and expressed by kinetic modeling.

$$\mathrm{WL}\ (\%) = \frac{W_i - W_d}{W_i} \times 100 \tag{2}$$

where W_i is the initial weight of AmB-gel and W_d the weight of gel at different times.

2.3.2. Porosity Study

The porosity percentage (P) was calculated by displacement of the solvent. The method consisted of immersing the previously dried AmB-gel in absolute ethanol for 2 min and then weighing after the excess ethanol on the surface was blotted. The porosity percentage was calculated using the following equation.

$$\mathrm{P} = \frac{w2 - w1}{\rho \times V} \times 100 \tag{3}$$

where, $w1$ represents the weight of the dried AmB-gel to be immersed in ethanol, $w2$ represents the weight of AmB-gel after being immersed in ethanol, ρ is the density of absolute ethanol, and V is the volume of the gel.

2.4. *Stability Study*

The AmB-gel was stored at two temperatures: 4 °C and 25 °C. The pH values of formulation were measured in a Crison 501 digital pH/mV-meter (Crison Instruments, Barcelona, Spain) for a period of

90 days (1, 30, 60, and 90 days) at both temperatures. Values were reported as the mean ± standard deviation (SD) of six replicates.

For the chemical stability studies, the formulation was suspended in *N,N*–dimethylformamide: methanol:water (55:15:30, *v*/*v*/*v*) and the amount of drug was quantified by a previously validated method of High Performance Liquid Chromatography (HPLC) (Waters, Milford, MA, USA) [12].

The short-term stability of AmB-gel was studied for a period of 90 days at 4 °C and 25 °C. A TurbiScan Lab®® (Formulaction Co., L'Union, France) was used to analyze the destabilization phenomena by transmission and light retrodispersion using a pulsed near-infrared light source (γ = 880 nm) at 25 °C over a span of 90 days.

2.5. *Rheological Studies*

The rheological measurements were performed using a Thermo Scientific Haake Rheostress 1 rotational rheometer (Thermo Fisher Scientific, Kalsruhe, Germany) equipped with cone plate geometry (60 mm diameter, 2° angle) with mobile upper cone Haake C60/2° Ti (0.105 mm gap). Viscosity and flow curves were rehearsed at 4 °C and 32 °C in triplicate. The shear rate ramp program included: 0→50 s^{-1} (3 min), 50 s^{-1} (1 min), and 50→0 s^{-1} (3 min). Obtained data were then fitted to different mathematical models: Newton, Bingham, Ostwald-de Waele, Cross, Casson, and Herschel–Bulkley.

2.6. *Gelation Time and Spreadability Test*

Ten milliliters of AmB-gel was added to a transparent vial with a magnetic bar and placed in a low temperature water bath. The solution was then heated to 37 ± 0.1 °C while being stirred (400 rpm). The gelation time was measured in triplicate once the magnetic bar stopped moving due to gelation.

The spreadability of AmB-gel was determined in triplicate as follows; 0.5 g of formulation was placed within a 1 cm diameter circle previously marked on a glass plate, after which a second glass plate was subsequently placed without sliding. A series of weights (15, 22, 27, 29, 32, and 37 g) were successively added and allowed to rest for 2 min each at 4 °C. The same operation was repeated at 32 °C but using different weights (100, 200, and 300 g). The diameters (cm) of the circle spreads were measured and recorded as comparative values. Experimental data were then fitted to mathematical models using GraphPad Prism®® version 6.0 (GraphPad Software Inc., San Diego, CA, USA).

2.7. *In Vitro Release and Kinetic Evaluation*

In vitro release studies were performed in vertical diffusion Franz cells (FDC-400, Vidra-Foc, Barcelona, Spain) using nylon membranes.

DMSO solution continuously stirred at 32 ± 1 °C was used as the receptor medium to accomplish sink conditions. An aliquot of 1.3 mL of the AmB-gel was placed in the donor phase. Aliquots of 300 µL were collected from the receptor compartment at different times for 24 h and replaced with an equal volume of tempered DMSO kept under stirring at 600 rpm. AmB was quantified by previously validated HPLC [12]. Results are reported as the mean ± SD of six replicates.

Experimental data were fitted to five kinetic models (zero-order, first-order, Peppas–Korsmeyer, Higuchi, and Weibull function) by nonlinear least squares regression using GraphPad Prism®® version 5.01. The best fit was selected based on the Akaike's Information Criterion (AIC) and coefficient determination (r^2).

2.8. *Ex Vivo Permeation Studies: Skin and Vaginal Mucosa*

Ex vivo permeation studies were performed as described in Section 2.7 using skin samples with thicknesses of 400 µm or Vaginal porcine mucosae as membranes. Transcutol P®® was used as the receptor medium which was kept at 32 ± 0.5 °C (Human skin) and 37 ± 1 °C (Vaginal porcine mucosa). The experiment was performed with a diffusion area of 0.64 cm^2. The human skin was obtained from the abdominal region of a healthy woman after abdominal plastic surgery. The experimental protocol was approved by the Bioethics Committee of Barcelona SCIAS Hospital (Barcelona, Spain) (ref: BEC/001/16) and written informed consent was provided by the volunteer. Integrity of skin was evaluated by measuring the transepidermal water loss (TEWL) with a DermaLab® module (Cortex Technology, Hadsund, Denmark), exhibiting values below 10 $g/m^2 \cdot h$.

Vaginal porcine mucosae were obtained under veterinary supervision, from three- to four-month-old pigs after sacrifice using an overdose of sodium thiopental at the Animal Facility at Bellvitge Campus of Barcelona University (Barcelona, Spain) in accordance with protocols prescribed by the Animal Experimentation Ethics Committee of the University of Barcelona, Spain (CEEA-UB). Mucosa was placed into of Hank's balanced salt solution (HBSS) and refrigerated until use. The experiments were carried out for 36 h (Human skin) and 6 h (Vaginal porcine mucosae), respectively.

At the end of the permeation study, the human skin and porcine vaginal mucosa were removed from the Franz diffusion cell, cleaned with a dodecyl sulfate solution 0.05% and washed in distilled water. AmB retained in the skin and vaginal mucosa was extracted with DMSO for a period of 20 min under cold sonication in an ultrasound bath. The resulting samples were measured by HPLC.

2.9. *Antifungal Efficacy*

The minimal inhibitory concentration (MIC), defined as the lowest concentration of an antimicrobial agent that inhibits the growth of a microorganism, was calculated by the broth microdilution method against *C. albicans* ATCC 10231, *C. glabrata* ATCC 66,032, and *C. parapsilosis* ATCC 22,019 strains (American Type Culture Collection, Manassas, VA, USA) following the procedure outlined by the European Committee for Antimicrobial Susceptibility Testing Guidelines (EUCAST) [19] and the Reference method CLSI M27-A3 [20].

This Standards Method provides a valid procedure for testing the susceptibility of glucose-fermenting yeasts to antifungal agents by determining the MIC. A synthetic medium containing RPMI-1640, glutamine, pH indicator without bicarbonate, and glucose 2% *w/v*: RPMI-1640 2% G (Invitrogen, Madrid, Spain) was used for working cultures. pH was adjusted to 7.0 with 1 M sodium hydroxide and the resulting solution was filtered using a 0.22 μm filter. As samples were not sterile, chloramphenicol was added to the RPMI medium at a final concentration of 500 μg/mL. The yeast strain was first cultured on Sabouraud Dextrose agar (Invitrogen, Madrid, Spain) at 30 °C for 48 h before testing. The inoculums were prepared by suspending colonies in sterile distilled water to achieve a density equivalent to 2 McFarland standards, the counting of which took place in a Neubauer Chamber shortly afterwards (1 to 5×10^6 Colony Forming Unit, CFU/mL). Working suspension was prepared by diluting the standardized suspension in sterile distilled water (1:10) in order to prepare 1 to 5×10^5 CFU/mL. The test was performed using 96-well polystyrene sterile microdilution plates. Serial dilutions from 75 to 0.009 μg/mL of the following forms were compared. (1) Free-AmB (AmB solution first dissolved in DMSO at 300 μg/mL and afterwards in RPMI-1640 double strength at 150 μg/mL). (2) AmB-gel (AmB gel dissolved in RPMI-1640 double strength at 150 μg/mL). (3) Blank-gel (Blank-gel dissolved in RPMI-1640 double strength at 12.5–0.00075%).

Finally, 100 μL of inoculum was added to all the wells. In addition, 3 posts were reserved in each plate for both the positive control (300 μL of the inoculum) and negative control (300 μL of the culture broth). The plates were read at t_0 and then at 24 h and 48 h after incubation at 30 °C, with a microplate reader model 680 (Bio-Rad, Madrid, Spain) at $\lambda = 620$ nm.

2.10. *Atomic Force Microscopy (AFM)*

2.10.1. Images

C. albicans cells were exposed to AMB-gel and Blank-gel during a period of 4 h. The cells were collected by centrifugation and washed three times with PBS solution (pH 7.40) in order to obtain a final suspension of 1×10^6 yeast cells/mL. The suspension was filtered through SMWP01300 Millipore® filters (Merck Chemical and Life Science, S.A, Madrid, Spain) with a pore size similar to the yeast size followed by gentle rinsing with PBS in order to clean the filter from non trapped cells, then subsequently cut and attached to a steel disk using a small piece of double-sided adhesive tape. Finally, the sample was transferred to the AFM liquid cell while avoiding dewetting. Throughout the procedure, MSNL-10, V shaped silicon nitride cantilevers (Bruker AFM Probes, Camarillo, CA, USA) with a nominal spring constant of 0.03 N/m were used.

Prior to measuring the nanomechanics the spring constants of the cantilevers were determined by thermal noise method. AFM images were acquired in contact mode by minimizing the force during the scan and continuously adjusting the set point with a 0° scan angle at a scan rate of 1.5 Hz. Images were processed using NanoScope®® analysis software (Bruker, AXS Co., Madison, WI, USA).

2.10.2. Force-Distance Curves

Mechanical properties were measured by recording arrays of 32 × 32 force curves, using a maximum force of 0.5–1 nN to avoid sample damage, a contact time of 100 ms, and approach and retract speeds of 1.0 μm/s. The Young's modulus of the yeast cells was determined as a first approximation by using the Hertz model.

2.11. *In Vivo Tolerance Study by Evaluating Biomechanical Properties of Human Skin*

Ten female volunteers between 25 and 35 years old with healthy skin participated in the study. The study was approved by the CEEA-UB according to the recommendations outlined in the Declaration of Helsinki (ref: IRB00003099) and all volunteers provided written informed consent [21]. All participants were requested not to use skin care cosmetics on the test areas of application for two days prior to the study. Skin temperature, transepidermal water loss (TEWL), and stratum corneum hydration (SCH) were determined using a thermometer ST500, a Tewameter TM 300, and a Corneometer CM 825 (Courage-Khazaka electronic GmbH, Cologne, Germany), respectively [22]. The measurements of these parameters were made before applying the AmB-gel (basal readings), immediately after the application of 0.5 mL/cm^2 (t_0) and after 2 h of application on the flexor side of the left forearm.

2.12. *In Vivo Tolerance Study by Draize Assay and Histological Analysis*

The tolerance of the formulation was evaluated using scarified rabbit skin. The blank-gel and AmB-gel were tested on New Zealand albino male rabbits (2 kg) according to the guidelines provided by the CEEA-UB. The rabbits were acclimated over a 5-day period before the study and were classified into three groups (n = 3/group): Group A (Blank-gel), Group B (Skin scarified-control group), and Group C (AmB-gel). The surrounding area of the dorsal trunk was shaved with clippers where a square was drawn for scarification with a razor before beginning the assay. After 30 min, a volume of 0.5 mL of either Blank-gel or AmB-gel was topically applied on the scarified skin of each corresponding group while group B was not exposed to any treatment. This area was protected with gauze and secured with hypoallergenic sticking plaster for 48 h. The signal of edema and erythema were determined after 24 h and 48 h of exposure. Both scores were established according to the degree of severity and the primary irritation index value was calculated. The treatment was classified according the reported specifications: "nonirritant" (<0.5), "irritant" [2–5], or "highly irritant" [5–8,23]. Afterwards, the rabbits were anesthetized and euthanized with sodium pentobarbital.

For histological analysis, the samples of back skin from the rabbits were cut and set up for 24 h in 4% buffered formaldehyde at room temperature. After fixation, all samples were paraffin embedded in paraffin blocks, cut into 5 μm sections, and mounted on microscope slides. Afterwards, the samples were stained with hematoxylin and eosin and finally viewed on blind coded samples under a light microscope (Olympus BX41 and Olympus XC50 camera) with 100× magnification for the evaluation of the tissue structure.

2.13. Statistical Analysis

Obtained experimental data were analyzed by one-way analysis of variance (ANOVA). Comparisons of findings were done by multiple comparison test. A p value < 0.05 was established as an indicator of statistically significant differences (SSD).

3. Results

3.1. Physicochemical Characterization

Figure 1, shows SEM micrographs of AmB-gel, which exhibited a heterogeneous structure with the formation of interconnected capillary channels in the form of holes similar to a porous sponge.

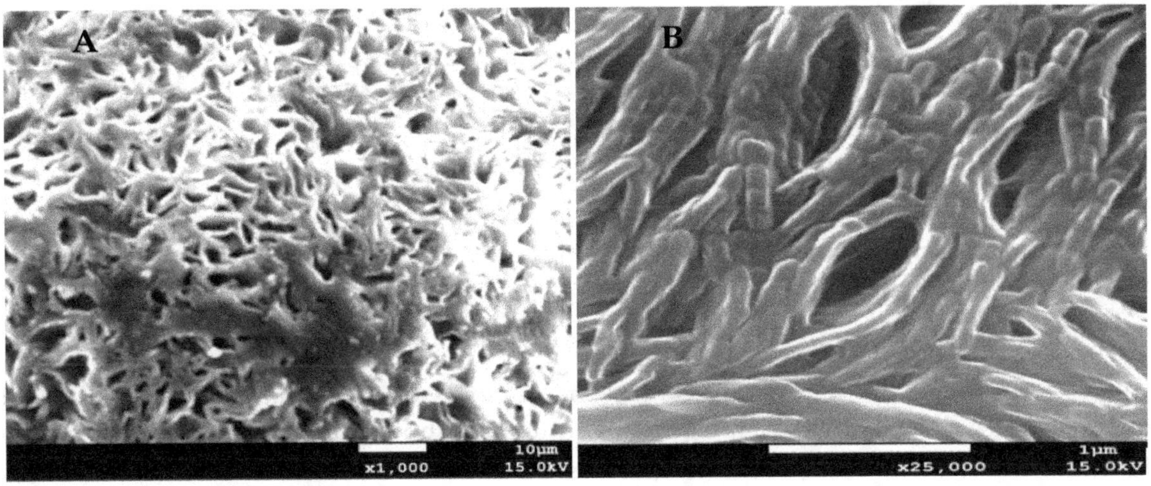

Figure 1. Morphological characterization by SEM. (**A**) AmB-gel porous sponge structure (×1000). (**B**) AmB-gel tubular appearance interconnected (×25,000).

The swelling process of AmB-gel followed a first-order kinetic model, which was represented by the kinetic constants k = 0.26 min^{-1} ($r^2 = 0.9986$) (Figure 2). The degradation process of AmB-gel was completed in 20 min and followed a hyperbola model with a kinetic constant of 0.15 min^{-1} ($r^2 = 0.9975$), whereas the percentage of P of AmB-gel was ~82.01 ± 0.5%.

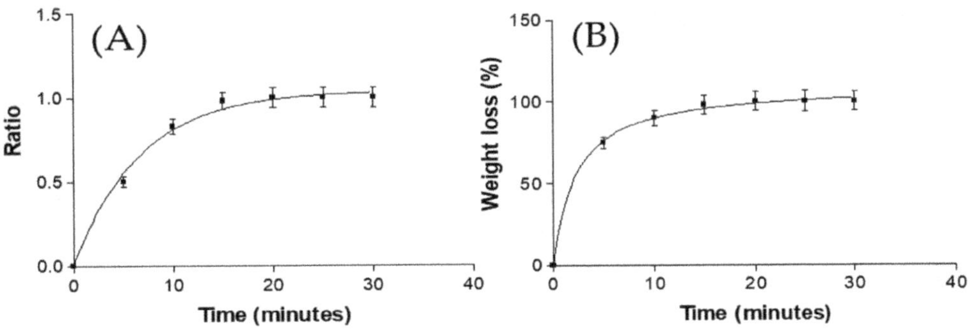

Figure 2. (**A**) Swelling ratio and (**B**) percentage of weight loss degradation of AmB-gel.

3.2. Stability Study

The pH value was suitable for application on the skin, ranging between 6.30 ± 0.05 and 6.70 ± 0.13 ($p > 0.05$) at 4 °C, and between 6.50 ± 0.13 and 6.67 ± 0.24 ($p > 0.05$) at 25 °C over a period of 90 days. The content of AmB present in the gel stored at 4 °C and 25 °C remained within the required margins of 90 to 100% during the first 90 days. With regards to the TurbiScan Lab®® analysis, Figure 3 shows the transmission profile of AmB-gel at 25 °C over a period of 90 days. The lower part of the vial is represented on the left side of the graph and the upper part on the right side. The peaks in the lower part and in the upper part of the vial correspond to the meniscus produced by the sample from contact with the glass. No sedimentation, flocculation, or coalescence phenomena were observed.

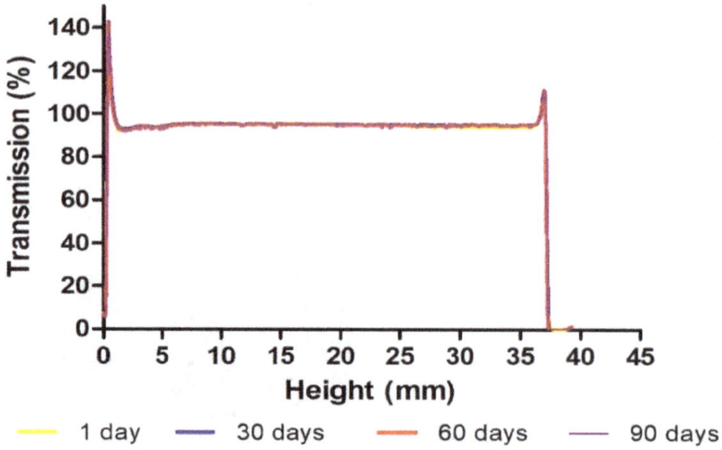

Figure 3. Transmission profile of AmB-gel obtained by Turbiscan Lab®® over 90 days at 25 °C. The left side of the curve corresponds to the bottom of the vial, whereas the right side corresponds to the sample behavior on the top.

3.3. Rheological Analysis

Figure 4A reproduces the flow curves and the viscosity curves obtained from the rheological characterization of AmB-gel. At 4 °C, the gel was liquid and showed a Newtonian behavior (constant viscosity under shear rate increase) adjusted by the Newton model ($r^2 = 1$) when under the programmed variations of shear rate. The viscosity at 4 °C was found to be $90.62 \pm 7.112 \times 10^{-2}$ mPa·s. Since AmB-gel transition is carried out as the temperature increases, at 32 °C a significantly sticky gel was formed which made it difficult to generate an adequate flow within the space between the conical plate. The rheogram (Figure 4B) showed a critical shear rate of ~10 s^{-1}. When above this value, the sample could not flow freely under the experimental conditions. As a result, the layout became quite irregular and the results were inconclusive. However, the valid curve portion showed non-Newtonian behavior with properties of shear thinning (pseudoplastic behavior), thus adjusting the Cross model ($r^2 = 0.981$). The punctual viscosity values at 10 s^{-1} and 32 °C determined from the ramp up period was ~3.8 Pa·s. The estimated viscosity of the gel at 32 °C and 50 s^{-1} was ~9.8 Pa·s.

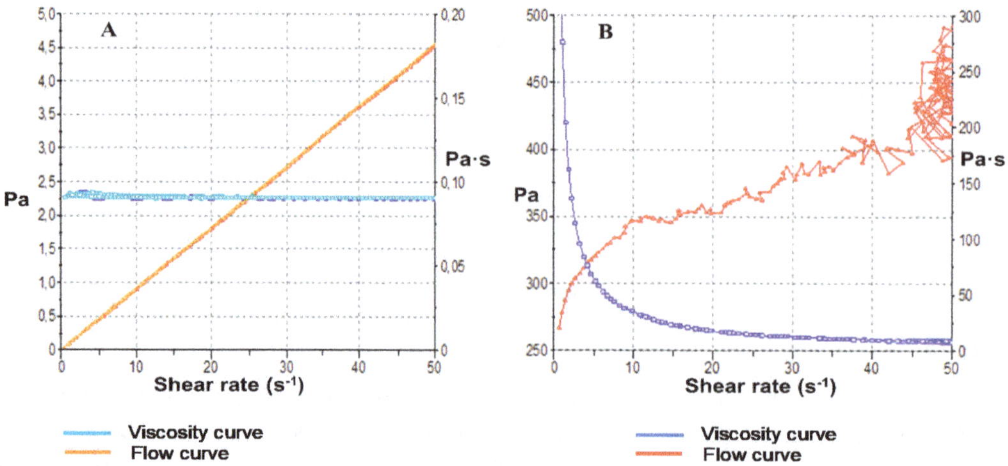

Figure 4. AmB-gel rheograms after 24 h: (**A**) Shear stress (Pa) and viscosity (Pa·s) curves at 4 °C and (**B**) Shear stress (Pa) and viscosity (Pa·s) curves at 32 °C.

3.4. Gelation Time and Spreadability

Gelation times of AmB-gel stored at 4 °C and 32 °C were 3 and 1.5 min, respectively. No differences in gelation times were evidenced between samples either with or without AmB. For AmB-gels stored for 3 months, the gelation times were even shorter at less than 1.5 min for 4 °C and 1 min 32 °C.

Figure 5 shows the results of spreadability test. The Boltzmann sigmoidal model for AmB-gel at 4 °C and hyperbola model for AmB-gel at 32 °C were the models that best fit the experimental data. At 4 °C, spreadability was greatly extended and with lower weight due to having lower viscosity at this temperature.

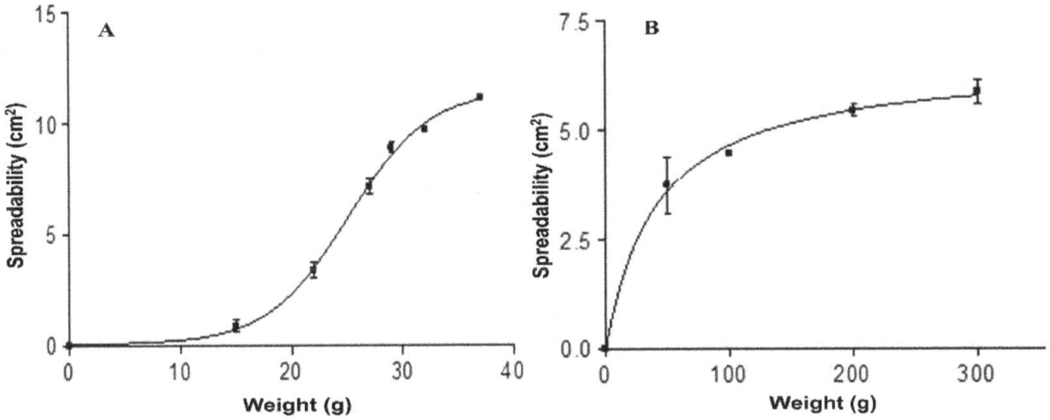

Figure 5. Spreadability charts of AmB-gel at different temperatures: (**A**) Spreadability curve at 4 °C; (**B**) Spreadability curve at 32 °C.

3.5. Release Studies

Figure 6 shows the release profile of AmB from the gel, where a sustained release exhibiting S-shaped behavior can be observed. After 24 h, more than 90% of the drug was released. The optimal kinetic model was fitted to the Boltzmann sigmoidal according to the following equation with AIC of 30.05 and r^2 of 0.999:

$$Y = Bottom + (Top - Bottom)/(1 + \exp\left(\frac{V50 - x}{Slope}\right) \quad (4)$$

where Y is the amount of drug released and *Top* and *bottom* are the initial and final values of drug release. *V50* is the time it takes to release half of the maximum amount susceptible for release and the slope of the curve indicates the steepness.

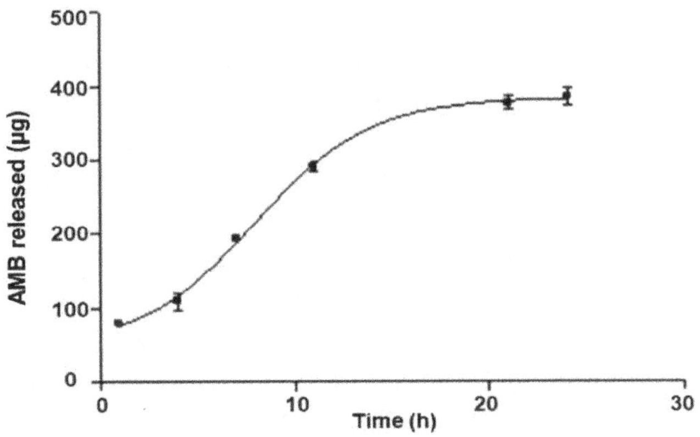

Figure 6. In vitro profile of AmB release from gel. The cumulative amount released was plotted against time. Data represent mean ± SD (n = 6).

3.6. Ex Vivo Permeation Studies of Skin and Vaginal Mucosa

No amount of AmB from gel was detected in the receptor chamber in either skin or vaginal mucosa. Thus, neither flux nor permeation parameters could be calculated. The amount of AmB retained in the skin was 960.0 μg/g/cm^2 and vaginal mucosa 737.52 μg/g/cm^2.

3.7. Antifungal Efficacy

The values from the susceptibility test after 48 h are reported in Table 1 as MIC values against strains of *C. albicans*, *C. glabrata*, and *C. parapsilosis*. It can be observed that AmB-gel exhibited the lowest MIC values (0.09, 0.37 and 0.19 μg/mL) compared with Free-AmB.

Table 1. MIC against different cultures of *Candida* spp., Free-AmB, AmB-gel, and Blank-gel after incubation at 30 °C for 48 h ($n = 3$).

Tested Species	Origin	MIC (μg/mL)		
		Free-AmB	AmB-gel	Blank-gel
C. albicans	ATCC 10,231	0.15	0.09	>250.000
C. glabrata	ATCC 66,032	0.60	0.37	>250.000
C. parapsilosis	ATCC 22,019	0.30	0.19	>250.000

3.8. Atomic Force Microscopy

Figure 7 shows the effect of a Blank-gel on *C. albicans* cell. Figure 7A shows the deflection image of a single yeast cell trapped in a pore which appears as the reddish region at the top-left of the image while the cell surface shows an extended region covered by filamentous structures. Figure 7B,C depicts magnified images of topographic and elasticity maps of this region prior to the addition of blank-gel to a final concentration of 6.5% (*w:v*) as well as Figure 7D,E after addition. The surface was quite smooth before the addition of the Blank-gel and some filamentous structures could be observed and differentiated by its different Young's modulus values with respect to the cell bulk structure (Figure 7B). After the addition of the blank-gel, the surface of the yeast cell became rougher and no filamentous structures could be observed any longer (Figure 7D). The elasticity map of the region (Figure 7E) evidences that it becomes more homogenous with the incorporation of polymer P407.

Figure 8 shows the effect of AmB-gel on *C. albicans* cells. Deflection, topographic and elasticity images (Figure 8A–C, respectively) of a single *C. albicans* yeast cell trapped in a pore are quite similar to those shown in Figure 6, although the filamentous structures are less evident in this case. The addition of AmB in the gel apparently altered the *C. albicans* cell. Figure 8D demonstrates that two different regions on cell surface can be clearly differentiated: (i) a reddish region (low region) that covers almost the 80% of the cell surface and (ii) a yellowish arched band (high region) crossing the surface from top-left to center-right of the cell surface protruding 40–80 nm over the reddish one. A close inspection of this yellowish band revealed a structure resembling a wrinkled sheet. Figure 8E,F shows the topographic and elasticity maps of the low region of Figure 8D. From these images, it is possible to recover the filamentous structures previously observed, although the differences in the Young's modulus values between the filaments and the bulk structure are not overly distinctive. Figure 8G,H shows the topographic and elasticity maps of the high region of Figure 8D. From the images, it is possible to observe two differentiated regions: (i) one diagonal from top-left corner to the bottom-right corner of Figure 8H (darker region) and (ii) a second region formed from the higher Young's values (lighter region) in Figure 8H occupying the bottom-left and top-right corners of the image with higher Young's modulus values than those of the low region. Considering that the darker region in Figure 8H is the higher region of the topographic image (Figure 8G), it is possible to identify these "wrinkled sheets" as regions with low elasticity modulus, thus suggesting that material in these structures is not as packed as those with blank-gel.

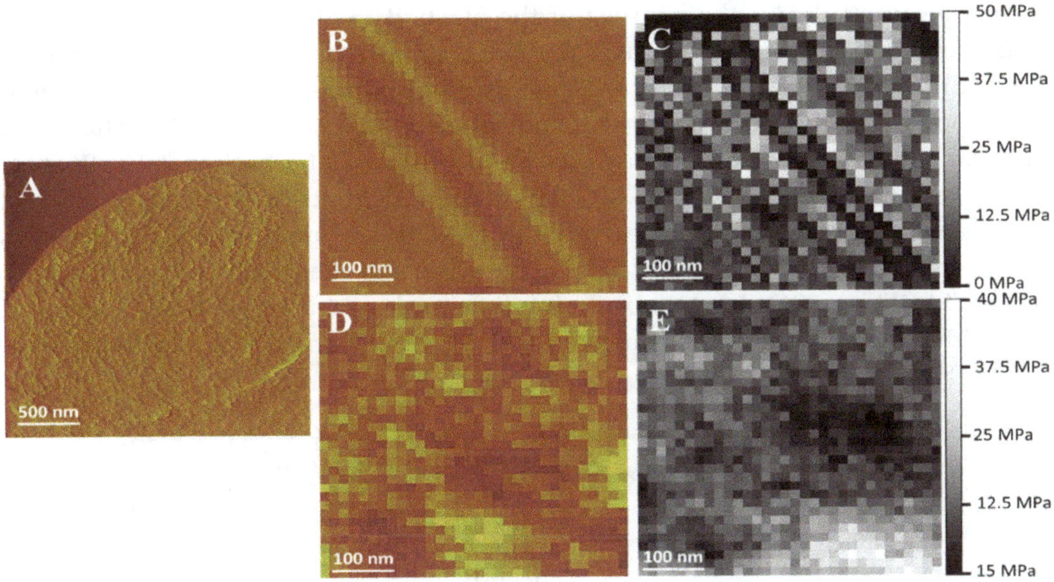

Figure 7. Effect of the Blank-gel on *C. albicans* cells. (**A**) Deflection image of a single yeast cell trapped in a pore. (**B**) Topographic map zoom image of the yeast cell before application of the Blank-gel. (**C**) Elasticity map zoom image of the yeast cell before application of the Blank-gel. (**D**) Topographic map zoom image of the cell yeast after application of the Blank-gel. (**E**) Elasticity map zoom image of the yeast cell after application of the blank-gel.

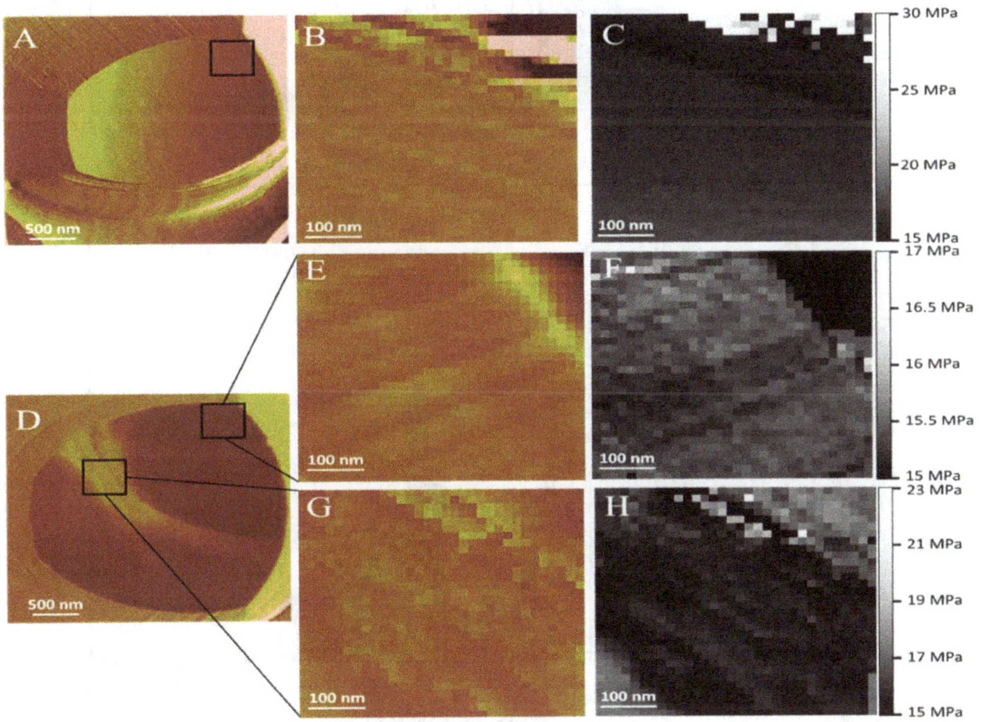

Figure 8. Effect of AmB-gel on *C. albicans* cells. (**A**) Deflection image of a single yeast cell trapped in a pore. (**B**) Topographic map zoom image of a single yeast cell trapped in a pore. (**C**) Elasticity map zoom image of a single yeast cell trapped in a pore. (**D**) A reddish region (low region) that covers almost the 80% of the cell surface and a yellowish arched band (high region) crossing the surface from top-left to center-right of the cell surface. (**E**) Topographic map zoom image of the low region. (**F**) Elasticity map zoom image of the low region. (**G**) Topographic map zoom image of the high region. (**H**) Elasticity map zoom image of the high region.

Conversely, Figure 9 shows the profiles of the elasticity values as a function of its frequency. Figure 9A represents the individual Young's modulus values as a function of its frequency before and after the addition of blank-gel. Before the addition of blank-gel, the yeast cell showed a wide distribution of Young's modulus values with a central value of 21.0 ± 0.4 MPa. After the addition of the blank-gel, the values distribution is narrower and centered at a higher value 26.29 × 0.08 MPa. Figure 9B shows a central peak around 18.48 MPa and a wide distribution function. The low region depicted in Figure 8D corresponds to a narrower peak with a Young's modulus mean value that is shifted towards smaller values (15.63 MPa). On the contrary, the protruding structure resembling "wrinkled sheets" in Figure 8D shows a bimodal distribution, one close to the values of the blank *C. albicans* cell with a mean Young's modulus value of 18.10 MPa and another shifted towards smaller values of 16.62 MPa.

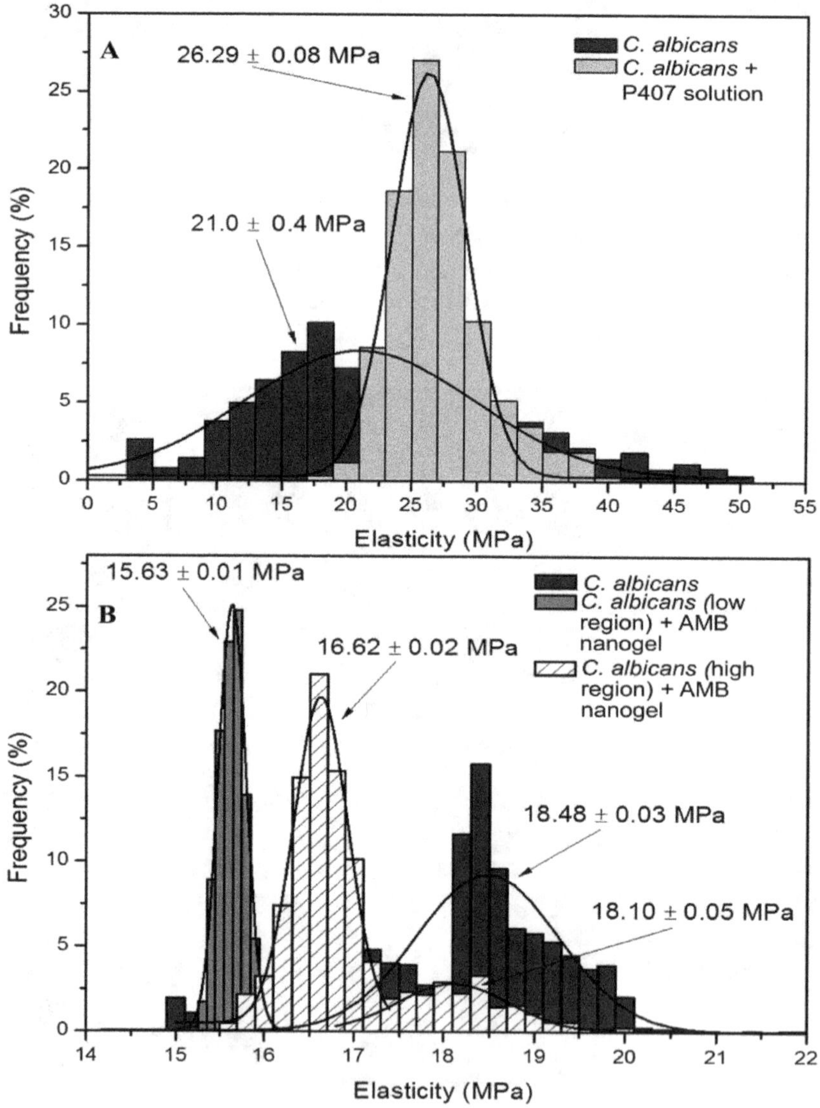

Figure 9. Individual Young's modulus values as a function of its frequency on *C. albicans* cells. (**A**) Individual Young's modulus values before and after the addition of Blank-gel. (**B**) Individual Young's modulus values before and after the addition of the AmB-gel.

3.9. In Vivo Tolerance Study by Evaluating Biomechanical Properties of Human Skin

The results of evaluated biomechanical parameters are depicted in Figure 10. No statistically significant changes of TEWL or skin temperature were observed between Blank-gel and AmB-gel or when compared with baseline measurements ($p > 0.05$). However, a significant decrease in SCH values was observed in the Blank-gel immediately after application (0 h) and at 2 h as well as in the AmB-gel after 2 h, with respect to the basal state (Figure 10E,F).

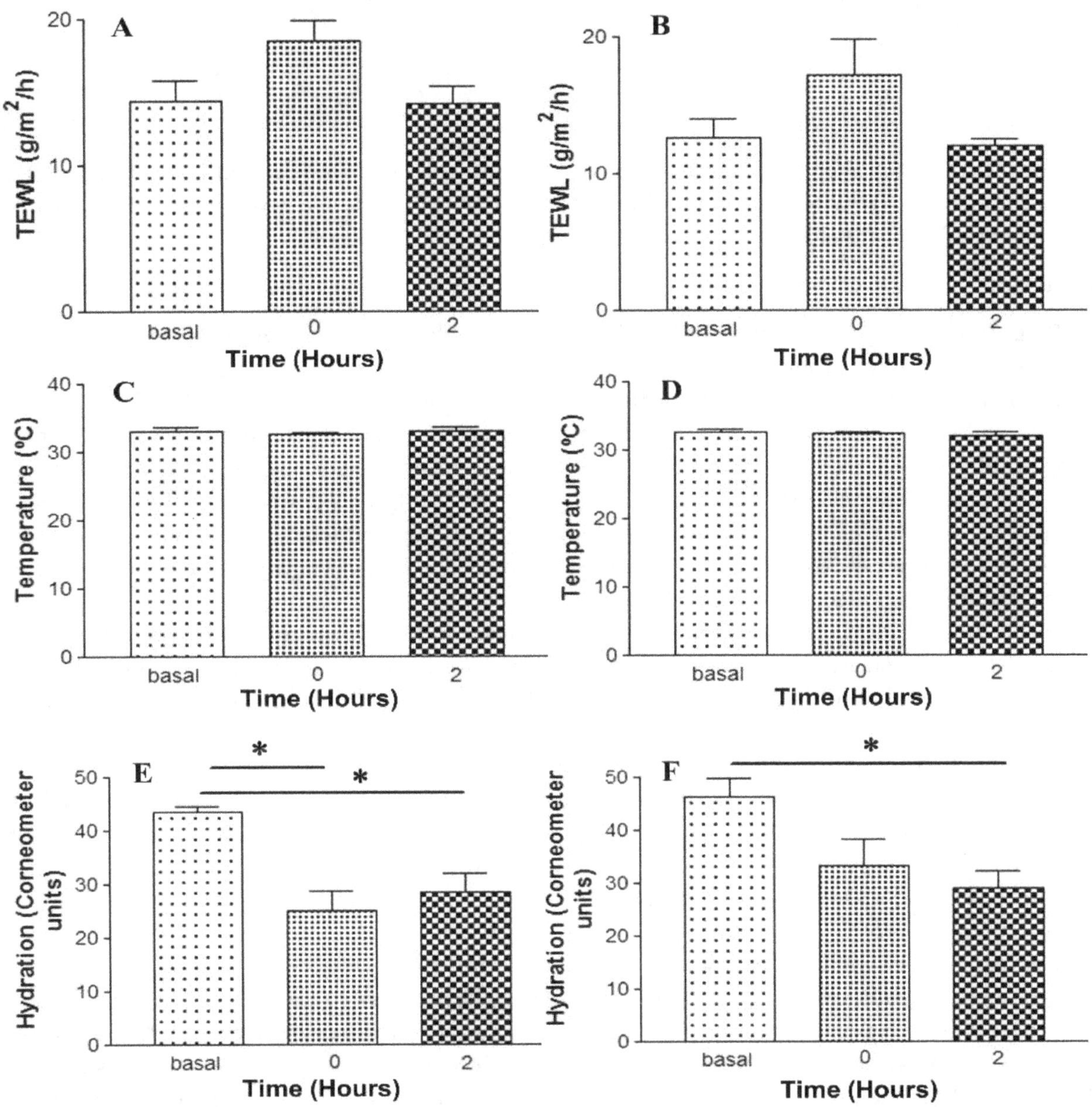

Figure 10. Biomechanical parameters evolution monitored before the application (basal), immediately after application (0 h) and 2 h after application. (**A**) TEWL values of blank-gel. (**B**) TEWL values of AmB-gel. (**C**) Skin temperature values of blank-gel. (**D**) Skin temperature values of AmB-gel. (**E**) SCH values of blank-gel. (**F**) SCH values of AmB-gel. * Statistically significant differences ($p < 0.05$).

3.10. *In Vivo Tolerance Study on Scarified Rabbit Skin by Draize Assay and Histological Analysis*

The Draize test was carried out in order to evaluate the skin irritation potential of AmB-gel. After 48 h, the resulting primary irritation index value for Blank-gel and AmB-gel was 0.38 and 0.45, respectively. This result indicates that both blank-gel and AmB-gel are nonirritants.

Regarding the histological evaluation, micrographs revealed that scarification caused histological alterations and the presence of nonspecific inflammatory cells in the skin (Figure 11B) while the topical application of Blank-gel (Figure 11A) and AmB-gel (Figure 11C) notably repaired these alterations, resulting in a less pronounced inflammatory process than that of the control group (Figure 11B).

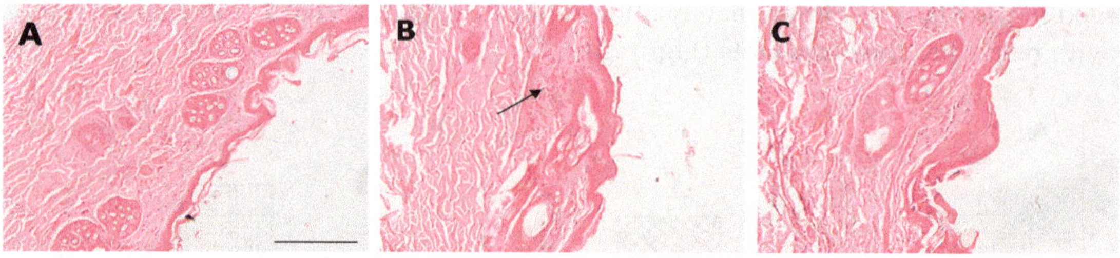

Figure 11. Optical microscopic images of skin. Blank-gel (**A**), skin-scarified control group (**B**), and AmB-gel (**C**). Hematoxylin and eosin stains nuclei blue/black while keratin and cytoplasm are stained red. Scale bar = 200 µm.

4. Discussion

P127 gels are used as the vanguard of drug delivery systems development due to the improved therapeutic efficacy and adherence to the recipient [24]. They have been used as vehicles for various routes of administration of drugs, including oral and topical [25], intranasal [18,26], vaginal and rectal [27], ocular [28], and parenteral [29]. In this study, AmB-gel was developed with 5% of DMSO as an optimal solubilizing agent and 25% of P127 to confer thermoreversible character. For the physicochemical characterization, SEM images were obtained, thus confirming that AmB-gel has a dense and well-oriented tubular appearance along with reticular networks. This type of structure has been reported in other studies [30,31], therefore supporting the postulation that a porous structure could help in the controlled release of drug.

The swelling of AmB-gel is a parameter dependent on the critical micelle concentration (CMC), given that P127-gels show two forms: gel form at 25 °C and liquid form at 4 °C, with liquid form showing thermoreversible behavior. Once the AmB-gel is poured into the swelling medium (PBS), a concentration of P407 decreases rapidly below CMC, thus producing swelling and solubilization in ~19 min. In the present study, 25% of P127 was used and at this concentration the SR followed a first-order kinetic model. Additionally, the degradation process was complete at 20 min, which is a typically rapid rate of degradation for these kinds of systems, as previous studies have also found [32]. On the other hand, the AmB-gel percentage of P was about 82.01 ± 0.5% corroborated with the SEM image which showed a high porosity structure.

The pH value of skin formulations is an important factor to consider in order to avoid skin irritation, particularly when under mycosis infections. AmB-gel showed pH levels to be slightly acidic, therefore biocompatibility with the natural acidity of the skin assures suitability for skin application [30]. What is more is that the AmB content in the gel was maintained between 90 and 100% over a span of 3 months while the superimposed graphs of transmission (Figure 3) showed variations below 10%, which indicates that the product will remain physically stable for a minimum of three months [33–35].

As expected, the rheological characteristics of AmB-gel were temperature-dependent (Figure 4). It is vital to evaluate rheological characterization because rheology can modulate biopharmaceutical properties such as release rates in addition to the widespread application on affected areas [36]. The viscosity at 4 °C was fairly low at ~90 mPa·s, which is an important value at the time of packaging because greater liquescence can lead to optimal forms of delivery, such as spray or roll-on applications, which help prevent the spread of mycotic infections. Once in contact with the affected skin at 32 °C, the solubility of the PPO chains decreases, subsequently forming micelles and assuming hexagonal and/or cubic structures, thus drastically increasing viscosity. The estimated viscosity of the AmB-gel at 32 °C and 50 s^{-1} was ~9.8 Pa·s, which is nearly 100 times higher than the viscosity at 4 °C. This thermal gelation of P407 can form and sustain a drug depot in this area and subsequently increase the contact time, which can then produce desirable drug release characteristics and prolong pharmacological action [37]. The thermal gelation process did not seem to be affected by the presence of AMB. All the results suggested that gel state would be reached after application on the skin and also gain viscosity instantaneously to increase residence time of the formulation on the application area [13].

The data obtained from release studies demonstrated that the AmB-gel provided a sustained release for approximately 24 h. Model fitting showed that release mechanism followed a sigmoidal model. This faster release could be attributed to the highly porous structure and the rapid degradation of P407-gel. Moreover, this mathematical model has been associated with these types of gels due to the fact that they are used to simulate the transport and reaction of fluid in porous media [38].

Ex vivo permeation studies revealed that AmB did not permeate through human skin nor porcine vaginal mucosa. Similar results were reported in previous studies in which no AmB from a nanoemulsion was detected in the ex vivo permeation study using human skin or pig's ear skin [12,39], which might be explained by the great molecular weight (926 D) and high hydrophobicity of AmB, effectively limiting its ability to pass through the aqueous structure of the vaginal mucosa and the hydrophilic barrier of the dermis. However, it was observed that AmB had high retention in the skin and vaginal mucosa with values of 960 $\mu g/g/cm^2$ and 737 $\mu g/g/cm^2$, respectively. This result confirms that AmB succeeded in crossing the SC and was distributed to both the epidermis and dermis. Furthermore, it was able to permeate into the vaginal mucosa without reaching the systemic circulation, which was confirmed with the high amount of drug retained in the tissue and is indicative of the formulation favoring a local effect on the target area with no side effects. This high drug retention capacity in both tissues could be due to the presence of P407 in the formulation, since the chemical structure of this polymer allows it to act as a surfactant that enhances the diffusion ability of drug, resulting in increased drug concentrations in the tissue layer that leads to efficiently provide a local effect [18]. These results suggest that the AmB in this formulation could be successfully implemented in order to achieve a local effect on the skin or vaginal mucosa without adverse systemic effects.

The antifungal action of AmB-gel was clearly observed (Table 1) with a MIC value lower than Free-AmB in all tested Candida species and thus was highly effective—essentially confirming the adequacy of the formulation due to its improved effectiveness against fungus and yeast infections, which is likely due to the synergistic effects reported between the formulations of poloxamers and antifungal agents [40]. On the other hand, Blank-gel did not have any effect against Candida strains and produced values consistent with those reported in previous studies [12]. These results were subsequently observed by AFM images (Figures 7 and 8) which evidenced the alterations on the surface of Candida yeast cells that were induced by AmB-gel. In an equivocal manner, the mean values of Young's modulus (Figure 9) demonstrate the destructuring effect of AmB-gel on the outer membrane of the yeast cell.

The tolerance of the formulation was studied by evaluating the biomechanical properties of skin, since parameters such as TEWL and SCH are important indicators of skin integrity. Thus, any changes in these parameters could be directly related to an alteration of the functionality of the skin barrier [41]. From the results of this noninvasive in vivo method, no statistically significant differences were observed in temperature or TEWL values of volunteers after treatment with AmB-gel or with blank-gel when compared with baseline measurements (Figure 10), whereas SCH values showed a significant reduction in both AmB-gel and blank-gel with respect to the basal state. This decrease in the hydration levels in the area of application of the final product could be due to the ability of the gel to absorb moisture produced by the sweat glands. When the formulation containing P407 dries on the surface of the skin, it forms a film that captures moisture and does so in a state of relative equilibrium with ambient humidity. This effect would be especially suitable in skin candidiasis because it could prevent the proliferation of microorganisms around the affected area [42,43]. Moreover, when comparing the values of the biomechanical parameters evaluated for AmB-gel and blank-gel, the incorporation of the AmB does not significantly modify the properties of the gel. Furthermore, none of the volunteers exhibited side effects of burning or itching after the application. Therefore, the AmB-gel did not alter the biophysical properties of the skin of volunteers throughout the course of the study.

Finally, the tolerability of the formulation was evaluated by in vivo model using scarified rabbit skin in order to simulate the damage of the skin barrier caused by the fungal infection. The irritation index values for AmB-gel and Blank-gel were less than 0.5 and can therefore be classified as nonirritant formulations. This result was consistent with histological analysis, which showed that both formulations did not cause any alteration of the skin architecture but, on the contrary, they actually repaired the ulcerated skin. According to this finding the ability of P407 to reduce wounds in burn patients while simultaneously stimulating the proliferation of collagen fibers, consequently increasing scarring and generating new tissue, have all been reported in previous studies [44]. In conjunction, these effects might favor the healing and alleviation of wounds caused by Candida. In conclusion, AmB-gel represents a promising therapeutic option to treat these types of infections via dermal application.

5. Conclusions

The focus of the present study was on the incorporation of AmB in a copolymer P407-based gel designed for application on both the skin and vaginal mucosa, specifically for the treatment of candidiasis. P407 has shown great potential as a support system in the administration of hydrophilic and hydrophobic drugs, as is the case of AmB. P407 is suitable due to its thermoreversible capacity, low toxicity, and permeation-enhancing properties. During the experimental phase, AmB-gel remained stable for at least 3 months, thereby demonstrating pH values suitable for both skin and vaginal application. Due to its low viscosity at predetermined temperatures and its porous structure which facilitates rapid drug release, AmB-gel can also be used in aerosol form in order to avoid contact with areas infected by the fungus and thus prevent the spread of infection to other anatomical sites while minimizing the risk of a subsequent superinfection. No drug was quantified in the receptor compartments of the Franz cells, which indicates nonabsorption of AmB and therefore avoids adverse systemic effects. None of volunteers exhibited burning or itching after application and the histological images of rabbit skin displayed high tolerability of the formulation. Furthermore, AmB-gel did not alter the biophysical properties of skin, thus confirming adequate safety as topical agents. According to the values of the amount of drug retained in the skin and vaginal mucosa, along with the MIC values and the images obtained by AFM, it can be concluded that AmB-gel provides a satisfactory antifungal effect across various Candida species.

Author Contributions: L.S. carried out the experiments and analyzed and wrote the results of the manuscript. A.C.C. conceived the idea and analyzed the results. M.S.-A. analyzed the results and wrote and edited the manuscript. M.R. and L.C.E. participated in the methodologic analysis and editing of the manuscript. M.J.R.-L. realized the histological studies. N.B. carried out the microbiological efficacy. O.D. performed the force atomic experiments and analyzed the results. B.C. conceived the idea and edited the manuscript. All authors read the manuscript and agreed with the submission.

Acknowledgments: We appreciate the help of Jonathan Proctor for the revision of the use of the English language. The authors are grateful to Lyda Halbaut for the help with rheological studies.

References

1. Havlickova, B.; Czaika, V.A.; Friedrich, M. Epidemiological trends in skin mycoses worldwide. *Mycoses* **2008**, *51*, 2–15. [CrossRef] [PubMed]
2. Sawant, B.; Khan, T. Recent advances in delivery of antifungal agents for therapeutic management of candidiasis. *Biomed. Pharm.* **2017**, *96*, 1478–1490. [CrossRef] [PubMed]
3. Sanchez, D.A.; Schairer, D.; Tuckman-Vernon, C.; Chouake, J.; Kutner, A.; Makdisi, J.; Friedman, J.M.; Nosanchuk, J.D.; Friedman, A.J. Amphotericin B releasing nanoparticle topical treatment of Candida spp. in the setting of a burn wound. *Nanomedicine* **2014**, *10*, 269–277. [CrossRef] [PubMed]

4. Qasim, M.; Baipaywad, P.; Udomluck, N.; Na, D.; Park, H. Enhanced therapeutic efficacy of lipophilic amphotericin B against Candida albicanswith amphiphilic poly(N-isopropylacrylamide) nanogels. *Macromol. Res.* **2014**, *22*, 1125–1131. [CrossRef]
5. Yapar, N. Epidemiology and risk factors for invasive candidiasis. *Clin. Risk Manag.* **2014**, *10*, 95–105. [CrossRef]
6. Cannon, R.D.; Lamping, E.; Holmes, A.R.; Niimi, K.; Baret, P.V.; Keniya, M.V.; Tanabe, K.; Niimi, M.; Goffeau, A.; Monk, B.C. Efflux-mediated antifungal drug resistance. *Clin. Microbiol. Rev.* **2009**, *22*, 291–321. [CrossRef] [PubMed]
7. Canuto, M.M.; Rodero, F.G. Antifungal drug resistance to azoles and polyenes. *Lancet Infect. Dis.* **2002**, *2*, 550–563. [CrossRef]
8. Morio, F.; Jensen, R.H.; Le Pape, P.; Arendrup, M.C. Molecular basis of antifungal drug resistance in yeasts. *Int. J. Antimicrob. Agents* **2017**, *50*, 599–606. [CrossRef]
9. Miceli, M.H.; Díaz, J.A.; Lee, S.A. Emerging opportunistic yeast infections. *Lancet Infect Dis.* **2011**, *11*, 142–151. [CrossRef]
10. Cannon, R.D.; Lamping, E.; Holmes, A.R.; Niimi, K.; Tanabe, K.; Niimi, M.; Monk, B.C. Candida albicans drug resistance another way to cope with stress. *Microbiology* **2007**, *153*, 3211–3217. [CrossRef]
11. Vincent, B.M.; Lancaster, A.K.; Scherz-Shouval, R.; Whitesell, L.; Lindquist, S. Fitness trade-offs restrict the evolution of resistance to amphotericin B. *PLoS Biol.* **2013**, *11*, e1001692. [CrossRef] [PubMed]
12. Sosa, L.; Clares, B.; Alvarado, H.L.; Bozal, N.; Domenech, O.; Calpena, A.C. Amphotericin B releasing topical nanoemulsion for the treatment of candidiasis and aspergillosis. *Nanomedicine* **2017**, *13*, 2303–2312. [CrossRef] [PubMed]
13. Tutaj, K.; Szlazak, R.; Szalapata, K.; Starzyk, J.; Luchowski, R.; Grudzinski, W.; Osinska-Jaroszuk, M.; Jarosz-Wilkolazka, A.; Szuster-Ciesielska, A.; Gruszecki, W.I. Amphotericin B-silver hybrid nanoparticles: Synthesis, properties and antifungal activity. *Nanomedicine* **2016**, *12*, 1095–1103. [CrossRef] [PubMed]
14. Perez, A.P.; Altube, M.J.; Schilrreff, P.; Apezteguia, G.; Celes, F.S.; Zacchino, S.; de Oliveira, C.I.; Romero, E.L.; Morilla, M.J. Topical amphotericin B in ultradeformable liposomes: Formulation, skin penetration study, antifungal and antileishmanial activity in vitro. *Colloids Surf. B Biointerfaces* **2016**, *139*, 190–198. [CrossRef] [PubMed]
15. Atiyeh, B.S.; Gunn, S.W.; Hayek, S.N. State of the art in burn treatment. *World J. Surg.* **2005**, *29*, 131–148. [CrossRef] [PubMed]
16. Giuliano, E.; Paolino, D.; Fresta, M.; Cosco, D. Mucosal application of polaxamer 407-based hydrogels: An overview. *Pharmaceutics* **2018**, *10*, 159. [CrossRef] [PubMed]
17. Dumortier, G.; Grossiord, J.L.; Agnely, F.; Chaumeil, J.C. A review of poloxamer 407 pharmaceutical and pharmacological characteristics. *Pharm. Res.* **2006**, *23*, 2709–2728. [CrossRef]
18. Espinoza, L.C.; Silva-Abreu, M.; Clares, B.; Rodríguez-Lagunas, M.J.; Halbaut, L.; Cañas, M.A.; Calpena, A.C. Formulation Strategies to Improve Nose-to-Brain Delivery of Donepezil. *Pharmaceutics* **2019**, *11*, 64. [CrossRef]
19. Subcommittee on Antifungal Susceptibility Testing (AFST) of the ESCMID European Committee for Antimicrobial Susceptibility Testing (EUCAST). EUCAST Definitive Document EDef 7.1: Method for the determination of broth dilution MICs of antifungal agents for fermentative yeasts. *Clin. Microbiol. Infect.* **2008**, *14*, 398–405. [CrossRef]
20. Clinical and Laboratory Standards Institute, CLSI. *Reference Method for Broth Dilution Antifungal Susceptibility Testing of Yeast*, 3rd ed.; document M27-A3; Clinical and Laboratory Standards Institute: Villanova, PA, USA, 2008; Volume 28, ISBN 1-56238-666-2, ISSN 0273-3099.
21. World Medical Association Declaration of Helsinki. Clinical Review and Education. 2013. Available online: https://www.wma.net/wp-content/uploads/2016/11/DoH-Oct2013-JAMA.pdf (accessed on 2 May 2019).
22. Du Plessis, J.; Stefaniak, A.; Eloff, F.; John, S.; Agner, T.; Chou, T.C.; Nixon, R.; Steiner, M.; Franken, A.; Kudla, I.; et al. International guidelines for the in vivo assessment of skin properties in non-clinical settings: Part 2. transepidermal water loss and skin hydration. *Ski. Res. Technol.* **2013**, *19*, 265–278. [CrossRef]
23. Draize, J.H.; Woodward, G.; Calvery, H.O. Methods for the study of irritation and toxicity of substances applied topically to the skin and mucous membranes. *J. Pharmacol. Exp. Ther.* **1944**, *82*, 377–390.
24. Wertheimer, A.I.; Santella, T.M.; Finestone, A.J.; Levy, R.A. Drug delivery systems improve pharmaceutical profile and facilitate medication adherence. *Adv. Ther.* **2005**, *22*, 559–577. [CrossRef] [PubMed]
25. Padilla, M.; Clark, G.T.; Merrill, R.L. Topical medications for orofacial neuropathic pain: A review. *J. Am. Dent. Assoc.* **2000**, *131*, 2. [CrossRef]

26. Jain, N.K.; Shah, B.K.; Taneja, L.N. Nasal absorption of metoprolol tartrate. *Indian J. Pharm. Sci.* **1991**, *53*, 16–19.
27. Ryu, J.M.; Chung, S.-J.; Lee, M.-H.; Chang-Kook, K.; Chang-Koo, S. Increased bioavailability of propanolol in rats by retaining thermally gelling liquid suppositories in the rectum. *J. Control. Release* **1999**, *59*, 163–172. [CrossRef]
28. Li, H.; Sung, K.C. Carbopol/pluronic phase change solutions for ophthalmic drug delivery. *J. Control. Release* **2000**, *69*, 379–388.
29. Koller, C.; Buri, P. Propriétés et intérêtpharmaceutique des gels thermoréversibles à base de poloxamers et poloxamines. *STP Pharma* **1987**, *3*, 115–124.
30. Yeh, M.Y.; Zhao, J.Y.; Hsieh, Y.R.; Lin, J.H.; Chen, F.Y.; Chakravarthy, R.D.; Chung, P.C.; Lin, H.C.; Hung, S.C. Reverse thermo-responsive hydrogels prepared from Pluronic F127 and gelatin composite materials. *RSC Adv.* **2017**, *7*, 21252. [CrossRef]
31. Rangabhatla, A.S.L.; Tantishaiyakul, V.; Boonrat, O.; Hirun, N.; Ouiyangkul, P. Novel in situ mucoadhesive gels based on Pluronic F127 and xyloglucan containing metronidazole for treatment of periodontal disease. *Iran. Polym. J.* **2017**, *26*, 851–859. [CrossRef]
32. Mallandrich, M.; Fernández-Campos, F.; Clares, B.; Halbaut, L.; Alonso, C.; Coderch, L.; Garduño-Ramírez, M.L.; Andrade, B.; Del Pozo, A.; Lane, M.E.; et al. Developing transdermal Application of Ketorolac Tromethamine Entrapped in Stimuli Sensitive Block Copolymer Hydrogels. *Pharm. Res.* **2017**, *34*, 1728–1740. [CrossRef]
33. Sierra, A.F.; Ramirez, M.L.; Campmany, A.C.; Martinez, A.R.; Naveros, B.C. In vitro and In vivo evaluation of the use of a newly developed melatonin loaded emulsion combined with UV filtres as a protective agent against skin irradiation. *J. Derm. Sci.* **2013**, *69*, 202–214. [CrossRef] [PubMed]
34. Alvarado, H.L.; Abrego, G.; Souto, E.B.; Garduño-Ramírez, M.L.; Clares, B.; García, M.L.; Calpena, A.C. Nanoemulsions for dermal controlled release of oleanolic and ursolic acids: In vitro, ex vivo and in vivo characterization. *Colloids Surf. B Biointerfaces* **2015**, *130*, 40–47. [CrossRef] [PubMed]
35. Abrego, G.; Alvarado, H.L.; Egea, M.A.; Gonzalez-Mira, E.; Calpena, A.C.; Garcia, M.L. Design of nanosuspensions and freeze-dried PLGA nanoparticles as a novel approach for ophthalmic delivery of pranoprofen. *J. Pharm. Sci.* **2014**, *103*, 3153–3164. [CrossRef] [PubMed]
36. Fernandez-Campos, F.; Clares Naveros, B.; Lopez Serrano, O.; Alonso Merino, C.; Calpena Campmany, A.C. Evaluation of novel nystatin nanoemulsion for skin candidosis infections. *Mycoses* **2013**, *56*, 70–81. [CrossRef] [PubMed]
37. Lenaerts, V.; Triqueneaux, C.; Quartern, M.; Rieg-Falson, F.; Couvreur, P. Temperature-dependent rheological behavior of Pluronic F-127. *Int. J. Pharm.* **1987**, *39*, 121–127. [CrossRef]
38. Navarro-Verdugo, A.L.; Goycoolea, F.M.; Romero-Melendez, G.; Higuera-Ciaparad, I.; Arguelles-Monal, W. A modified Boltzmann sigmoidal model for the phase transition of smart gels. *Soft Matter* **2011**, *7*, 5847. [CrossRef]
39. Moraes Santos, C.; Barbosa de Oliveira, R.; Arantes, V.T.; Rodrigues-Caldeira, L.; De Oliveira, M.C.; Tabosa-Egito, E.S.; Miranda-Ferreira, L.A. Amphotericin B-Loaded Nanocarriers for Topical Treatment of Cutaneous Leishmaniasis: Development, Characterization, and In Vitro Skin Permeation Studies. *J. Biomed. Nanotechnol.* **2012**, *8*, 322–329.
40. Banov, D. Synergistic Effect of Poloxamer-based Composition and Itraconazole on Fungus and Yeast. U.S. Patent 9,763,934B2, 19 September 2017.
41. Mohammed, D.; Hirata, K.; Hadgraft, J.; Lane, M.E. Influence of skin penetration enhancers on skin barrier function and skin protease activity. *Eur. J. Pharm. Sci.* **2014**, *51*, 118–122. [CrossRef]
42. Gilbert, J.; Richardson, J.; Pallin, K.J.; Hadgraft, J.T. The effect of solutes and polymers on the gelation properties of Pluronic F-127 solution for controlled drug delivery. *J. Control. Release* **1987**, *5*, 113–118. [CrossRef]
43. Grove, G.L.; Allenby, K.; Houser, T. DFD-01 Reduces Transepidermal Water Loss and improves skin hydration and flexibility. *Dermatol. Ther.* **2017**, *7*, 507–514.
44. Kant, V.; Gopal, A.; Kumar, D.; Gopalkrishnana, A.; Pathaka, N.N.; Kurade, N.P.; Tandana, S.K.; Dinesh, K. Topical pluronic F-127 gel application enhances cutaneous wound healing in rats. *Acta Histochem.* **2013**, *116*, 5–13. [CrossRef] [PubMed]

4

The Fungal Defensin Family Enlarged

Jiajia Wu, Bin Gao and Shunyi Zhu *

Group of Animal Innate Immunity, State Key Laboratory of Integrated Management of Pest Insects and Rodents, Institute of Zoology, Chinese Academy of Sciences, 1 Beichen West Road, Chaoyang District, Beijing 100101, China

* Author to whom correspondence should be addressed; Zhusy@ioz.ac.cn.

Abstract: Fungi are an emerging source of peptide antibiotics. With the availability of a large number of model fungal genome sequences, we can expect that more and more fungal defensin-like peptides (fDLPs) will be discovered by sequence similarity search. Here, we report a total of 69 new fDLPs encoded by 63 genes, in which a group of fDLPs derived from dermatophytes are defined as a new family (fDEF8) according to sequence and phylogenetic analyses. In the oleaginous fungus *Mortierella alpine*, fDLPs have undergone extensive gene expansion. Our work further enlarges the fungal defensin family and will help characterize new peptide antibiotics with therapeutic potential.

Keywords: peptide antibiotic; gene duplication; exon-intron structure; cysteine-stabilized α-helical and β-sheet motif

---

1. Introduction

Fungal defensin-like peptides (fDLPs) are emerging as attractive anti-infective agents due to their therapeutic efficacy, low toxicity and high serum stability [1,2]. On the basis of a combined analyses of sequence, structural, and phylogenetic data, we has identified seven fDLP families [2,3], in which three members (plectasin, micasin and eurocin), classified as ancient invertebrate-type defensins (AITDs) [1,2,4,5], have been structurally and functionally characterized. These fDLPs exhibit activity against several antibiotic-resistant clinical isolates with significant therapeutic potential [1,2,5,6]. Some efforts have been taken to improve antimicrobial efficacy and to reduce undesirable side effects of fDLPs. For example, an improved mutant of plectasin (NZ2114) is superior to two conventional antibiotics (vancomycin and daptomycin) in inhibiting methicillin-resistant *Staphylococcus aureus* (MRSA) with even more enhanced serum stability and extended *in vivo* half-life [7–9]. In this work, we describe 69 new fDLPs in terms of their sequences, structural characteristics, and phylogenetic relationship. This provides an array of candidates for development of new anti-infective agents against antibiotic-resistant human pathogens.

2. Discovery of New fDLPs

The database search strategy used here has been described previously [3]. Through an exhaustive search of 26 fungal species, we retrieved a total of 69 new fDLPs. As previously stated, overall this class of molecules exhibits a taxa-specific distribution pattern in the fungus kingdom, of which 21 fDLPs are derived from *Ascomycota*, 39 from *Zygomycota*, eight from *Basidiomycota* and one from *Glomeromycota*. In the basal fungi (*Microsporidia* and *Chytridiomycota*), no typical fDLP has been identified (Figure 1). The general features of these peptides are listed in Tables 1 and 2. They can be grouped into six families based on sequence similarity, five of which are classified into the previously known families (fDEF1, fDEF2, fDEF3, fDEF4, and fDEF6) [3] (Figures 2 and 3). This grouping is consistent with the phylogenetic analysis supported by high bootstrap values (Figure 4).

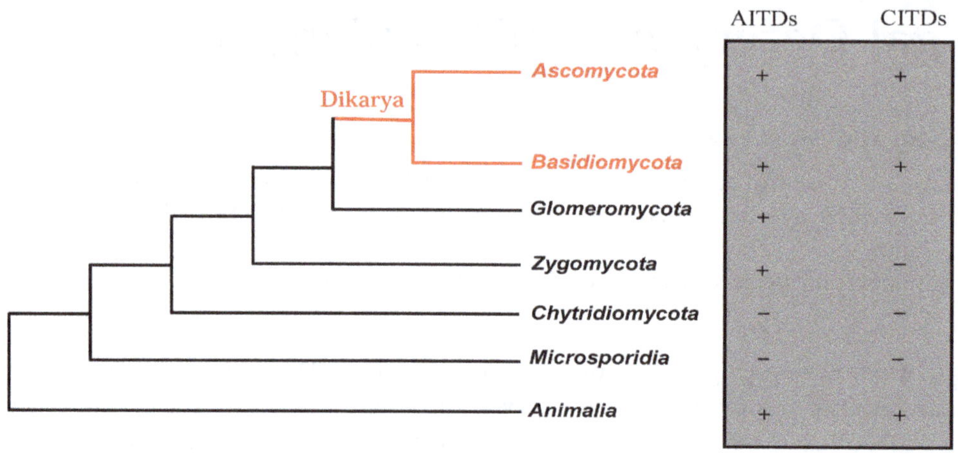

Figure 1. Phylogenetic distribution of fDLPs. The left: A parsimony tree of fungal species, animalia is used as an outgroup. This tree is a modification of the SSU and LSU r-RNA analyses of Lutzoni *et al.* for the fungal kingdom [10]. The right: "+" means presence and "−" means absence.

All the fDLPs characterized here have a signal peptide located in the N-terminus. In comparison with fDEF1 and fDEF2 that possess a propeptide located between signal and mature peptides, fDEF6 and fDEF8 lack a propeptide. Five precursors (maglosin, beauvesin2, manisin, pochlasin2 and asosin) could release two defensins from a single precursor after the removal of a spacer propeptide (Figure 5). The malpisin family from *Mortierella alpine* exhibits two types of precursor organization: (1) the first type contains 10 members, all having a propeptides identified by its acidic feature and single or two basic amino acids at their ends as putative cleavage site of proprotein convertase [11]; (2) the second type contains 14 members that lack a propeptide and thus no further processing step is needed (Figure S1).

Table 1. Sources and characteristics of newly discovered non-*Mortierella* fDLPs.

Name I Accession No.	Class	Species (phylum: subphylum: class)	Size	MW	NC
Pyronesin1 I CATG01000243 (G)		*Pyronema omphalodes* (Ascomycota: Pezizomycotina: Pezizomycetes)	40	4317	+1.2
Pyronesin2 I CATG01000243 (G)		*P. omphalodes*	40	4402	+0.2
Pyronesin3 I CATG01000243 (G)		*P. omphalodes*	40	4389	+1.2
Pyronesin4 I CATG01000243 (G)		*P. omphalodes*	40	4416	+2.2
Pyronesin5 I CATG01000243 (G)	fDEF1	*P. omphalodes*	40	4375	+1.2
Pyronesin6 I CATG01000243 (G)		*P. omphalodes*	40	4291	+2.4
Abisin1 I AEOK01000166 (G)		*Agaricus bisporus* (Basidiomycota: Agaricomycotina: Agaricomycetes)	40	4097	-3.8
Abisin2 I AEOK01000166 (G)		*A. bisporus*	40	4097	-3.8
Abisin3 I AEOK01000166		*A. bisporus*	39	3926	-2.8
Beauvesin1 I ADAH01000714 (G)		*Beauveria bassiana* (Ascomycota: Pezizomycotina: Sordariomycetes)	52	5475	+2.9
Pyrelysin I GAJI01023341 (T)		*Pyrenochaeta lycopersici* (Ascomycota: Pezizomycotina: Dothideomycetes)	55	5858	+5.4
Risin I JAQX01005622		*Rhizophagus irregularis* (Glomeromycota: Glomeromycetes)	55	5972	+6.1
Trimensin I FG132536 (E)		*Trichophyton mentagrophytes* (Ascomycota: Pezizomycotina: Eurotiomycetes)	38	4156	+2.2
Lecasin I AWYC01000479		*Lecanosticta acicola* (Ascomycota: Pezizomycotina: Dothideomycetes)	42	4314	−4.8

Table 1. *Cont.*

Name I Accession No.	Class	Species (phylum: subphylum: class)	Size	MW	NC
Pochlasin1 I AOSW01002431		*Pochonia chlamydosporia* (Ascomycota: Pezizomycotina: Sordariomycetes)	43	4339	−3.5
Perisin I AFRD01000258	fDEF2	*Periglandula ipomoeae* (Ascomycota: Pezizomycotina: Sordariomycetes)	43	4080	−1.5
Masysin I CANK01000016		*Malassezia sympodialis* (Basidiomycota: Ustilaginomycotina: Exobasidiomycetes)	35	3432	+2.2
Maglosin1N I AAYY01000039 (G)		*Malassezia globosa* (Basidiomycota: Ustilaginomycotina: Exobasidiomycetes)	40	3980	+1.2
Maglosin2N I AAYY01000024 (G)		*M. globosa*	40	4022	+0.2
Maglosin1C I AAYY01000039 (G)		*M. globosa*	41	3910	+2.7
Maglosin2C I AAYY01000024 (G)		*M. globosa*	40	3835	+2.7
Beauvesin2C I ADAH01000123 (G)		*B. bassiana*	41	4243	+0.9
ManisinC I ADNJ01000735	fDEF3	*Metarhizium anisopliae* (Ascomycota: Pezizomycotina: Sordariomycetes)	41	4211	−0.1
Pochlasin2C I AOSW01005877		*P. chlamydosporia*	41	4381	+0.2
AsosinC I BACA01000303		*Aspergillus sojae* (Ascomycota: Pezizomycotina: Eurotiomycetes)	38	4002	−1.0
Beauvesin2N I ADAH01000123 (G)		*B. bassiana*	48	5067	+2.9
ManisinN I ADNJ01000735	fDEF4	*M. anisopliae*	46	4921	+0.2
Pochlasin2N I AOSW01005877		*P. chlamydosporia*	49	5185	+2.9
AsosinN I BACA01000303		*A. sojae*	49	5140	−1.1
Rhimisin1 I ANKS01000620		*Rhizopus microsporus* (Zygomycota: Mucoromycotina: Mucorales)	45	4867	+10.0
Rhimisin2 I ANKS01000620		*R. microsporus*	44	4638	+3.4
Rhimisin3 I ANKS01001486		*R. microsporus*	44	4768	+1.5
Rhimisin4 I ANKS01001486	fDEF6	*R. microsporus*	45	4811	+8.0
Rhidesin1 I AACW02000043		*Rhizopus delemar* (Zygomycota: Mucoromycotina: Mucorales)	55	5885	+10.4
Rhidesin2 I AACW02000259		*R. delemar*	48	5270	+0.5
Mirresin I AZYI01000143		*Mucor irregularis* (Zygomycota: Mucoromycotina: Mucorales)	60	6424	+13.4
Mucisin I AOCY01001156 (G)		*Mucor circinelloides* (Zygomycota: Mucoromycotina: Mucorales)	53	5548	+2.2
Phycomysin I EX863311 (E)		*Phycomyces blakesleeanus* (Zygomycota: Mucoromycotina: Mucorales)	50	5342	+9.4
TritoDLP I ACPI01000196 (G)		*Trichophyton tonsurans* (Ascomycota: Pezizomycotina: Eurotiomycetes)	41	4323	+3.7
TrequiDLP I ABWI01000729 (G)	fDEF8	*Trichophyton equinum* (Ascomycota: Pezizomycotina: Eurotiomycetes)	41	4323	+3.7
TriveDLP I ACYE01000402		*Trichophyton verrucosum* (Ascomycota: Pezizomycotina: Eurotiomycetes)	42	4403	+4.7
ArgyDLP I ABQE01000293		*Arthroderma gypseum* (Ascomycota: Pezizomycotina: Eurotiomycetes)	41	4247	+3.7
ArbeDLP I ABSU01000004		*Arthroderma benhamiae* (Ascomycota: Pezizomycotina: Eurotiomycetes)	42	4493	+4.7
TriruDLP I ACPH01000567 (G)		*Trichophyton rubrum* (Ascomycota: Pezizomycotina: Eurotiomycetes)	42	4479	+4.7
MicaDLP I ABVF01000093		*Arthroderma otae* (Ascomycota: Pezizomycotina: Eurotiomycetes)	43	4745	+3.2

Note: MW: molecular weight; NC (net charge) is estimated at pH 7.0 with protein calculation V3.4. "E" means peptides from the Expressed Sequence Tags (EST) database and "T" means peptides from the Transcriptome Shotgun Assembly (TSA) database. "G" means proteins currently annotated in the GenBank database as hypothetical proteins (http://www.ncbi.nlm.nih.gov/) [12].

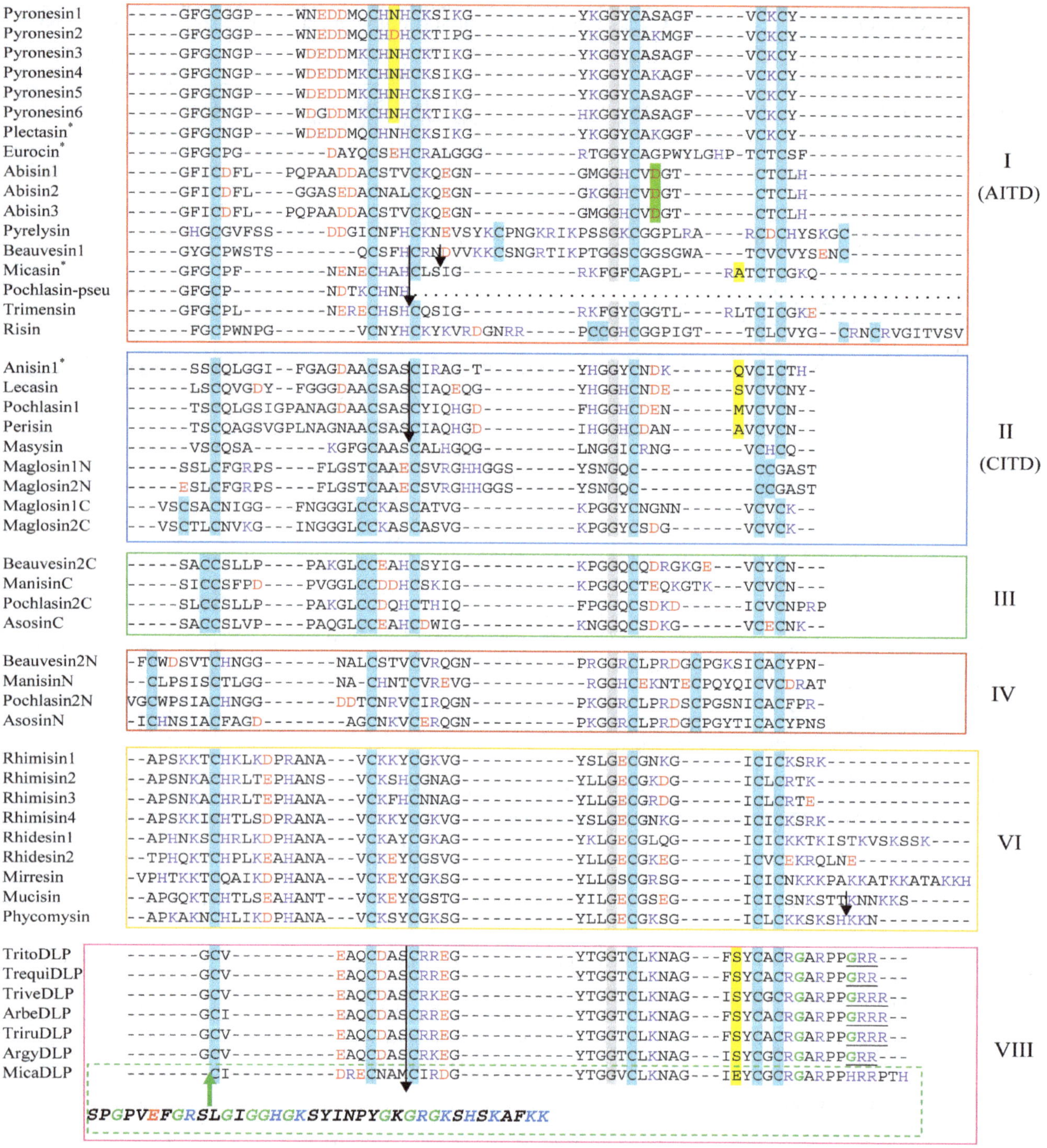

Figure 2. Multiple sequence alignment of fDLPs. Cysteines are shadowed in cyan. Conserved glycines are highlighted in grey. Negatively (D and E) and positively (R, K and H) charged residues are boldfaced in red and blue, respectively. Introns are shown by arrows (phase 0) or small boxes (green: phase 1, yellow: phase 2). Functionally characterized fDLPs were indicated by "*". The N-terminal extension sequence in micaDLP belonging to the family fDEF8 is italicized. Defensins from *Pyronema omphalodes* have been predicted and investigated by RNA-seq [13]. Extra residues for C-terminal amidation are underlined once.

Table 2. Sources and characteristics of the malpisin family.

Name ǀ Accession No.	Organism	Scaffold (Contig)	Range	Size	MW	NC
Malpisin1-1 ǀ AZCI01001104			55070–55405	41	4048	−0.0
Malpisin1-2 ǀ AZCI01001104			55870–56127	48	5166	−3.3
Malpisin1-3 ǀ AZCI01001104		jtg7180000084593 f_7180000084594f	56393–56635	45	5047	+0.7
Malpisin1-4 ǀ AZCI01001104			63869–64117	39	4117	−1.0
Malpisin1-5 ǀ AZCI01000882	*Mortierella alpina* B6842		22045–22248	37	4259	-2.8
Malpisin1-6 ǀ AZCI01000882			25851–26051	39	4543	−3.5
Malpisin1-7 ǀ AZCI01000882		Contig 7180000084767	42456–42677	33	3624	−1.0
Malpisin1-8 ǀ AZCI01000882			43573–43800	47	5078	+1.7
Malpisin1-9 ǀ AZCI01000882			45037–45261	48	5203	+3.0
Malpisin1-10 ǀ AZCI01000882			45559–45738	35	3914	−0.0
Malpisin1-11 ǀ AZCI01000882			46707–46913	43	4941	+5.4
Malpisin1-12 ǀ AZCI01001135		jtg7180000084204f_7 180000084205f_7180000084206f	135437–135676	44	4722	−0.0
Malpisin1-13 ǀ AZCI01001084		jtg7180000084699f_7180000084700f	362415–362627	47	4919	−1.8
Malpisin1-14 ǀ AZCI01001006		jtg7180000084769f_7180000084770f_7 180000084771f_7 180000084772f	179488–179673	38	4188	+0.2
Malpisin2-1 ǀ ADAG01001070			9785–10114	39	4105	+1.0
Malpisin2-2 ǀ ADAG01001070		Contig 1070	10532–10792	48	5187	−2.3
Malpisin2-3 ǀ ADAG01001070			11052–11297	44	4783	−0.0
Malpisin2-4 ǀ ADAG01001070	*Mortierella alpina* ATCC 32222		11773–12021	39	4052	−1.8
Malpisin2-5 ǀ ADAG01000791		Contig 791	4894–5097	37	4259	−2.8
Malpisin2-7 ǀ ADAG01000903			13145–13357	33	3899	+1.2
Malpisin2-8 ǀ ADAG01000903		Contig 903	14223–14450	47	5065	+1.7
Malpisin2-9 ǀ ADAG01000903			15634–15852	45	4917	+4.0
Malpisin2-10 ǀ ADAG01000903			16158–16337	35	3937	+0.2
Malpisin2-11 ǀ ADAG01000903			17264–17446	39	4531	+5.0

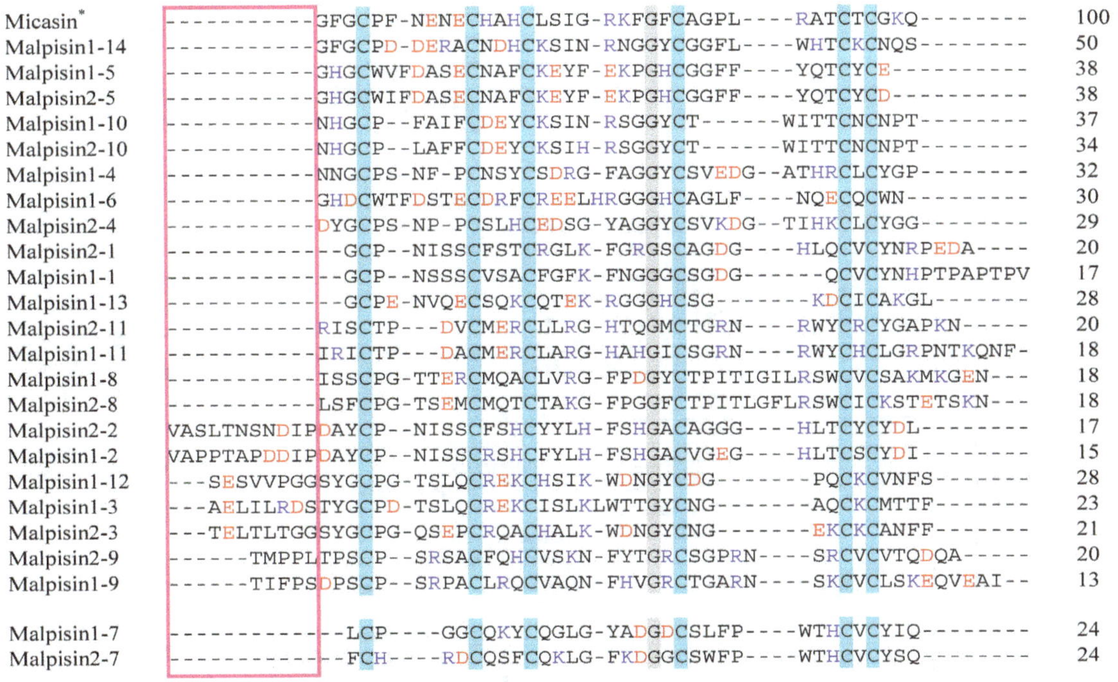

Figure 3. Multiple sequence alignment of malpisins. Color codes and symbol notes used here are the same as those in Figure 2. Pink box indicates the N-terminus of DLPs with variable length. Sequence identity (%) to micasin is shown on the right.

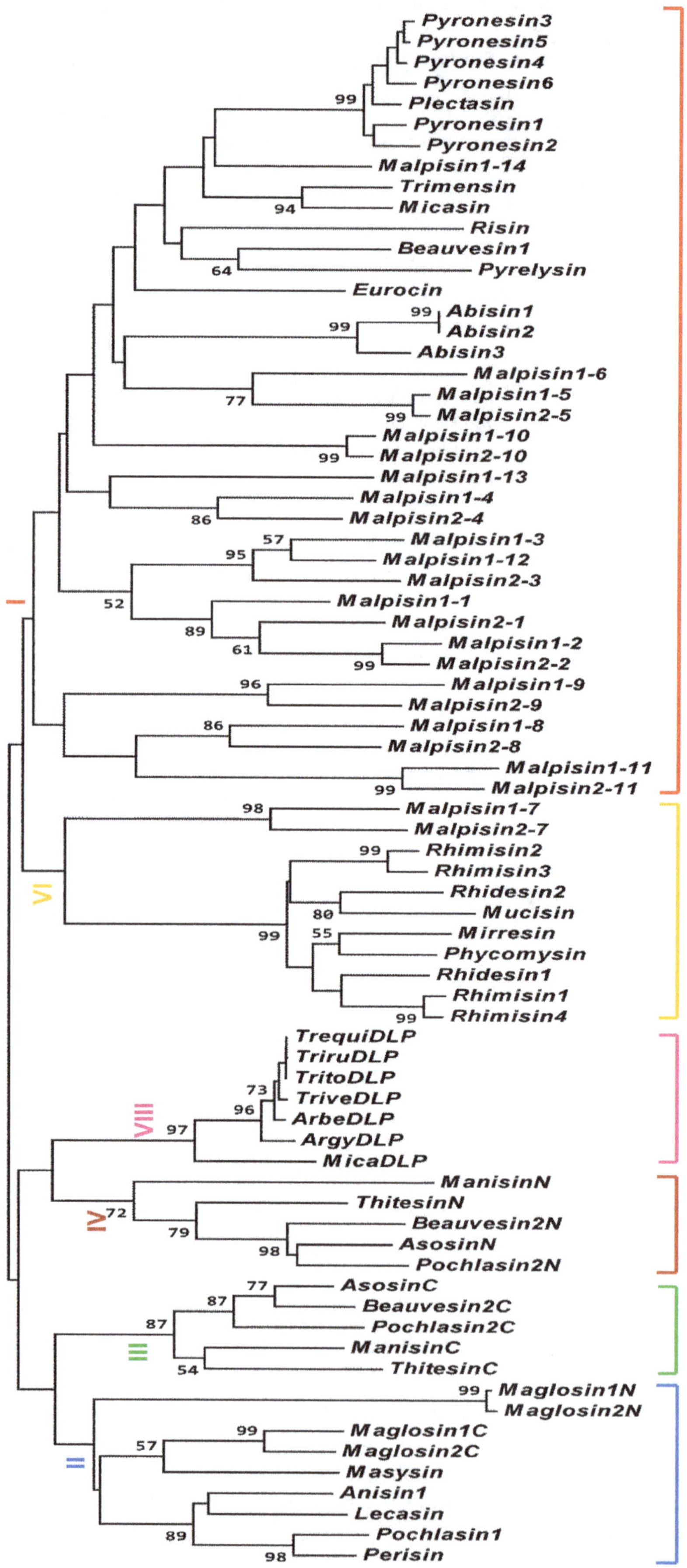

Figure 4. Phylogenetic tree of fDLPs. The tree was constructed from the aligned amino acid sequences presented in Figures 2 and 3 with the neighbor-joining method. The numbers on nodes represent bootstrap values, and only values ≥50% are shown.

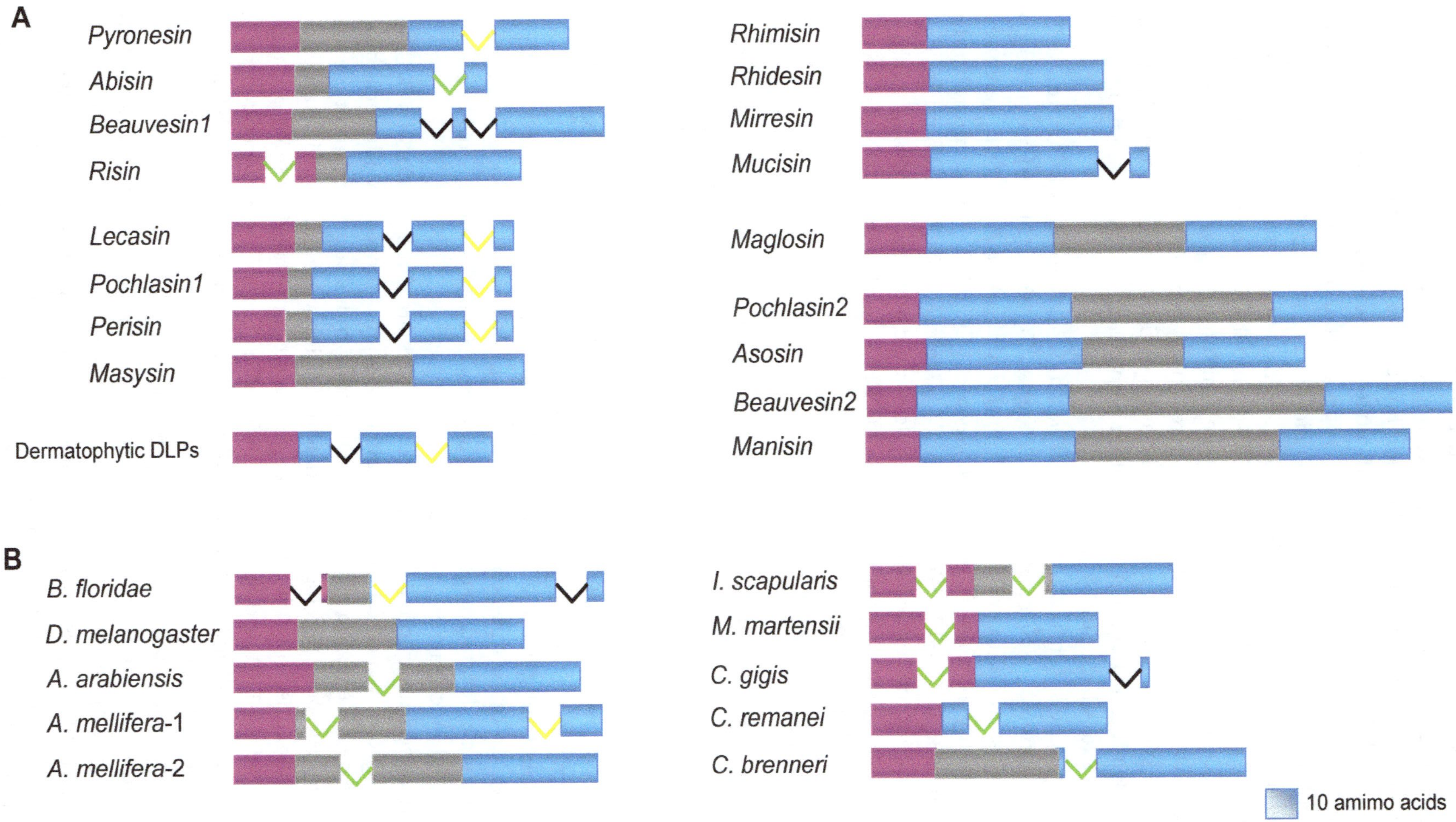

Figure 5. Comparison of precursor organization and exon-intron structures between fDLPs and animal defensins. (**A**) fDLPs; (**B**) Animal defensins. Signal, pro- and mature peptides are shown in pink, grey and blue, respectively. Intron phases are shown in the same colors as Figure 2. Representative animal defensins are derived from *Branchiostoma floridae*, *Drosophila melanogaster*, *Anopheles arabiensis*, *Apis mellifera*, *Ixodes scapularis*, *M. martensii*, *Crassostrea gigas*, *Caenorhabditis remanei*, and *C. brenneri*.

Peptides in fDEF8, all derived from dermatophytes, are characterized as a new family with a short N-terminus and an extra C-terminal extension rich in arginines, prolines and glycines (Figure 2). The C-terminal extension has been considered as a common mechanism for the complexity increase of some invertebrate antimicrobial peptides (AMPs). For example, the hymenopteran defensin-1 subfamily has an extended C-terminus relative to its ancestral defensin-2 subfamily by a so-called intron exonization-mediated mechanism [14,15]. It thus appears that fungal and invertebrate defensins both convergently evolved their C-termini. The extension of a C-terminal sequence via convergent evolution was also recently observed in interleukin 6 (IL-6), a class-I helical cytokine, of two leporids (*Oryctolagus* and *Pentalagus*) [16]. The presence of C-terminal Gly-Arg or Gly-Arg-Arg in some dermatophyte-derived fDLPs suggest that they may be amidated, as previously observed in some animal toxins, e.g., the *Mesobuthus* α-toxins [17]. Interestingly, the mature peptide of micaDLP is larger in size than that of other members in this family, as identified by an N-terminal extension of 38 amino acids (Figure 2). High content of glycines together with a cationic characteristic hints a putative antimicrobial role of this extended unit.

M. alpine is a saprophytic species of *Mucoromycotina*, known as an oleaginous fungus [18]. The draft genome sequences of two *M. alpina* isolates (B6842 and ATCC 32222) [18,19] provide a possibility to undertake comparative study of their fDLPs. We found that the *M. alpine* B6842 genome encodes 14 fDLPs (Figure 3) but only 10 were found in *M. alpine* ATCC 32222. The failure to detect the four homologs (*i.e.*, malpisin1-6, 1-12, 1-13, 1-14) in *M. alpine* ATCC 32222 could be due to the incompletely-assembled genome sequences. Our phylogenetic analysis divides all malpisins into fDEF1 and fDEF6 (Figure 4). Some malpisin members of fDEF1 extended their N-termini with diverse sequences and variable lengths (Figure 3).

3. Gene Duplication of fDLPs

Gene duplication extensively occurs in antimicrobial peptides from insects to humans [15,20,21]. In fungi, initial annotation of defense molecules of *Pyronema omphalodes* also identified gene duplication as a minor multigene family of fDLPs (herein termed pyronesin1 to pyronesin6) [13]. These fDLPs are highly similar to plectasin (Figure 6A). Our studies revealed new gene duplication event in other fungal species. Malpisin is a representative example of gene duplication. As mentioned previously, there are 14 and 10 members in *M. alpine* B6842 and *M. alpine* ATCC 32222, respectively. Malpisin1-1, 1-2, 1-3 and 1-4 are tandem located on one contig (jtg7180000084593f _7180000084594f), and malpisin1-5 to malpisin1-11 on another contig (Contig 7180000084767). In addition, malpisin1-12, malpisin 1-13 and malpisin 1-14 reside on other three contigs, as shown in Figure 6B. In *M. alpine* ATCC 32222, malpisin2-1 to malpisin2-4 are located on contig 1070 and malpisin2-7 to malpisin2-11 on contig 903. Only malpisin2-5 is located on contig 791.

In the widely cultivated mushroom *Agaricus bisporus*, there are three paralogous fDLPs (abisin1 to abisin3) (Figure 6C), two of which (abisin1 and abisin3) share completely identical amino acid sequences in the mature peptide region but exhibit four synonymous substitutions at the nucleotide level. In the *Pochonia chlamydosporia* paralogues, pochlasin1 is highly similar to CITDs and pochlasin2 possesses two defensin-domains. In addition, a putative pseudogene (herein named pochlasin-pseu) was also identified in scaffold 1191 and assigned to AITDs in view of its high sequence similarity to micasin in the first exon. Pochlasin1 and pochlasin-pseu share a conserved phase 0 intron within the α-helical region. The loss of the last two exons (2 and 3) results in the lack the last four cysteines involved in the Csαβ folding of a mature peptide (Figure 2).

Gene duplication also occurs in the *Mucorales*-derived fDLPs, which leads to four and two gene copies in *Rhizopus microsporus* (Figure 6D) and *R. delemar*, respectively. In a Neighbor-Joining (NJ) tree, rhimisin1 and rhimisin4 (*R. microsporus*) constitutes a single clade clustering with the other three fDLPs (rhidesin1 from *R. delemar*, phycomycin from *Phycomyces blakesleeanus* and mirresin from *Mucor irregularis*) whereas rhimisin2 and rhimisin3 (*R. microsporus*) cluster with rhidesin2 (*R. delemar*) and mucisin (*M. circinelloides*) (Figure 4), suggesting that the gene duplication event could have occurred in the ancestor of the *Mucorales* prior to their speciation.

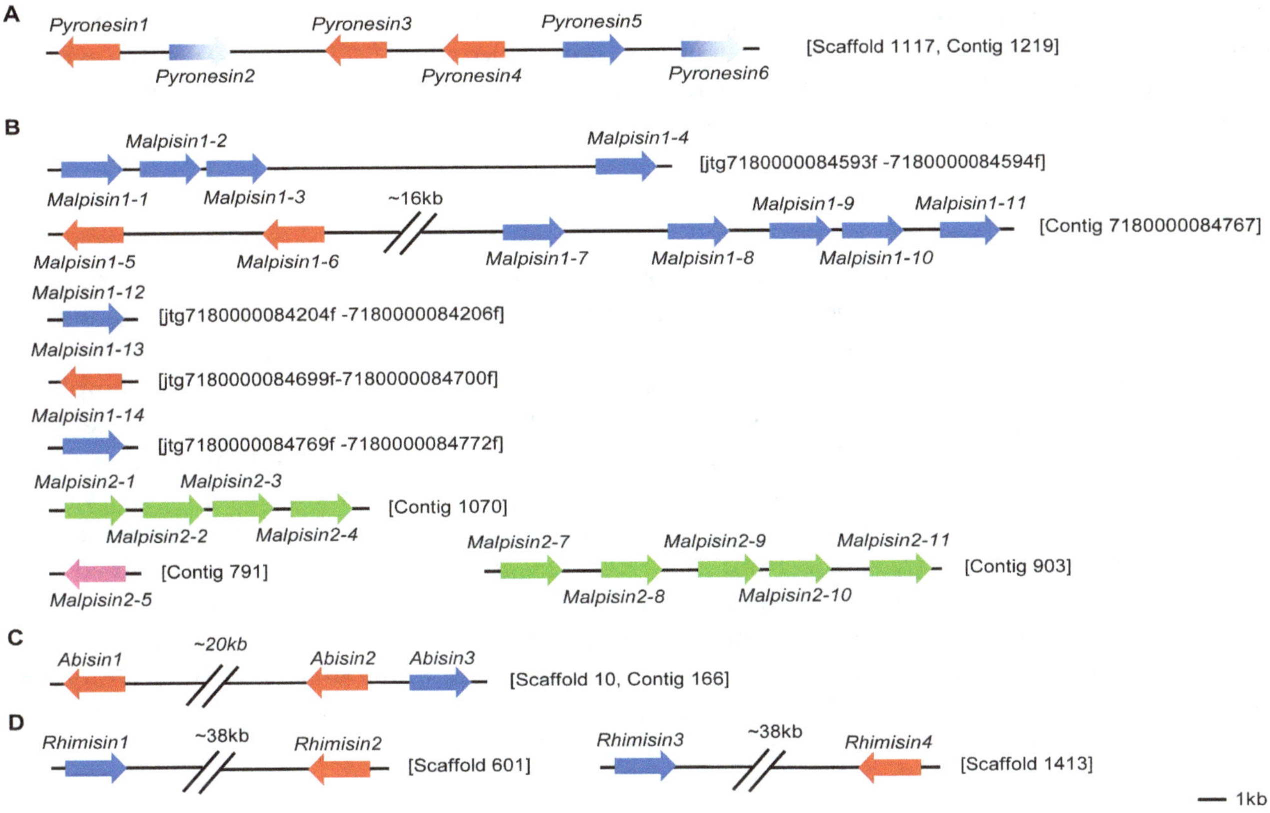

Figure 6. The arrangement of defensin genes in chromosomes. Color arrows refer to different orientation of the genes. **A** to **D** represent the genome location of defensins in four species: *Pyronema omphalodes*, *Mortierella alpine*, *Agaricus bisporus* and *Rhizopus microsporus*. Malpisins in *M. alpine* B6842 is indicated in red and blue while in pink and green in *M. alpine* ATCC 32222. Pseudogenes of pyronesins are shown in gradient blue.

4. Variable Gene Structures of fDLPs

Analysis of the exon-intron structures of the newly-discovered fDLPs revealed their variability that can be described as follows: (1) all the fDLPs retain the integrity of the signal peptide except risin (*Rhizophagus irregularis*) and malpisin1-1 (or malpisin2-1) that have a phase 1 or phase 0 intron disrupting their signal peptides; (2) all of the genes in fDEF8 and three genes in fDEF2 (*i.e.*, lecasin, pochlasin1 and perisin) have the same gene organization as previously identified dermatophytic defensins (micasin, arbesin, trivesin, tritosin and trirusin) and they contain two introns: the first intron (phase 0) disrupting the α-helical region; the second intron (phase 2) disrupting the c-loop; (3) the pyronesin and abisin multi-gene family in fDEF1 have only one intron disrupting either the α-helical or the c-loop region; (4) In addition to these intron-containing fDLP genes, there are some members without introns (Figures 2 and 5).

The highly variable gene structures in fDLPs are reminiscent of invertebrate defensins that also exhibit diverse gene structures [22,23] (Figure 5 and Figure S2). Compared with invertebrate defensins of 5'-biased intron positions, introns of fDLPs occur preferentially in the 3'-end of the precursor-coded sequences. Because all eukaryotic Csαβ-type defensins are hypothesized to be originated from a common bacterial ancestor [24], it is reasonable to infer that considerable intron gains might have occurred in defensins from some eukaryotic lineages, and later they differentially lost in some specific species. Such a dynamic intron evolution thus shapes the biased intron location pattern between fDLPs and animal DLPs after the animal-fungi split. It is also worth mentioning that some recognizable orthologues of defensins in *Branchiostoma floridae* [25,26], the basal chordate amphioxus, also contain a phase 0 intron located in their c-loop (Figure 5 and Figure S2). Given a remote evolutionary distance between fungi and amphioxus, their intron position conservation could be a consequence of convergent insertion in a similar position due to the existence of "protosplice sites" [27,28]. However, the evolution via ancestral origin can be not completely ruled out in the case of the lack of gene structure information in many animal defensins from different lineages.

5. Conclusions

It is estimated that there are as many as 1.5 million species of fungi in this world. However, only a small fraction has been described and even fewer have been sequenced. To date, only about six hundred genomes were being sequenced or completely sequenced. Fungal genome project (FGP) allows us to systematically exploit peptide antibiotics instead of accidental discovery or complicated biochemical screening. This work sheds light on the persistent discovery of fDLPs from model fungal genome data. Despite this, in the lack of experimental data, it cannot be stated that all these fDLPs possess antibacterial function because in fact a classical insect-type fungal defensing - pechrysin was found to lack antibacterial activity [29] likely due to the absence of cationic residues on its molecular surface. In addition, anisin1, a DLP from *Aspergillus giganteus*, was found to be involved in the fitness of the species by linking stress signaling with developmental regulation [30]. Recent studies have also shown that although some peptides of fungal origin contain a similar defensin structure, they exhibit diverse or alternative biological functions beyond antimicrobial activity. An interesting overview is given by Hegedüs and Marx [31]. Therefore, further biochemical characterization of these newly-discovered fDLPs will help evaluate their potential as human medicines.

Acknowledgments: This work was supported by the National Basic Research Program of China (2010CB945300), the National Natural Science Foundation of China (31221091), and the State Key Laboratory of Integrated Management of Pest Insects and Rodents (Grant No. ChineseIPM1307).

Author Contributions: J.W. and S.Z. discovered all fDLP genes described here. J.W. and S.Z. wrote the paper. B.G. revised the paper.

References

1. Mygind, P.H.; Fischer, R.L.; Schnorr, K.M.; Hansen, M.T.; Sonksen, C.P.; Ludvigsen, S.; Raventos, D.; Buskov, S.; Christensen, B.; De Maria, L.; *et al.* Plectasin is a peptide antibiotic with therapeutic potential from a saprophytic fungus. *Nature* **2005**, *437*, 975–980. [CrossRef]
2. Zhu, S.; Gao, B.; Harvey, P.J.; Craik, D.J. Dermatophytic defensin with antiinfective potential. *Proc. Natl. Acad. Sci. USA* **2012**, *109*, 8495–8500. [CrossRef]
3. Zhu, S. Discovery of six families of fungal defensin-like peptides provides insights into origin and evolution of the CSαβ defensins. *Mol. Immunol.* **2008**, *45*, 828–838. [CrossRef]
4. Schneider, T.; Kruse, T.; Wimmer, R.; Wiedemann, I.; Sass, V.; Pag, U.; Jansen, A.; Nielsen, A.K.; Mygind, P.H.; Raventos, D.S.; *et al.* Plectasin, a fungal defensin, targets the bacterial cell wall precursor Lipid II. *Science* **2010**, *328*, 1168–1172. [CrossRef]
5. Oeemig, J.S.; Lynggaard, C.; Knudsen, D.H.; Hansen, F.T.; Norgaard, K.D.; Schneider, T.; Vad, B.S.; Sandvang, D.H.; Nielsen, L.A.; Neve, S.; *et al.* Eurocin, a new fungal defensin: Structure, lipid binding, and its mode of action. *J. Biol. Chem.* **2012**, *287*, 42361–42372. [CrossRef]
6. Hara, S.; Mukae, H.; Sakamoto, N.; Ishimoto, H.; Amenomori, M.; Fujita, H.; Ishimatsu, Y.; Yanagihara, K.; Kohno, S. Plectasin has antibacterial activity and no affect on cell viability or IL-8 production. *Biochem. Biophys. Res. Commun.* **2008**, *374*, 709–713. [CrossRef]

7. Xiong, Y.Q.; Hady, W.A.; Deslandes, A.; Rey, A.; Fraisse, L.; Kristensen, H.H.; Yeaman, M.R.; Bayer, A.S. Efficacy of NZ2114, a novel plectasin-derived cationic antimicrobial peptide antibiotic, in experimental endocarditis due to methicillin-resistant *Staphylococcus aureus*. *Antimicrob. Agents Chemother.* **2011**, *55*, 5325–5330. [CrossRef]

8. Ostergaard, C.; Sandvang, D.; Frimodt-Moller, N.; Kristensen, H.H. High cerebrospinal fluid (CSF) penetration and potent bactericidal activity in CSF of NZ2114, a novel plectasin variant, during experimental pneumococcal meningitis. *Antimicrob. Agents Chemother.* **2009**, *53*, 1581–1585. [CrossRef]

9. Andes, D.; Craig, W.; Nielsen, L.A.; Kristensen, H.H. *In vivo* pharmacodynamic characterization of a novel plectasin antibiotic, NZ2114, in a murine infection model. *Antimicrob. Agents Chemother.* **2009**, *53*, 3003–3009. [CrossRef]

10. Lutzoni, F.; Kauff, F.; Cox, C.J.; McLaughlin, D.; Celio, G.; Dentinger, B.; Padamsee, M.; Hibbett, D.; James, T.Y.; Baloch, E.; *et al.* Assembling the fungal tree of life: Progress, classification, and evolution of subcellular traits. *Am. J. Bot.* **2004**, *91*, 1446–1480. [CrossRef]

11. Seidah, N.G.; Chrétien, M. Proprotein and prohormone convertases: A family of subtilases generating diverse bioactive polypeptides. *Brain Res.* **1999**, *848*, 45–62.

12. Benson, D.A.; Karsch-Mizrachi, I.; Lipman, D.J.; Ostell, J.; Wheeler, D.L. GenBank. *Nucleic Acids Res.* **2008**, *36*, D25–30. [CrossRef]

13. Traeger, S.; Altegoer, F.; Freitag, M.; Gabaldon, T.; Kempken, F.; Kumar, A.; Marcet-Houben, M.; Poggeler, S.; Stajich, J.E.; Nowrousian, M. The genome and development-dependent transcriptomes of *Pyronema confluens*: A window into fungal evolution. *PLoS Genet.* **2013**, *9*, e1003820. [CrossRef]

14. Tian, C.; Gao, B.; Fang, Q.; Ye, G.; Zhu, S. Antimicrobial peptide-like genes in *Nasonia vitripennis*: A genomic perspective. *BMC Genomics* **2010**, *11*, 187. [CrossRef]

15. Zhang, Z.; Zhu, S. Comparative genomics analysis of five families of antimicrobial peptide-like genes in seven ant species. *Dev. Comp. Immunol.* **2012**, *38*, 262–274. [CrossRef]

16. Neves, F.; Abrantes, J.; Pinheiro, A.; Almeida, T.; Costa, P.P.; Esteves, P.J. Convergent evolution of IL-6 in two leporids (*Oryctolagus* and *Pentalagus*) originated an extended protein. *Immunogenetics* **2014**. [CrossRef]

17. Zhu, S.; Peigneur, S.; Gao, B.; Lu, X.; Cao, C.; Tytgat, J. Evolutionary diversification of *Mesobuthus* α-scorpion toxins affecting sodium channels. *Mol. Cell. Proteomics* **2012**. [CrossRef]

18. Wang, L.; Chen, W.; Feng, Y.; Ren, Y.; Gu, Z.; Chen, H.; Wang, H.; Thomas, M.J.; Zhang, B.; Berquin, I.M.; *et al.* Genome characterization of the oleaginous fungus *Mortierella alpina*. *PLoS ONE* **2011**, *6*, e28319. [CrossRef]

19. Etienne, K.A.; Chibucos, M.C.; Su, Q.; Orvis, J.; Daugherty, S.; Ott, S.; Sengamalay, N.A.; Fraser, C.M.; Lockhart, S.R.; Bruno, V.M. Draft genome sequence of *Mortierella alpina* isolate CDC-B6842. *Genome Announc.* **2014**, *2*, e01180-13.

20. Schutte, B.C.; Mitros, J.P.; Bartlett, J.A.; Walters, J.D.; Jia, H.P.; Welsh, M.J.; Casavant, T.L.; McCray, P.B., Jr. Discovery of five conserved β-defensin gene clusters using a computational search strategy. *Proc. Natl. Acad. Sci. USA* **2002**, *99*, 2129–2133. [CrossRef]

21. Semple, C.A.; Rolfe, M.; Dorin, J.R. Duplication and selection in the evolution of primate β-defensin genes. *Genome Biol.* **2003**, *4*, R31. [CrossRef]

22. Froy, O.; Gurevitz, M. Arthropod and mollusk defensins - evolution by exon-shuffling. *Trends Genet.* **2003**, *19*, 684–687. [CrossRef]

23. Rodriguez de la Vega, R.C.; Possani, L.D. On the evolution of invertebrate defensins. *Trends Genet.* **2005**, *21*, 330–332. [CrossRef]

24. Gao, B.; Rodriguez Mdel, C.; Lanz-Mendoza, H.; Zhu, S. AdDLP, a bacterial defensin-like peptide, exhibits anti-*Plasmodium* activity. *Biochem. Biophys. Res. Commun.* **2009**, *387*, 393–398. [CrossRef]

25. Yu, J.K.; Wang, M.C.; Shin-I, T.; Kohara, Y.; Holland, L.; Satoh, N.; Satou, Y. A cDNA resource for the cephalochordate amphioxus *Branchiostoma floridae*. *Dev. Genes Evol.* **2008**, *218*, 723–727. [CrossRef]

26. Zhu, S.; Peigneur, S.; Gao, B.; Umetsu, Y.; Ohki, S.; Tytgat, J. Experimental conversion of a defensin into a neurotoxin: implications for origin of toxic function. *Mol. Biol. Evol.* **2014**, *31*, 546–559. [CrossRef]

27. Sverdlov, A.V.; Rogozin, I.B.; Babenko, V.N.; Koonin, E.V. Reconstruction of ancestral protosplice sites. *Curr. Biol.* **2004**, *14*, 1505–1508. [CrossRef]

28. Rogozin, I.B.; Sverdlov, A.V.; Babenko, V.N.; Koonin, E.V. Analysis of evolution of exon-intron structure of eukaryotic genes. *Brief. Bioinformatics* **2005**, *6*, 118–134. [CrossRef]
29. Wu, Y.; Gao, B.; Zhu, S. Fungal defensins, an emerging source of anti-infective drugs. *Chin. Sci. Bull.* **2014**, *59*, 931–935. [CrossRef]
30. Eigentler, A.; Pocsi, I.; Marx, F. The anisin1 gene encodes a defensin-like protein and supports the fitness of *Aspergillus nidulans*. *Arch. Microbiol.* **2012**, *194*, 427–437. [CrossRef]
31. Hegedus, N.; Marx, F. Antifungal proteins: more than antimicrobials? *Fungal Biol. Rev.* **2013**, *26*, 132–145. [CrossRef]

5

Human Antimicrobial Peptides and Proteins

Guangshun Wang

Department of Pathology and Microbiology, College of Medicine, University of Nebraska Medical Center, 986495 Nebraska Medical Center, Omaha, NE 68198-6495, USA; gwang@unmc.edu;

Abstract: As the key components of innate immunity, human host defense antimicrobial peptides and proteins (AMPs) play a critical role in warding off invading microbial pathogens. In addition, AMPs can possess other biological functions such as apoptosis, wound healing, and immune modulation. This article provides an overview on the identification, activity, 3D structure, and mechanism of action of human AMPs selected from the antimicrobial peptide database. Over 100 such peptides have been identified from a variety of tissues and epithelial surfaces, including skin, eyes, ears, mouths, gut, immune, nervous and urinary systems. These peptides vary from 10 to 150 amino acids with a net charge between −3 and +20 and a hydrophobic content below 60%. The sequence diversity enables human AMPs to adopt various 3D structures and to attack pathogens by different mechanisms. While α-defensin HD-6 can self-assemble on the bacterial surface into nanonets to entangle bacteria, both HNP-1 and β-defensin hBD-3 are able to block cell wall biosynthesis by binding to lipid II. Lysozyme is well-characterized to cleave bacterial cell wall polysaccharides but can also kill bacteria by a non-catalytic mechanism. The two hydrophobic domains in the long amphipathic α-helix of human cathelicidin LL-37 lays the basis for binding and disrupting the curved anionic bacterial membrane surfaces by forming pores or via the carpet model. Furthermore, dermcidin may serve as ion channel by forming a long helix-bundle structure. In addition, the C-type lectin RegIIIα can initially recognize bacterial peptidoglycans followed by pore formation in the membrane. Finally, histatin 5 and GAPDH(2-32) can enter microbial cells to exert their effects. It appears that granulysin enters cells and kills intracellular pathogens with the aid of pore-forming perforin. This arsenal of human defense proteins not only keeps us healthy but also inspires the development of a new generation of personalized medicine to combat drug-resistant superbugs, fungi, viruses, parasites, or cancer. Alternatively, multiple factors (e.g., albumin, arginine, butyrate, calcium, cyclic AMP, isoleucine, short-chain fatty acids, UV B light, vitamin D, and zinc) are able to induce the expression of antimicrobial peptides, opening new avenues to the development of anti-infectious drugs.

Keywords: antimicrobial chemokines; antimicrobial neuropeptides; antimicrobial proteins; cathelicidin LL-37; defensins; dermcidin; hepcidins; histatins; RNases

---

1. Introduction

Host defense antimicrobial peptides (AMPs) are key components of the innate immune system shared by both invertebrates and vertebrates. Invertebrates such as insects and crustaceans do not have adaptive immune systems and innate defense systems serve as the only protective mechanism. It is now appreciated that innate immune systems also play an indispensable role in vertebrates by directly killing invading microbes in the early stage. Later, vertebrate AMPs can also help augment the adaptive immune system to further handle infections. Thus, host defense peptides may have dual role: rapid microbial killing and subsequent immune modulation [1–6].

The universality of AMPs is evidenced by the identification of these molecules in a variety of organisms. Over 2,300 such peptides have been isolated and characterized according to the online updated Antimicrobial Peptide Database (APD) [7,8]. As of April 2014, there are 233 AMPs from bacteria (*i.e.*, bacteriocins), six from protozoa, 12 from fungi, 306 from plants, and 1,801 host defense peptides from animals. AMPs are usually gene-coded and can be constitutively expressed or induced to fend off invading pathogens. In addition, some bacteria use a second mechanism to assemble peptide antibiotics by using a multiple-enzyme system, leading to distinct chemical modifications not observed in gene-coded cases. Most of the AMPs are cationic and short with less than 50 amino acids. Such features are ideal to target the negatively charged surface of bacteria [1–6].

AMPs also protect humans from microbial infection. They have been identified in a variety of exposed tissues or surfaces such as skin, eyes, ears, mouth, airways, lung, intestines, and the urinary tract. While human cathelicidin LL-37 is detected in the skin of new born infants [9], human beta-defensin 2 (hBD-2) is frequently expressed in older individuals. Human S100 proteins, hBD-2, human beta-defensin 3 (hBD-3), and cathelicidin are significantly higher in fetal keratinocytes than in postnatal skin cells [10]. In addition, psoriasin (S100A7), RNase 7, and hBD-3 are differentially expressed in healthy human skin [11]. When the skin barrier is broken, psoriasin is up-regulated [12]. Lysozyme and lactoferrin have been found in human tears [13]. In addition, β-defensins are expressed in human middle ear epithelial cells [14]. Drosomycin-like defensin (DLD) [15] is produced in human oral epithelial cells as part of host defense against fungal infection. Defensins, cathelicidins, and histatins are important in preventing oral cavity [16]. Apart from antimicrobial activity, human AMPs such as cathelicidins and defensins possess other functions such as immune modulation, apoptosis, and wound healing [1–6]. It is now recognized that certain defensins also play a critical role in sperm fertilization [17–19]. By the time this manuscript was completed, 103 human AMPs were found in the APD [7,8]. A selected set of these peptides is provided in Table 1. The lengths of these human peptides range from 10 (neurokinin A) to 149 amino acids (RegIIIα). Their net charges vary from −3 (β-amyloid peptide) to +20 (antimicrobial chemokine CXCL9). On average, human AMPs have 55 amino acids with a net charge of +5.6. Thus, both the average length and net charge for the current list of human AMPs are higher than those averages from all the AMPs (32.4 residues and net charge +3.2). An important reason for this is the inclusion of human antimicrobial proteins (> 100 amino acids) with high net charges (on average +10). The sequence diversity of human AMPs directly determines their structural and functional diversity. This review article highlights the discovery, activity, structure, mechanism of action, and therapeutic strategies of human host defense peptides selected from the APD.

Table 1. Discovery timeline of select human antimicrobial peptides and proteins [1].

Year	Name	Sequence	Source	Activity [2]	Ref.
1922	Lysozyme	KVFERCELARTLKRLGMDGYRGISL ANWMCLAKWESGYNTRATNYNAG DRSTDYGIFQINSRYWCNDGKTPGA VNACHLSCSALLQDNIADAVACAKR VVRDPQGIRAWVAWRNRCQNRDV RQYVQGCGV	saliva, tears, intestine	G, F	[20]
1985	α-Defensin HNP-1	ACYCRIPACIAGERRYGTCIYQGRL WAFCC	Neutrophils, bone marrow	G, V, F, P, C	[21]
1985	α-Defensin HNP-2	CYCRIPACIAGERRYGTCIYQGRL WAFCC	Neutrophils, bone marrow	G, V, F, C	[21]
1985	α-Defensin HNP-3	DCYCRIPACIAGERRYGTCIYQGRLW AFCC	Neutrophils, bone marrow	G, V, F, C	[21]
1988	Histatin 1	DSHEKRHHGYRRKFHEKHHSH REFPFYGDYGSNYLYDN	saliva	F	[22]

Table 1. *Cont.*

Year	Name	Sequence	Source	Activity [2]	Ref.
1988	Histatin 3	DSHAKRHHGYKRKFHEKHHSHR GYRSNYLYDN	saliva	G, F	[22]
1989	α-Defensin HNP-4	VCSCRLVFCRRTELRVGNCLIGGVSFT YCCTRV	neutrophils	G, V, F	[23]
1990	RNase 2	KPPQFTWAQWFETQHINMTSQQCTNA MQVINNYQRRCKNQNTFLLTTFANVVN VCGNPNMTCPSNKTRKNCHHSGSQVP LIHCNLTTPSPQNISNCRYAQTPANMFY IVACDNRDQRRDPPQYPVVPVHLDRII	eosinophils	V, P	[24]
1990	RNase 3 (Eosinophil cationic protein, ECP)	RPPQFTRAQWFAIQHISLNPPRCTIAM RAINNYRWRCKNQNTFLRTTFANVVN VCGNQSIRCPHNRTLNNCHRSRFRVPL LHCDLINPGAQNISNCTYADRPGRRFY VVACDNRDPRDSPRY PVVPVHLDTTI	neutrophils	G, V, P	[24]
1992	α-Defensin HD-5	ATCYCRTGRCATRESLSGVCEISGRL YRLCCR	Paneth cells/intestine, female reproductive system	G, V, F	[25]
1993	α-Defensin HD-6	AFTCHCRRSCYSTEYSYGTCTVM GINHRFCCL	Paneth cells/intestine	V, F	[26]
1995	β-Defensin hBD-1	DHYNCVSSGGQCLYSACPIFTKIQ GTCYRGKAKCCK	Kidney, Skin, salivary glands	G, F, C	[27]
1995	Cathelicidin LL-37	LLGDFFRKSKEKIGKEFKRIVQRIK DFLRNLVPRTES	neutrophils; skin	G, V, F, P, C	[28–30]
1997	β-Defensin hBD-2	GIGDPVTCLKSGAICHPVFCPRRY KQIGTCGLPGTKCCKKP	skin, lung, epithelia, uterus, salivary glands	G, V, F	[31]
1998	Granulysin	GRDYRTCLTIVQKLKKMVDKPTQRS VSNAATRVCRTGRSRWRDVCRNFM RRYQSRVTQGLVAGETA QQICEDLR	cytolytic T and NK cells	G, F, P, C	[32]
1999	Ubiquicidin	KVHGSLARAGKVRGQTPKVAKQEK KKKKTGRAKRRMQYNRRFVNVVPT FGKKKGPNANS	macrophages	G	[33]
2000	Thrombocidin-1 (TC-1)	AELRCMCIKTTSGIHPKNIQSLEVIG KGTHCNQVEVIATLKDGRKICLDPD APRIKKIVQKKLAGDES	human blood platelets	G, F	[34]
2000	Hepcidin 25 (LEAP-1)	DTHFPICIFCCGCCHRSKCGMCCKT	plasma, Urine/Liver	G, F	[35]
2000	Neuropeptide α-MSH	SYSMEHFRWGKPV	brain	G+, V, F	[36]
2001	β-Defensin hBD-3	GIINTLQKYYCRVRGGRCAVLSCL PKEEQIGKCSTRGRKCCRRKK	Skin, salivary glands	G, V, F	[37]
2001	β-Defensin hBD-4	FELDRICGYGTARCRKKCRSQEYRI GRCPNTYACCLRKWDESLLNRTKP	testis, lung, kidney, neutrophils	G	[38]
2001	Dermcidin	SSLLEKGLDGAKKAVGGLGKLGK DAVEDLESVGKGAVHDVKDVLDSV	eccrine sweat/skin	G, F	[39]
2002	RNase 7	KPKGMTSSQWFKIQHMQPSPQACN SAMKNINKHTKRCKDLNTFLHEPFSS VAATCQTPKIACKNGDKNCHQSHGA VSLTMCKLTSGKYPNCRYKEKRQNK SYVVACKPPQKKDSQQFHLVPVHLDRVL	urinary tract; respiratory tract; skin	G, F	[40]
2003	RNase 5 (angiogenin)	QDNSRYTHFLTQHYDAKPQGRDDR YCESIMRRRGPTSPCKDINTFIHGNK RSIKAICENKNGNPHRENLRISKSSFQ VTTCKLHGGSPWPPCQYRATAGFRN VVVACENGLPVHLDQSIFRRPRP	Liver, skin, intestine	G+, F	[41]

Table 1. *Cont.*

Year	Name	Sequence	Source	Activity [2]	Ref.
2003	Chemokine CCL20	SNFDCCLGYTDRILHPKFIVGFTRQL ANEGCDINAIIFHTKKKLSVCANPK QTWVKYIVRLLSKKVKNM	skin	G, F, P	[42]
2003	Chemokine CXCL9	TPVVRKGRCSCISTNQGTIHLQSLK DLKQFAPSPSCEKIEIIATLKNGVQT CLNPDSADVKELIKKWEKQVSQKK KQKNGKKHQKKKVLKVRKSQRSR QKKTT	blood	G, P	[42]
2005	Psoriasin (S100A7)	MSNTQAERSIIGMIDMFHKYTRRD DKIDKPSLLTMMKENFPNFLSACD KKGTNYLADVFEKKDKNEDKKID FSEFLSLLGDIATDYHKQSHGAA PCSGGSQ	Skin, salivary glands, breast	G-	[43]
2006	RegIIIα	EEPQRELPSARIRCPKGSKAYG SHCYALFLSPKSWTDADLACQ KRPSGNLVSVLSGAEGSFVSSL VKSIGNSYSYVWIGLHDPTQG TEPNGEGWEWSSSDVMNYFA WERNPSTISSPGHCASLSRSTAF LRWKDYNCNVRLPYVCKFTD	intestine	G+	[44]
2008	Substance P	RPKPQQFFGLM	the nervous system	G, F	[45]
2008	Drosomycin-like defensin (DLD)	CLAGRLDKQCTCRRSQPSRRS GHEVGRPSPHCGPSRQCGCHMD	oral epithelial cells, skin	F	[46]
2009	Elafin	AQEPVKGPVSTKPGSCPIILIRCA MLNPPNRCLKDTDCPGIKKCCE GSCGMACFVPQ	γδ T cells	G, F, V	[47]
2010	β-amyloid peptide 1-42	DAEFRHDSGYEVHHQKLVFFAE DVGSNKGAIIGLMVGGVVI	brain	G, F	[48]
2011	Chemerin	ELTEAQRRGLQVALEEFHKHPP VQWAFQETSVESAVDTPFPAGI FVRLEFKLQQTSCRKRDWKKP ECKVRPNGRKRKCLACIKLGS EDKVLGRLVHCPIETQVLREAE EHQETQCLRVQRAGEDPHSFY FPGQFAFS	skin	G, F	[49]
2012	Amylin	KCNTATCATQRLANFLVHSS NNFGAILSSTNVGSNTY	pancreatic β-cells	G	[50]
2012	KDAMP	RAIGGGLSSVGGGSSTIKY	eyes	G-	[51]
2013	DEFB[114]	DRCTKRYGRCKRDCLESEKQ IDICSLPRKICCTEKLYEEDDMF	epididymis	G, F	[19]

[1] Data from the APD [7,8]. For a complete list of human AMPs, please visit the APD website (*http://aps.unmc.edu/AP*) and search in the name field using "human". [2] In the APD, antimicrobial activities against different types of microbes are annotated as below: G, bacteria; G+, Gram-positive bacteria only; G-, Gram-negative bacteria only; F, fungi; V, viruses; P, parasites; C, cancer cells.

2. Identification of Human Antimicrobial Peptides

Antimicrobial substances might have been noticed long time ago [1–6]. Human lysozyme (130 amino acids), discovered in saliva by Alexander Fleming in 1922 [20], is recognized as the first antimicrobial protein [6]. However, the isolation and characterization of many more AMPs with defined amino acid sequences did not start until the 1980s (please refer to the annual AMP discovery plot in ref. [52]). Two major methods were utilized for AMP identification. Initially, chromatographic approaches were used to isolate and characterize new peptides. With the recognition of peptide sequence motifs, bioinformatic approaches were later developed to identify AMPs at the genomic level. In the following, we describe the discovery of the major families of human antibacterial peptides identified during 1985 and 2013.

2.1. Human Defensins

Host defense peptides are usually expressed as precursor proteins and the mature form is released by protease processing. In 1985, the Lehrer group isolated a family of the mature form of α-defensins from human blood [21]. Based on the source, property and size, these peptides were named as human neutrophil peptides (HNP-1, HNP-2, and HNP-3). The three defensins have nearly identical amino acid sequences (Table 1). Compared to HNP-2, both HNP-1 and HNP-3 contain only one additional amino acid residue at the N-terminus: alanine for HNP-1 and aspartate for HNP-3. This additional acidic residue in HNP-3 may make HNP-3 less active than HNP-1 or HNP-2 in killing *Staphylococcus aureus*, *Pseudomonas aeruginosa*, and *Escherichia coli*. A fourth human neutrophil defensin, HNP-4, was reported in 1989 [23]. It was also purified to homogeneity by chromatographic methods. HNP-4 has a distinct peptide sequence with 33 amino acids. *In vitro*, purified HNP-4 was shown to kill *E. coli*, *Streptococcus faecalis*, and *Candida albicans*. Lehrer and colleagues found that HNP-1, HNP-2, and HNP-3 are abundant in bone marrow, and can be detected in peripheral blood leukocytes, spleen and thymus by RT-PCR [53].

In 1989, Ouellette and colleagues identified α-defensin genes from mouse Paneth cells [54]. Bevins hypothsized that such orthologs also exist in human epithelial cells as part of the host defense mechanism. A genetic approach was developed to map additional defensin genes based on the high conservation of the nucleotide sequences in the signal coding region as well as the untranslated 5′ region. Using the probes from the conserved regions, they cloned the gene of HD-5 from human Paneth cells [25]. Likewise, HD-6 was identified [26]. These peptides are tissue-specific as they are only expressed in the Paneth cells of human intestines. The six human α-defensins (Table 1) share the same disulfide bond pattern. If we number the six cysteines in Roman numbers: I, II, III, to VI, the three disulfide bonds in α-defensins are C^{I}–C^{VI}, C^{II}–C^{IV}, and C^{III}–C^{V}. Interestingly, alpha defensins have been found in the neutrophils of rabbits, rats, hamsters, and guinea pigs, but not in mice or pigs [55].

Members from the human β-defensin family were discovered in the 1990s. Different from α-defensins, the three disulfide bonds in β-defensins are C^{I}–C^{V}, C^{II}–C^{IV}, and C^{III}–C^{VI}. Also, β-defensins have a slightly longer sequence to allow for an additional helical region. The first human β defensin (hBD-1) was reported by Bensch *et al.* from human plasma in 1995 [27]. Quantitative mRNA analysis revealed kidney as the major source for hBD-1 [56]. In addition, different truncated forms of hBD-1 were also isolated and found to be active against *E. coli*. The activity of hBD-1 might have been compromised in cystic fibrosis (CF) lung due to its salt-sensitive activity against *P. aeruginosa* [57]. Subsequently, hBD-2 was identified from lesional psoriatic skin using the whole *E. coli* affinity column [32]. This material was selected for AMP isolation based on the fact that patients with lesional psoriatic skin have fewer skin infections than expected. This peptide is effective in killing Gram-negative bacteria *E. coli*, *P. aeruginosa*, and yeast *C. albicans*, but is only bacteriostatic against Gram-positive *S. aureus*. Like hBD-1, the activity of HBD-2 is also salt-sensitive [58]. In 2001, both hBD-3 and hBD-4 were documented [37,38]. Based on this disulfide bond linkage pattern, hBD-3 was also identified by using a bioinformatic approach [59,60]. In contrast to hBD-1 and hBD-2, hBD-3 remained active against *S. aureus* and vancomycin-resistant *Enterococcus faecium* at physiological salt concentrations [37]. Bioinformatic studies led to the identification of 28 additional human and 43 mouse β-defensin genes in the respective genome [61]. Several of these β-defensins (hBD-6, hBD-26, hBD-27, hBD-28, and DEFB114) are indeed antimicrobial *in vitro* [62–64]. This sequence motif-based peptide prediction may be applied to any other species with a completed genome.

In insects, the activation of TOLL directly leads to the expression of drosomycin against fungal infection [65]. In 2008, human drosomycin-like defensin was detected in oral mucosa [46,66], indicating that this ancient innate defense mechanism is conserved. Sequence alignment in the APD revealed 40% similarity to insect drosomycin, which comprises one α-helical and three β-strands. Therefore, such a combined structure resembles human β-defensins to some extent. This peptide appears to be specifically effective against filamentous fungi (e.g., *Aspergillus* spp) as it did not kill tested yeast, Gram-positive or Gram-negative bacteria. Although the connection pattern of the six cysteines has not yet elucidated, the resulting three disulfide bonds are critical for the antifungal activity of human drosomycin-like defensing [46].

It is interesting to mention that a different type of defensins (called θ-defensins) has been identified from non-human primates [66,67]. These 18-residue defensins are circular due to the formation of a peptide bond between the N- and C-terminal ends. Like α- and β-defensins, they are also stabilized by three sets of disulfide bonds (C^{I}–C^{VI}, C^{II}–C^{V}, and C^{III}–C^{IV}). These defensins are generated by liganding two truncated α-defensins. These genes are not expressed in humans due to the existence of a premature stop codon. Like monkey θ-defensins, synthetic peptides corresponding to these human counterpart pseudogenes are HIV-1 inhibitory [68–70]. It is uncertain whether the loss of θ-defensins made humans generally more susceptible to HIV-1 infection.

2.2. Human Histatins: Two Genes Multiple Peptides

Histatins are a family of AMPs rich in histidines. In 1988, histatins 1, 3, and 5 were isolated from human saliva by size-exclusion chromatography followed by HPLC separation [22]. All three histatins exhibit the ability to kill the pathogenic yeast, *C. albicans*. Subsequently, other histatins were also isolated [71]. However, only histatins 1 and 3 are gene encoded [22,72], since others are the cleaved products of these two peptides. The histatin genes are located on chromosome 4, band q13 and exclusively expressed in human salivary secretions [73].

2.3. Human Cathelicidins: One Gene Multiple Peptides

The significance of cathelicidins in protecting humans from infection is established by data from animal models [74–76]. Cathelicidin peptides were first isolated in 1989 [77]. The precursor proteins of cathelicidins share a highly conserved N-terminal "cathelin" domain, but have drastically different antimicrobial sequences, ranging from Pro- and Arg-rich peptides, helical peptides, to disulfide-linked sequences [78]. The word "cathelicidin" was originally used to refer to the entire precursor protein. However, it is now accepted as the family name for mature AMPs from the C-terminal region. Another term hCAP-18 is abbreviated from human cationic protein of 18 kDa, representing the precursors prior to the release of cathelicidin peptides. However, these terms are interchangeably used in the literature.

Based on the conserved sequences in the cathelicidin precursors, Agerberth and colleagues cloned the only human cathelicidin gene and predicted the antimicrobial peptide as FALL-39 in analogy to PR-39 discovered in cattle [28]. Using the probes designed based on rabbit CAP-18, Larrick *et al.* also cloned the C-terminal antimicrobial peptide [29]. In the same year, Cowland *et al.* isolated a 19 kDa precursor protein hCAP-18 from human neutrophils [30]. Subsequently, the European group isolated the natural form of the mature human cathelicidin peptide from neutrophils [79]. Since the isolated peptide contains 37 amino acids and starts with a pair of leucines, it was named LL-37, which is two residues shorter than the initially predicted peptide FALL-39 [28]. Interestingly, ALL-38, another form of human cathelicidin peptides, was also characterized in 2003 [80]. This alterative form contains one more alanine at the N-terminus than LL-37. ALL-38 was generated in female vagina due to the action of gastricsin on sperm hCAP-18. Antimicrobial assays revealed a similar activity spectrum for LL-37 and ALL-38 against a panel of bacteria, including *E. coli*, *S. aureus*, *P. aeruginosa*, and *Bacillus megaterium*. Thus, ALL-38, as well as other active peptides such as SgI-29 [81], plays a defense role in the human reproductive system. In addition, LL-37 fragments were isolated from human skin by chromatographic approaches [82]. These fragments have varying activities compared to intact LL-37. Hence, a single human cathelicidin gene has been processed into different forms of active peptides [83]. This phenomenon, however, is not unique to humans. There is precedence that multiple AMPs are programmed in a single plant gene [84]. One possibility for this is that different cathelicidin fragments provide a means to expanding the functional space of the single human cathelicidin gene. A different model is utilized by sheep, horses, and cattle, which produce multiple cathelicidins with varying functions [85–88].

2.4. Human Dermcidin

Besides human cathelicidin LL-37 [89], dermcidin, an anionic defense peptide, was found in human sweat [39]. Unlike human defensins and cathelicidins that are induced under inflammatory and injured conditions, dermcidin is constitutively expressed in human sweat [90]. Furthermore, dermcidin variants as well as fragments were also detected. It appears that the level of dermcidin did not vary between healthy people and infected patients [91]. In addition, dermcidin may be related to other human diseases such as cancer and atherosclerosis [92,93].

2.5. Human Hepcidins

Human liver expressed antimicrobial peptide-1 (LEAP-1) was discovered from human blood ultrafiltrate in 2000 [35]. The same peptide was also found by Ganz *et al.* from human urine and named as hepcidin 25 [94]. This liver-synthesized peptide is especially rich in cysteines (32%), leading to four disulfide bonds in a 25-residue peptide. In 2009, the connection pattern of the four disulfide bonds was revised to C7–C22, C10–C13, C11–C19, and C14–C22 [95]. This antimicrobial peptide also plays an important role in ferrous use [96] and single-residue mutations in this molecule are associated with severe juvenile hemochromatosis, a genetic disease of severe iron overload [97]. Unlike LEAP-1, antimicrobial peptide LEAP-2, however, is not involved in the regulation of iron use [98].

2.6. Human AMPs Derived from Known Proteins

Some AMPs are derived from known proteins. Park *et al.* isolated buforin I from amphibians in 1996 [99]. Sequence comparison revealed that buforin I is a cleaved fragment of histone H2A. Of interest, this mRNA was also detected in humans, suggesting a possible role of this peptide in antimicrobial defense [100].

The human airways are essential for the exchange of molecules with the environment. It is necessary to guard this channel to prevent the infection of microbes in the air. In 2001, Ganz and colleagues isolated calcitermin primarily targeting Gram-negative bacteria. This 15-residue peptide is derived from the C-terminus of calgranulin C (a S100 protein). It contains three histidines (His9, His11, and His13) at the N-terminus and has the potential to adopt a helical conformation in membranes. These histidines may explain its enhanced activity in acidic buffers (pH 5.4) and in the presence of micromolar concentrations of $ZnCl_2$ [101].

Another example for protein-derived AMPs is KDAMP, keratin-derived AMPs, which were identified from bactericidal lysate fractions of human corneal epithelial cells. These molecules are rich in glycines [51]. The glycines appear to be important for killing *P. aeruginosa* as substitution of a string of glycines with alanines reduced peptide potency. A search of the APD reveals that glycine-rich (>25%) AMPs have also been identified in bacteria, plants, insects, spiders, nematodes, crustaceans, fish, and amphibians. Thus, glycine-rich peptides constitute a common molecular design for host defense [102–110].

2.7. Antimicrobial Chemokines and AMPs from Human Immune Cells

The fact that some AMPs possess chemotactic effects inspired the evaluation of antimicrobial activity of chemokines, which are known for chemotaxis. In 2000, Krijgsveld *et al.* found antimicrobial thrombocidins, peptides derived from CXC chemokines in human blood platelets [34]. In 2003, Oppenheim and colleagues identified 20 antimicrobial chemokines [42] and additional two members (CCL27 and CCL28) were also reported by Hieshima and colleagues [111]. In 2011, antimicrobial activity of chemotactic chemerin was also reported [49]. Further studies are required to establish the *in vivo* relevance of the *in vitro* activity of these chemokines. The common nature of chemokines and AMPs, however, bridges the innate and adaptive immune systems.

Antimicrobial peptides have also been found in other immune cells. In 1999, Hiemstra *et al.* identified ubiquicidin from ribosomal protein S30 in various tissues. This peptide is active against *Listeria monocytogenes, S. aureus, Salmonella typhimurium, and E. coli.* Considering the fact that *L. monocytogenes* can live within cells, the expression of ubiquicidin in macrophages would limit the replication of this bacterium. Interestingly, ribosomal protein S30 is identical in rats, mice and humans [33]. In 1998, granulysin (74 amino acids) was detected in human cytotoxic T cells and natural killer (NK) cells [32]. Similar proteins called NK-lysins are found in other animals [112]. Granulysin is active against Gram-positive and Gram-negative bacteria, and fungi, including mycobacteria. Thus, the human adaptive immune system has incorporated an innate defense molecule for direct disruption of tumor cells or invading microbes. In addition, human $\gamma\delta$ T cells produce antimicrobial peptide elafin [47]. Like human secretory leucoprotease inhibitor (SLPI), elafin was initially identified as a protease inhibitor. Elafin shows an inhibitory effect on bacteria, fungi, and viruses [113].

2.8. *Antimicrobial Neuropeptides*

Antibacterial peptides were also isolated from the neuroendocrine system from cattle. Secretolytin corresponds to the C-terminal fragment (residues 614–626) of bovine chromogranin B [114]. This peptide displayed activity against *M. luteus* and reduced the growth of *B. megaterium*. Vasostatin-1 is a 76-residue N-terminal fragment of bovine chromogranin A. This peptide is active against both Gram-positive bacteria and fungi [115]. It is conserved in humans, pigs, horses, mice, rats, and frogs. Catestatin is a 21-residue AMP derived from human chromogranin A [116]. Subsequently, cattle enkelytin, the C-terminal fragment corresponding to residues 209–237 of proenkephalin-A was also found to be antibacterial [117]. A similar proenkephalin system exists in humans although the processing machinery can differ [118]. Thus, these neuropeptides also play a communication role between neuroendocrine and the immune system [119].

In 1998, human neuropeptide Y (36 residues) was demonstrated to have antimicrobial activity [120]. Interestingly, the antifungal activity of this peptide against *C. albicans* increased several folds by truncating N-terminal 12 residues, implying the importance of the helical region 14–32. A more recent study, however, only observed activity against *E. coli,* but not *C. albicans* [121]. Future studies will clarify whether the peptide has direct antimicrobial effects. In 1999, adrenomedullin, usually expressed on surface epithelial cells, was reported to have antibacterial activity against all the tested bacteria, but not *C. albicans* [122]. Alpha-MSH was added to the human AMP list in 2000 as well [36]. These findings extended host defense peptides to the nervous system [123]. Since then, more antimicrobial neuropeptides have been documented [45,124]. Some of these neuropeptides may become leads for developing new antibiotics. For example, alarin is a human brain neuropeptide with activity against only Gram-negative bacteria such as *E. coli,* but not Gram-positive bacteria such as *S. aureus* [124]. In particular, α-MSH showed *in vitro* antifungal activity against *C. albicans* at fM to pM [125], much lower than nM for some bacterial lantibiotics and μM for many cationic peptides.

2.9. *Beta-Amyloid Peptides*

Beta-amyloid peptides have long been thought to be the culprit of Alzheimer's disease. It is believed that the β-sheet form, not the helical form of the peptide, is toxic. A recent demonstration of antimicrobial activity for β-amyloid peptides adds a new research dimension to this worrisome disease [48]. Further studies along this line could be useful to provide novel insight into the mechanism of this human disease. In 2012, amylin (human islet amyloid polypeptide, hIAPP) was found bactericidal, too [50]. Transformation of amylin into toxic fibrils can disrupt cell membranes and lead to β-cell death, perhaps one of the causative factors of type 2 diabetes mellitus. The aggregated form of amylin is likely to exert its cytotoxicity by damaging cell membranes [126]. It is noticeable that, when in excess, bacteria microcin E492 can form fibrils as a storage form and lose antimicrobial activity [127]. Is there anything in common here from bacteria to humans? Perhaps, this is one mechanism that nature attempts to remove the toxic effects of an over expressed protein, including antimicrobial peptide.

2.10. Human Antimicrobial Proteins

There are 14 antimicrobial proteins (>100 amino acids) in the APD database as of March 2014 [8]. This includes the first antimicrobial protein lysozyme [20]. Several eosinophil proteins were purified in 1990. Both eosinophil-derived neurotoxin (EDN, or RNase 2) and eosinophil cationic protein (ECP, or RNase 3) possess anti-parasitic activity against *Brugia pahangi* and *Brugia malayi* [24]. These two ribonucleases are also active against respiratory syncytial virus (RSV) with a single-stranded RNA [128]. In addition, RNase 3 has a unique bacterial agglutinating activity [129]. In 2002, RNase 7 was identified from human skin [40]. Remarkably, it is active against bacteria such as *Mycobacterium vaccae* and yeast, even at 4 °C [130]. Recombinant RNase 7 exhibited antimicrobial activity against uropathogens (*E. coli, P. aeruginosa, Klebsiella pneumonia, Proteus mirabilis, E. faecalis,* and *Staphylococcus saprophyticus*) [131,132]. In fact, RNase 7 is the most abundant innate defense peptide in the human urinary tract [132], although the contributions of other human AMPs cannot be ignored [56,133–135]. Human RNase 5, (also known as angiogenin or ANG) with weak RNase activity, is initially implicated in angiogenesis. It appears that the nucleus location is necessary for angiogenesis [136]. In 2003, RNase 5 was found to have a toxic effect on Gram-positive bacteria and fungi [41]. However, another study found little activity using a commercial material [137]. In 2006, RNase 8 was found to inhibit *M. vaccae* [138,139]. Therefore, of the eight human ribonucleases, RNases 2, 3, 5, 7, and 8 appear to play a role in host defense.

Psoriasin is another human protein with multiple functions. It is identical to S100A7, a protein member of the S100 family. Psoriasin was initially characterized as a Ca^{2+} binding protein with chemotactic property from human skin psoriatic lesions [140,141]. Subsequently, psoriasin was found in cancer lesions, making it a potential cancer biomarker [142]. However, the antimicrobial activity of psoriasin against *E. coli* was not demonstrated until 2005 [43].

Three RegIII (regenerating gene family protein III) proteins were initially identified in mice [143]. RegIIIα, a RegIIIγ homolog protein, was found in humans. Different from RegIIIβ from mice, human RegIIIα only inhibited the growth of Gram-positive bacteria such as *L. monocytogenes, Listeria innocua,* and *E faecalis* [44].

3. Antimicrobial and Anticancer Activities of Human Antimicrobial Peptides

3.1. Antibacterial Activities

Antibacterial activities of human AMPs have been mentioned in the preceding section. This section provides an overview of the activity spectrum of these peptides. Based on the APD [8], the majority of human AMPs (90 out of 103) can inhibit the growth of bacteria. They display a broad-spectrum activity against a variety of Gram-positive and Gram-negative bacteria. However, three human AMPs kill primarily Gram-positive bacteria. RNase 5 has an effect on *S. pneumonia* [41], while α-MSH is inhibitory to *S. aureus* [36]. A third AMP, RegIIIα, is active against *L. monocytogenes, L. innocua,* and *E. faecalis* [44]. In addition, ten human AMPs are inhibitory mainly to Gram-negative bacteria. These include hBD-26, hBD-27, human calcitermin, psoriasin/S100A7, CCL8, CCL13, CCL19, alarin, HMGN2, and KDAMP peptides [42,43,51,63,101]. They may control different Gram-negative pathogens. For example, both calcitermin and HMGN2 were active against *E. coli* and *P. aeruginosa* [101,144]. Alarin is active against *E. coli,* while the KDAMP peptides are primarily active against *P. aeruginosa.* Thus, these peptides may form the basis for developing new antimicrobials with a desired antibacterial activity spectrum.

3.2. Antiviral Activity

Of the 103 human AMPs, 16 are virucidal. They include the six well-characterized human α-defensins (HNP-1, HNP-2, HMP-3, HNP-4, HD-5, and HD-6), three β-defensins (hBD-1, hBD-2, and hBD-3), cathelicidin LL-37, histatin 5, α-MSH, elafin, SLPI, CXCL12, RNase 2, and RNase 3. Elafin is the major antiviral protein in cervicovaginal lavage fluid [113]. Both RNase 2 and RNase 3 inhibit respiratory syncytial viruses (RSV) [145,146]. SLPI levels in saliva and semen, but not breast milk, approximate the level required for HIV-1 inhibition *in vitro* [147]. Although HNP-1 is a lectin that binds to gp120 and CD4, it shows an inhibitory effect after HIV-1 entry [148]. It also inhibits non-enveloped BK virus infection by aggregating virions and blocks binding to host cells [149]. Of the four human β-defensins, hBD-2 and hBD-3 can be induced by viral infection and block HIV replication by directly neutralizing the virions and through modulation of the CXCR4 coreceptor [150]. Human cathelicidin LL-37 is also inhibitory to HIV-1 [151,152]. Wang *et al.* further dissected the active region of LL-37. While the central fragment GI-20 showed an optimal therapeutic index, the LL-37 core peptide FK-13 contains the minimal anti-HIV sequence [152]. In the histatin family, only a histatin-5-derived peptide has an effect on HIV-1 [153]. For a systematic review of AMPs with known anti-HIV activity, interested readers may refer to a recent review article [154].

3.3. Antifungal Activity

In the APD, 58 human AMPs are fungicidal [8]. Typical examples are human α-defensins, cathelicidin LL-37, hepcidins, and histatins. In the case of LL-37, protease processing into fragments such as KS-30 and RK-31 is essential in inhibiting *C. albicans* [155]. In addition, the antifungal activity of LL-37 depends on both media and pH. Both LL-25 and RK-31 can rapidily enter the cell cytoplasm [156]. It is likely that these LL-37 fragments target intracellular molecules. It appears that such cathelicidin fragments in human sweat play a role in human skin innate defense against fungal infection [155].

3.4. Antiparasitic Activity

Some human AMPs also have antiparasitic properties. These include HNP-1, LL-37, granulysin, CCL2, CCl20, CCL28, CXCL4 (hPF4), CXCL6, CXCL9, CXCL10, RNase 2, and RNase 3. RNases 2 and 3 might be the earliest AMP examples from humans that were demonstrated to have antiparasitic activity [24]. Other more recent examples are HNP-1 against the promastigotes and amastigotes forms of *Leishmania major* [157], chemokine CCL28 against *Leishmania mexicana* [158], LL-37 against *Entamoeba histol* ytica [159], and Platelet factor 4 (hPF4) against malarial parasite *Plasmodium falciparum* [160]. These examples verify that human defense peptides also play a role in controlling parasite infections.

3.5. Anticancer Activity

There is a growing interest in developing AMPs into anticancer peptides. Magainins, cecropins, and defensins were all shown to have anticancer effects [161–163]. Many other AMPs possess this activity as well and some were discussed in previous review articles [164–166]. A more complete and updated list of anticancer AMPs can be searched in the APD database [8]. The 166 anticancer peptides cover multiple sources, including animals (105 peptides), plants (48 AMPs), bacteria (seven bacteriocins), fungi (one peptide), and laboratory synthesis (five peptides).

The anticancer activities of human AMPs have not been widely evaluated since only six members are annotated as anticancer in the APD [8]. They are HNP-1, HNP-2, HNP-3, hBD-1, LL-37, and granulysin. Indeed, reduced expression of granulysin in patients is correlated with the progression of cancer [167]. However, the level of granulysin increased substantially in cancer cells [168]. Similar observations have been made with human defensins and LL-37. While HNP-1 inhibits the growth of human lung adenocarcinoma xenograft in nude mice [169], the same molecule can be overexpressed in tumors [170,171]. HBD-1 can suppress urological and prostate cancers [172,173]. In oral squamous cell carcinoma, hBD-1 also suppressed tumor proliferation, whereas hBD-2 and hBD-3 showed an opposite effect [174]. Likewise, human cathelicidin LL-37 is overexpressed in breast, ovarian, and lung cancers, but it suppresses tumorigenesis in gastric cancer [175]. Such a complex involvement of AMPs in various cancers deserves additional studies. In particular, it is important to elucidate the factors that trigger the overexpression of AMPs in certain cancer cells.

Our current knowledge, however, may be utilized to our advantage. For instance, the over-expression of human cathelicidin LL-37 or defensins may serve as useful biomarkers for cancer diagnosis [176–178]. In addition, the fragments of LL-37 with demonstrated anticancer effects *in vitro* [179] and *in vivo* [180] might constitute useful templates for designing new anti-tumor drugs, especially those resistant to existing therapeutics. Anticancer AMPs can work by different mechanisms. The effects may result from a direct bacterial killing when bacteria could be the culprit of cancer (e.g., gastric cancer) [175]. AMPs may selectively kill cancer cells in part due to exposed anionic phosphatidylserines (PS) [181]. It is also possible that some AMPs kill cancer cells indirectly by inducing apoptosis (see below).

3.6. *Cytotoxic Effects of Human AMPs*

It is accepted that many AMPs target bacterial membranes. While bacteria are abundant in anionic lipids such as phosphatidylglycerols (PG) and cardiolipin (CL) [83], human cells comprise zwitterionic phosphocholines (PC) and cholesterol. The differences in membranes of bacterial and human cells to a large extent determine cell selectivity of cationic AMPs. Indeed, among the 103 human AMPs, only three peptides are annotated to have cytotoxic effects on mammalian cells. In the case of LL-37, we found it possible to reduce the peptide cytotoxicity by decreasing peptide hydrophobicity [179,182]. The relatively low cytotoxicity of human AMPs makes them attractive templates for engineering new antimicrobials.

In addition to membrane differences, human cells could use other mechanisms to reduce or remove the potential toxic effect of AMPs on themselves. By expressing a peptide called p33 on the cell surface, the toxic effects of human LL-37 is masked [183]. Instread of directly secreting AMPs, humans also release exosomes (nanovesicles enriched in host defense peptides) into the urinary tract to keep it sterile [184]. It may be speculated that such exosomes, similar to artificial AMP-containing liposomes, could be an effective way to reduce cytotoxicity to human cells.

3.7. *Other Biological Functions of Human AMPs*

In addition to antimicrobial and anticancer activities, many human AMPs possess other functions such as chemotaxis, apoptosis, and wound healing:

Chemotactic activity. Currently, 35 human AMPs have chemotactic properties. Examples are defensins and cathelicidin LL-37. Antimicrobial chemokines were originally identified for chemotactic activity. A clear difference between chemokines and AMPs is the concentration needed for action. While the chemotactic effect needs peptides in the nM-pM range, antimicrobial action usually requires μM peptides [185]. Another difference between chemotactic and antimicrobial activities lies in the molecular target. While AMPs usually target membranes of invading bacteria, the chemotactic effects require the association of peptides to host cell receptors. As one example, human LL-37 achieves its chemotactic ability to monocytes, macrophages, neutrophils, and T cells by binding formyl peptide receptor-like 1 (FPRL-1) [186].

Apoptosis. Apoptosis is the process of programmed cell death. Different factors can trigger cell apoptosis. AMPs are one of these factors. Interestingly, apoptosis may be induced or suppressed by the same peptide depending on the biological context. Human LL-37 induces apoptosis in vascular smooth muscle cells, primary airway epithelial cells, oral squamous cell carcinoma SAS-H1 cells, intact rat aorta rings and cultured rat aorta smooth muscle cells, Jurkat T-cells and A549 cells [187–191], while it suppresses this process in keratinocytes and neutrophils [192,193]. As a consequence, elucidation of the mechanism to control apoptosis may offer new therapeutic strategies. A recent interesting finding is that inhibition of human LL-37-induced apoptosis by administrating urothelial glycosaminoglycan (GAG) analogs can prevent the development of interstitial cystitis (IC) in a mouse model [194]. LL-37 could suppress the lipopolysaccharides (LPS)-induced apoptosis of endothelial cells, thereby attenuating lethal sepsis/endotoxin shock [195]. In the case of colon cancer, however, activation of apoptosis suppresses tumorigenesis [196]. It seems that apoptosis requires the major antimicrobial region FK-16 (*i.e.*, corresponding to residues 17-32) of human cathelicidin LL-37 [179,180].

Wound healing. Human host defense peptides can also promote wound healing, a process of injury repairs. Salivary histatin 2 can enhance fibroblast cell migration, whereas human LL-37 at 1 μM can induce cell migration and promote proliferation [197]. It is proposed that these peptides play a role in fast wound coverage.

In summary, antimicrobial activity is a common property of human AMPs, although the *in vivo* relevance has not firmly established for each polypeptide. Furthermore, human AMPs can perform other functions depending on the biological context, peptide concentration, proteases, and the metabolic state. Under diseased conditions, AMPs may have an opposite effect (e.g., cancer suppression *vs.* progression). Understanding the elegant balance of AMPs in these processes in the healthy state as well as the factors that could tilt the balance to a diseased state may yield useful means for cancer treatment.

4. Three-Dimensional Structures of Human Antimicrobial Peptides

Three-dimensional structure of human host defense AMPs are helpful to understand the function of AMPs described above. Many short and linear antimicrobial peptides do not have a folded structure free in solution. However, they may become structured upon interactions with host cells by binding to a specific receptor to trigger the biological responses to microbial invasion. In addition, such AMPs may also adopt a defined structure upon association with bacterial targets such as membranes. The bound structure in either category is not trivial to determine. Membrane-mimetic models are normally utilized to determine the membrane-bound structures of receptors or AMPs. These models include organic solvents, detergent/lipid micelles, lipid bicelles, nanodiscs, and lipid bilayers [198,199]. The known 3D structures of these short peptides are primarily determined by multi-dimensional solution nuclear magnetic resonance (NMR) spectroscopy [199]. Some AMPs possess a folded structure in aqueous solutions primarily due to the structural stabilization of disulfide bonds. The structures of these small proteins can be determined by NMR or X-ray crystallographic methods. When both methods are applied, similar structures are usually found. In addition, NMR measurements can gain insight into protein dynamics (*i.e.*, motions). Among the 103 human AMPs annotated in the APD database, 42 have a known 3D structure (27 determined by NMR and 15 by X-ray) [8].

Although there are different classification schemes [1–6,200], the structures of natural AMPs fall into four large families (α, β, αβ, and non-αβ) [201]. Peptides in the α family contain α-helical structure as the major secondary structure. Typical examples are human cathelicidin LL-37, histatins, dermcidin, and granulysin. The β family is characterized by at least a pair of two β-strands in the structure. Human α-defensins, hepcidins, and SLPI use this type of structure. The αβ family contains both α and β secondary structures, whereas the non-αβ family has neither α nor β structure (also called extended structures). While there are multiple structural examples for the αβ family (Table 2), no structural example has been found for the non-αβ family of human AMPs. In the following, we highlight atomic structures of human AMPs from the α, β, and αβ families. These structures are annotated in the APD database [8] and structural coordinates can be obtained from the Protein Data Bank (PDB) [202] via the APD links.

Table 2. Properties of selected human antimicrobial peptides with known 3D structure [1].

APD ID	Peptide name	Length	Net charge	Pho%	Boman index	Structure class
2257	Lysozyme	130	+8	40	2.28	α
505	Histatin 5	24	+5	8	4.81	α
780	Lactoferricin	49	+10	36	3.14	α
310	LL-37	37	+6	35	2.99	α
433	Dermcidin	47	−2	38	1.11	α
1161	Granulysin	74	+11	33	3.5	α
2072	Psoriasin/S100A7	101	−1	32	2.3	α
1676	β-Amyloid peptide 1-42	42	−3	45	0.77	α
176	HNP-1	30	+3	53	1.07	β
177	HNP-2	29	+3	51	1.17	β
178	HNP-3	30	+2	50	1.42	β
179	HNP-4	33	+4	51	1.4	β

Table 2. *Cont.*

APD ID	Peptide name	Length	Net charge	Pho%	Boman index	Structure class
180	HD-5	32	+4	40	2.6	β
181	HD-6	32	+2	40	1.71	β
192	Hepcidin 20	20	+3	60	0.46	β
193	Hepcidin 25 (LEAP-1)	25	+2	52	0.89	β
2095	SLPI	107	+12	34	1.87	β
451	hBD-1	36	+4	36	1.3	αβ
524	hBD-2	41	+7	36	0.9	αβ
283	hBD-3	45	+11	33	2.87	αβ
811	LEAP-2	40	+4	40	2.94	αβ
2067	RNase 5	125	+11	28	2.99	αβ
2073	RNase 7	128	+16	32	2.16	αβ
2071	RegIIIα	149	+1	33	1.77	αβ
2085	CCL1	73	+10	41	2.25	αβ
2086	CCL8	75	+6	37	2.27	αβ
2088	CCL13	75	+11	36	1.89	αβ
2075	CCL20	69	+8	43	1.34	αβ
2187	CCL27	56	+1	41	1.57	αβ
2076	CXCL1	73	+6	38	1.51	αβ
2080	CXCL10	77	+11	36	2.25	αβ

[1] Obtained from the Antimicrobial Peptide Database (*http://aps.unmc.edu/AP*) [8]. Peptide hydrophobic amino acid content (percent) is represented by pho% in the table. Protein-binding potential [1] was re-named as Boman index in the APD database in 2003.

4.1. *The α-Helical Family: Histatins, Cathelicidins, Dermcidin, and Granulysin*

Histatins. Histatins 1, 3, and 5 are active against *C. albicans* and their candidacidal activities are in the following order: histatin 5 > histatin 3 > histatin 1 [203]. Rai *et al.* investigated the relationship between sequence length and activity using histatin 5 as the template. They found that the C-terminal sequence is important [204]. P-113 with 12 residues corresponding to residues 4–15 of histatin 5 retained anti-candida activity [205]. Using histatin 3 as a model, Zuo *et al.* found increased activity when the active sequence was expressed in tandem (repeated once) [206]. However, duplication of the functional domain of histatin 5 did not enhance candidacidal activity [207]. These results suggest that active domain duplication is not necessary a universal strategy for activity enhancement. Histatin 5 can adopt a helical conformation in the presence of membrane-mimetic agents [204]. However, this helical structure did not appear to be essential for candidacidal activity as peptides with a less helical structure (achieved by proline insertion) can be equally active [208]. Histatin 5 contains a consensus sequence, HEXXH, which is known to bind Zinc. Zinc binding can lead to vesicle fusion and helical conformation as well [209]. Zinc binding actually potentiates peptide activity against gram-positive bacteria *E. faecalis* [210]. An analog of histatin 5 was found to bind DNA and have nuclease activity due to the synergistic oxidative and hydrolytic activities of the metal-peptide complex [211].

Human cathelicidin LL-37. To understand the structural basis of antimicrobial activity, 3D triple-resonance NMR spectroscopy was used to solve a high-quality structure for human LL-37 in the presence of sodium dodecyl sulfate (SDS) micelles [182]. LL-37 has a long helix covering residues 2–31, whereas the C-terminal tail is disordered and does not superimpose well to each other (Figure 1A). This structure is fully consistent with the backbone dynamics measured by an independent NMR experiment. This amphipathic helical region determined in SDS micelles is responsible for binding to bacterial outer and inner membranes. Interestingly, the LL-37 tail appeared to be involved in peptide aggregation [212], which influences LL-37 activity [213]. The N-terminal region of LL-37 is less important for antibacterial activity since LL-23, a natural fragment of LL-37, is only active against susceptible *E. coli* or *S. aureus* strains. The weak activity of LL-23 is attributed to a hydrophilic residue Ser9 that splits the hydrophobic face into two clusters [214]. This Ser9 residue also segregates the hydrophobic surface of LL-37 into two hydrophobic domains. It is established that the central helix

(Figure 1B) of human LL-37 is critical for antibacterial, anti-biofilm, and antiviral activity (reviewed in ref [83]).

Dermcidin. Unlike cationic cathelicidin LL-37 (net charge +6), dermcidin (DCD-1) has a net charge of −2. This peptide also prefers anionic membranes, however. DCD-1L, a variant with one additional leucine at the C-terminus, showed an enhanced affinity for membranes than DCD-1. In the membrane bound state, DCD-1L has a helical conformation. It is located on the membrane surface and can aggregate in the presence of zinc [215]. This oligomeric structure of dermcidin has recently been determined by X-ray crystallography [216]. A hexameric helix-bundle structure (Figure 1C) is proposed to insert into bacterial membrane as an ion channel. In the crystal, the Zn^{2+} coordinates with a group of acidic amino acids. It should be pointed out that the 3D structure of DCD-1L was also determined previously by 3D NMR spectroscopy using a ^{15}N-labeled peptide in a 50% trifluoenthanol (TFE) solution. Four helical regions were identified (α1: 5–7; α2: 10–12; α3: 26–33; and α4: 36–45) [217]. In this case, TFE might have disrupted the oligomeric structure of dermcidin. There are precedents for such an effect of TFE. For example, the oligomeric structure of a K^+ channel did not survive in TFE but retained in membrane-mimetic micelles such as SDS (reviewed in ref. [198]). These examples emphasize the importance of determining the 3D structure of AMPs in a proper environment.

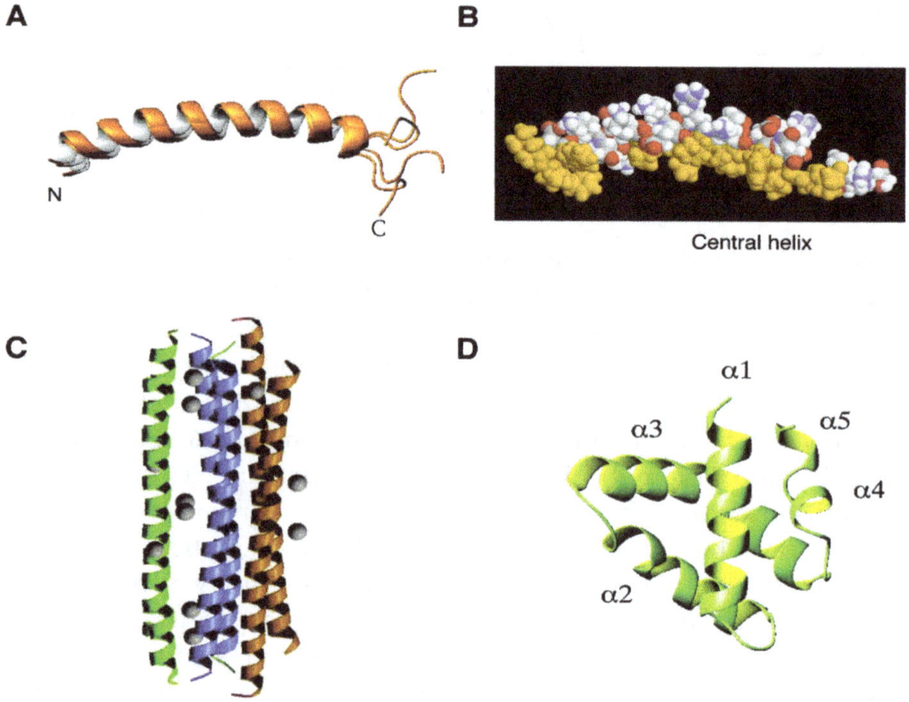

Figure 1. Three-dimensional structures of human antimicrobial peptides from the α-helical family: (**A**) and (**B**) human cathelicidin LL-37 determined by NMR spectroscopy (PDB ID: 2K6O); (**C**) dermcidin determined by X-ray crystallography (PDB ID, 2YMK); and (**D**) granulysin determined by X-ray diffraction (PDB ID: 1L9L). In the case of LL-37, an ensemble of five structures is shown to better view the disordered C-terminal tail (A), whereas a space-filling model is given to show the segregation of the hydrophobic surface (gold) into two domains (B) [182]. The longer one corresponds to the central helix which is important for antimicrobial, anti-biofilm and antiviral activities [83]. Images were generated by using the software MOLMOL [218]. Further details can be found in the text.

Granulysin. Incorporation of AMPs into cytotoxic T cells might have conferred the ability to lyse cells. The crystal structure of granulysin is shown in Figure 1D. There are five helical regions (α1: 2–17; α2: 23–35); α3: 39–61; α4: 66–69; α5: 71–73) [219]. The sequences of human granulysin (74 amino acids) and other NK-lysins share a low degree of similarity (~35%), but homologous modeling reveals antimicrobial features (active helices and basic residue positions) are conserved [112]. Although granulysin only contains two disulfide bonds, it belongs to the saposin-like protein family [220]. Saposin-like proteins comprise several helices usually stabilized by three disulfide bonds [221]. Twelve AMPs in the APD [8] from amoebozoa, nematodes, and large animals such as pigs are annotated to share the saposin-like protein fold [112]. To be antimicrobial, however, neither the entire sequence nor the protein fold is needed. For example, synthetic peptides and analogs derived from helices 3 and 4 are active against *Vibrio cholera* [222]. In addition, the peptide based on the helix-bend-helix motif (residues 31–50) displayed similar antimicrobial activity against Propionibacterium acnes (a key therapeutic target in acne) when synthesized entirely using D-amino acids [223]. Because short peptides can be readily synthesized, they provide useful alternatives for topical treatment of such bacterial infections.

4.2. The β Family: α-Defensins

Alpha-defensins. Structurally, α-defensins consist of three β-strands that form a β-sheet. In the crystal, a dimeric structure is found for human HNP-1, where two copies of the molecule pack together. HNP-2 and HNP-3 have a similar structure. Thus, it is primarily due to the single amino acid difference in these defensins (Table 1) that influences peptide activity. With a more hydrophobic sequence, HNP-4 is more potent against *E. coli* and *C. albicans* than other human α-defensins [23]. Using a kinetic 96-well turbidimetric procedure, the relative potencies of six human α-defensins were compared. In the case of Gram-positive *S. aureus*, the activity is in the following order: HNP-2 > HNP-1 > HNP-3 > HNP-4. In contrast, their relative potencies against Gram-negative *E. coli* is HNP-4 > HNP-2 > HNP-1 = HNP-3 [224]. Thus, the antibacterial activities of these defensins are also bacteria dependent. This likely reflects the distinct differences in membranes of these organisms. The poor antibacterial activity of HNP-3 is not surprising considering the presence of an acidic aspartate at the N-terminus of the peptide, making it unfavorable to target the negatively charged surface of bacteria. HD-5 displayed a rather potent activity, which is comparable to HNP-2 against *S. aureus* and HNP-4 against *E. coli*. The higher activities of HNP-4 and HD-5 against *E. coli* are correlated with their higher net charge of +4 (Table 2). HD-6 has a poor antibacterial activity. In the crystal, it forms a tetrameic structure (Figure 2B) [123].

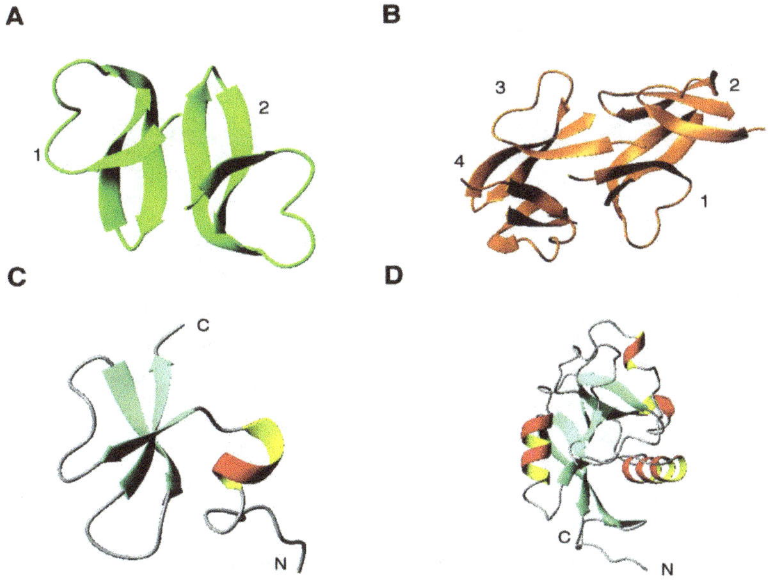

Figure 2. Select 3D structures of human antimicrobial peptides from the β and αβ families: (**A**) HNP-1 (dimeric crystal structure, PDB ID: 3GNY); (**B**) HD-6 (tetrameric crystal structure, PDB ID: 1ZMQ); (**C**) hBD-3 (NMR structure, PDB ID: 1KJ6) and RegIIIα (crystal structure, PDB ID: 4MTH). See the text for further details.

4.3. The αβ Family: β-Defensins, Antimicrobial Chemokines, RNases, and RegIIIα

Beta-defensins. Human β-defensins comprise both α and β structures in the same 3D fold. Figure 2C shows the NMR structure of human β-defensin 3 (hBD-3), which starts with a helical structure followed by three beta strands [225]. NMR translational diffusion studies revealed a dimer for hBD-3, but a monomer for both hBD-1 and hBD-2 in solution. The stronger antibacterial activity of hBD-3 than either hBD-1 or hBD-2 was attributed to the dimeric structure as well as higher charge density on the protein surface [225]. Interestingly, the disulfide-linked form of hBD-1 is poorly active and became highly potent against bacteria and fungus *C. albicans* under reduced conditions where the disulfide-linked structure was disrupted [226]. It seems that the folded hBD-1 is the stored form, which can be transformed into an active form when needed.

Antimicrobial chemokines. Chemokines interact with receptors to realize chemotactic functions. They share a similar fold consisting of a three-stranded sheet followed by one α-helix at the C-terminus [227–229]. The N-terminal region is frequently disordered (Figure 3A–C).

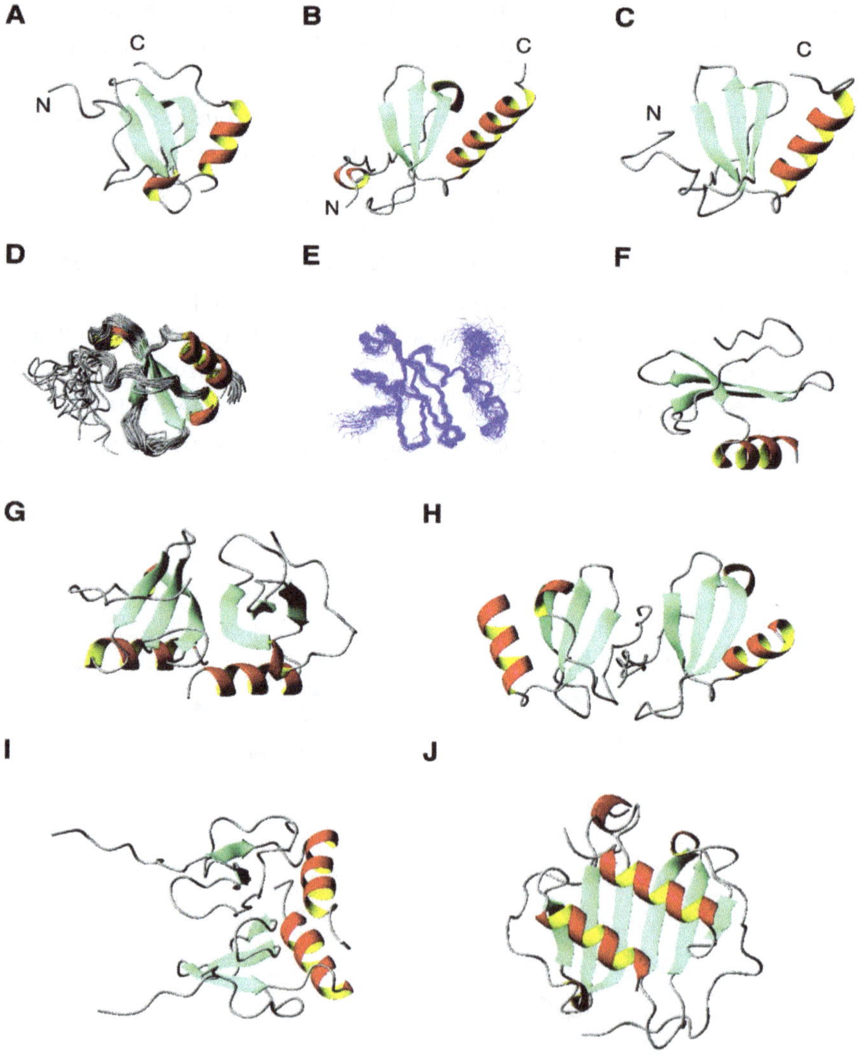

Figure 3. 3D structures of human chemokines with antimicrobial activity. Shown are (**A**) CCL1 (NMR structure, PDB ID: 1EL0); (**B**) CCL8 (crystal structure, PDB ID: 1ESR); (**C**) CCL11 (NMR structure, PDB ID: 2EOT); (**D**) CCL21 (NMR structure, PDB ID: 2L4N); (**E**) CCL27 (NMR structure, PDB ID: 2KUM); (**F**) CXCL12 (NMR structure, PDB ID: 2KOL); (G) CCL20 (crystal structure, PDB ID: 1M8A); (**H**) CCL13 (crystal structure, PDB ID: 2RA4); (**I**) CXCL1 (NMR structure, PDB ID: 1MSH); (**J**) CXCL10 (crystal structure, PDB ID: 1O80).

This can be best seen using a superimposed structural ensemble for CCL20 or CCL27 [230,231] determined by NMR (Figure 3D,E). The β-sheet appears to separate the N-terminal domain that interacts with cell receptors and the C-terminal domain that contains the antimicrobial helix for targeting bacterial membranes (Figure 3F) [232]. Some chemokines can also form oligomers. The dimeric forms of CCL20, CCL13, CXCL1, and CXCL10 [233–236] are shown in panels G to J of Figure 3. The dimer interface is normally composed of the C-terminal helix and strand 3. In the case of CCL13, however, it is the N-terminal region that occupies the interface (Figure 3H). Yung *et al.* found a direct binding of antimicrobial chemokines CXCL9 (net charge of +20) and CXCL10 (net charge +11) to the cell wall of *S. aureus* likely via the positively charged patches on these protein surfaces [237].

Under certain situations, the antimicrobial peptide is generated by further processing of a precursor protein. For example, antimicrobial thrombocidin-1 (TC-1) is produced by truncating two residues from the C-terminus of the parent protein NAP-2 (*i.e.*, neutrophil-activating peptide-2), which is poorly active. NMR analysis revealed that the C-terminus of TC-1 is mobile. In contrast, the C-terminus of NAP-2 is less mobile. It was proposed that the additional two residues locked the C-terminus via electrostatic interactions [238]. The additional Asp residue could have masked the positively-charged surface of the C-terminal helix that targets bacterial membranes. Likewise, insertion of an acidic Glu to the N-terminal region of GF-17, a peptide corresponding to the major antimicrobial region of human cathelicidin LL-37 [179], substantially reduced the peptide activity [239].

RNases. The structures of RNase 3 (Figure 4, panels A and B) and RNase 5 (panels C and D) were solved by both X-ray diffraction and multi-dimensional NMR spectroscopy. Although RNase 3 is dimeric in the crystal, the protein fold determined by the two techniques is similar. In addition, NMR studies revealed two conformations for His114 of RNase 5 in solution [240]. The structures of RNase 2 and RNase 7 are given in Figure 4 (panels E and F). Unlike chemokines discussed above, the antimicrobial region has been mapped to the N-terminus of RNase 7 [130,241]. In particular, a cluster of lysines were identified as key elements for antibacterial activity (bold in Table 1). It is proposed recently that the N-terminal antimicrobial function is conserved in the ribonuclease family [242]. One may wonder why a protein is created for bacterial defense if only part of the chain is required to kill pathogens. One possibility is the stability gain as part of the protein. Another possibility is that a folded protein structure allows for the incorporation of a variety of active sites on the protein surface. In certain cases, such functional sites may be overlapping [243]. In the case of RNase 7, the adjacent active site and antimicrobial residues allows us to propose a yet-to-be-proved "peel-and-kill" model. In other words, binding to bacteria by the cationic amino acids is followed by digestion of pathogenic nucleic acids. The multiple active sites also enable functional regulation. For example, an endogenous molecule can bind to RNase 7 and regulates its antimicrobial activity [244]. This could be one of the unique features of antimicrobial proteins distinct from small antimicrobial peptides.

Antimicrobial lectin RegIIIα. RegIIIα (or HIP/PAP) is a C-type lectin that binds peptidoglycan carbohydrates of Gram-positive bacterial cell walls. The structural basis of this binding has been elucidated (Figure 2D) [245]. Different from other C-type calcium-dependent lectins, the binding of RegIIIα to peptidoglycans is calcium independent (*i.e.*, lacking calcium-binding motif). The binding, however, requires the "EPN" motif and depends on sugar chain length. However, it seems that this peptidoglycan binding serves as an early recognition step for the peptide action as it can create a pore on bacterial membranes. The structure of the oligomeric form of the protein has recently been determined by combining X-ray structure and electron microscopy data, providing insight into the lethal step of bacterial killing by this intestine lectin [246].

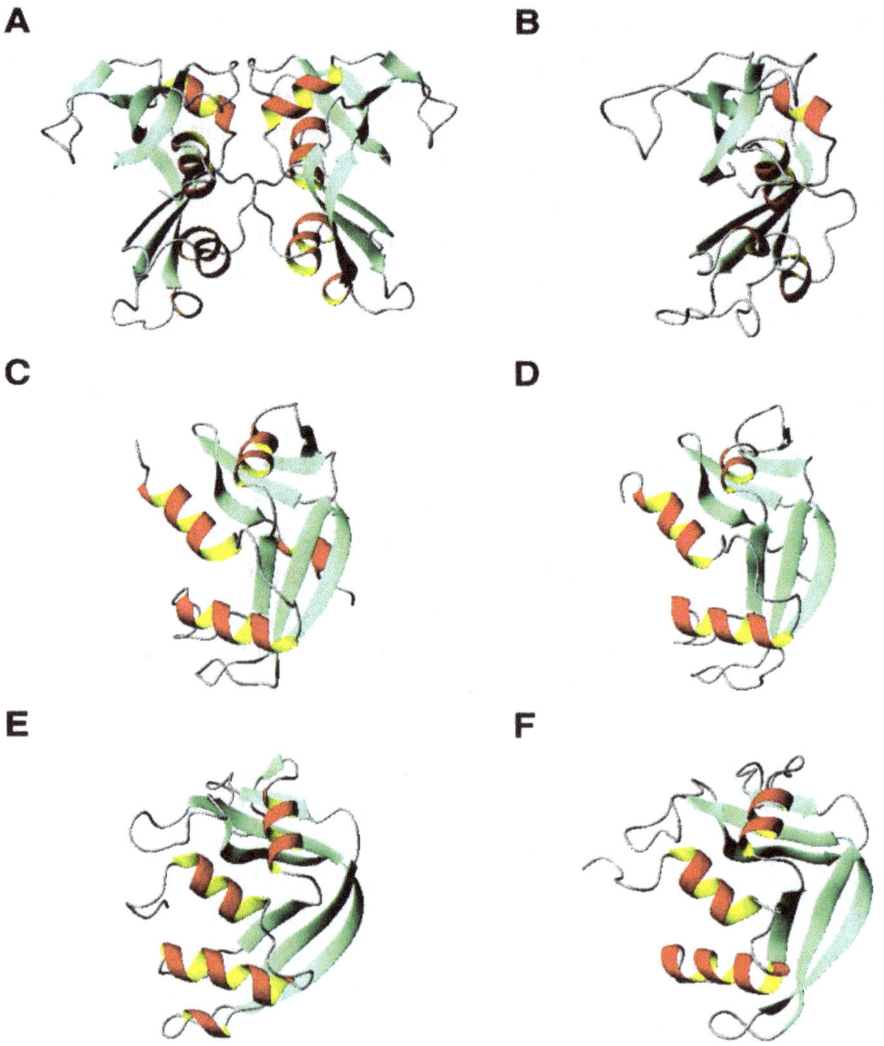

Figure 4. 3D structures of human ribonucleases with antimicrobial activity. Shown are (**A**) RNase 3 (dimeric crystal structure, PDB ID: 4A2O); (**B**) RNase 3 (NMR structure, PDB ID: 2KB5); (**C**) RNase 5 (crystal structure, PDB ID: 1B1I); (**D**) RNase 5 (NMR structure, PDB ID: 1AWZ); (**E**) RNase 2 (crystal structure, PDB ID: 2BZZ); and (**F**) RNase 7 (NMR structure, PDB ID: 2HKY).

5. Mechanism of Action of Human Antimicrobial Peptides

It is generally believed that cationic AMPs target anionic bacterial membranes. In the past years, significant advances have been made in elucidating the molecular targets of human AMPs. As described below, human AMPs can interact with a variety of molecular targets either on the cell surface (including membranes) or within the cells.

5.1. Targeting Bacterial Cell Wall

The molecular targets of AMPs are not limited to bacterial membranes. The assembly of HD-6 on bacterial surface entangles bacteria, providing a new defense mechanism for human innate immunity [123]. HNP-1 targets lipid II to block the biosynthesis of bacterial cell walls [247]. Böhling *et al.* found a close correlation of the hBD-3 activity with cell wall components [248]. A subsequent study corroborated the binding of hBD-3 to lipid II as well [249]. In the APD [7,8], there are 18 AMPs that use this mechanism to combat bacteria. Examples are nisins, mersacidin from bacteria, plectasin from fungi, Cg-Def, an oyster defensin [250–252]. Hence, blocking bacterial cell wall synthesis is a widely deployed innate defense mechanism. It is possible to identify small molecule mimetics that bind bacterial cell walls [253,254]. Although not discussed here, other defensins can directly recognize specific lipids in fungal membranes [255–257].

RegIII proteins are a family of lectins that can specifically recognize the carbohydrate portion of bacteria. While RegIIIα targets the peptidoglycan carbohydrate backbone for Gram-positive bacterial killing [245], mouse RegIIIβ associates with the lipid A portion of Gram-negative bacterial LPS [258]. In the case of murine RegIIIβ, amino acid residues in two structural motifs termed "loop 1" and "loop 2" are important for peptidoglycan and lipid A binding (Arg-135, Asp-142) and for the bactericidal activity (Glu-134, Asn-136, and Asp-142).

It is well known that human lysozyme not only binds a single peptidoglycan chain but also cuts the sugar repeats, thereby inhibiting bacterial cell wall synthesis [259]. In addition, some AMPs can associate with cell surface proteins to interfere with the docking and entry of viruses such as human immunodeficiency virus type 1 (HIV-1). For example, the association of SLPI with human annexin II can avoid the attachment of viral lipid phosphatidylserine (PS) to the same protein in human macrophages [260].

5.2. *Targeting Bacterial Inner Membranes*

Human cathelicidin LL-37 is a representative member in the helical family. It is proposed that LL-37 disrupts bacterial membranes. The membrane disruption of LL-37 involves at least three steps. First, the cationic peptide can recognize and coat the anionic surface of bacteria. With a classic amphipathic helical structure, this cationic peptide prefers to target anionic bacterial membranes. Second, LL-37 binds to the outer membranes and cross the outer membrane. Third, the peptide reaches the inner membrane. It initially binds to the inner membrane parallel to the surface, which is the basis for the carpet model [261]. At elevated concentrations, the peptide may disrupt the membranes by micellization. Alternatively, the peptide might take a vertical position to form a pore [262].

The ability of hepcidin 25 (hep-25) and its isoform hepcidin 20 (hep-20) to perturb bacterial membranes is markedly pH-dependent. The membrane disruption is more evident at acidic pH than at neutral pH. At acidic conditions, histidines become positively charged and more effective in membrane disruption [263].

While there is no agreement in the case of human LL-37 regarding the carpet or pore formation, recent structural determination of dermcidin provides evidence for possible pore formation in bacteria membranes. In the crystal structure [216], the peptide forms a hexamer, where two trimers are connected by zinc (Figure 1C). It is proposed that this structure might be directly inserted into bacterial membranes, serving as an ion channel.

In addition to α-defensins (HD-5 and HD-6), RegIII peptides are expressed to control the microbiota and keep the bacteria away from the epithelial surface of intestine. In particular, specific bacteria (e.g., *Bifidobacterium breve* NCC2950) can effectively induce the expression of RegIIIγ (an ortholog of human RegIIIα) in the intestine of mice via the MyD88-Ticam1 pathway [264]. RegIIIα is a lectin that binds to peptidoglycans of Gram-positive bacteria. However, it adopts a hexametic membrane-permeating pore structure to kill bacteria [246]. Such a pore is reminiscent of other pore structures solved for toxins [265–267]. The structure also provides a basis for selective killing of Gram-positive bacteria such as *L. monocytogenes*, *L. innocua*, and *E. faecalis* but not Gram-negative bacteria. This is because LPS, the major component of the outer membranes of Gram-negative bacteria, inhibits the pore-forming activity of RegIIIα [246].

5.3. *Cell-Penetrating Peptides and Intracellular Targets*

There are other AMPs that may work primarily by binding DNA. Buforin is such an example [83]. This is not surprising because this AMP was derived from DNA-binding histone 2A. In addition, SLPI, a small protein that inhibits elastase and cathepsin G, displayed antibacterial activity against *E. coli* by binding nucleic acids [268]. It is also likely that AMPs kill bacteria by more than one mechanism. For example, human LL-37 may first damage bacterial membranes followed by DNA binding, leading to the shutdown of bacterial machinery [83].

Unlike human LL-37, histatin 5 caused only small membrane damaging effects [269]. To interpret the killing effect of this peptide, two models have been proposed. In the first model, treatment of *C. albicans* with histatin 5 induces the efflux of ATP and increases cell permeability to small molecules, leading to ion imbalance. Thus, *C. albicans* cells respond by activating the osmotic stress responding pathways to minimize ion loss. This model is supported by the fact that knocking out the TRK1 gene that encodes a major K^+ uptake system made histatin 5 ineffective. A second model was also proposed based on the observation that the candida killing ability of histatin 5 is lost using a mitochondrial respiration mutant or after treatment with sodium azide that inhibits cellular metabolism [270]. In addition to the requirement of the mitochondrial respiration machinery [271], cellular internalization of histatins is also facilitated by peptide binding to heat shock protein Ssa2p on the surface of *C. albicans* [272]. This interference with mitochondrial respiration chain may be responsible for the formation of reactive oxygen species (ROS), leading to cell death [273]. Vylkova *et al.* performed a DNA microarray study of the effect of histatin 5 and found that these two models can be unified. This is because the oxidative stress could be produced as a secondary effect of osmotic stress. This proposal is in line with the observation that the killing of histatin 5 is facilitated in the presence of an osmotic agent sorbital but not an oxidant agent H_2O_2 [274]. It should be mentioned that human GAPDH(2–32), an antifungal peptide derived from the highly conserved protein GAPDH, can also enter *C. albicans* to induce apoptosis [275].

As a different mechanism to combat bacterial infection, some AMPs are reported to penetrate immune cells and activate them to boost immune response. For example, chromagranin A-derived peptides can penetrate neutrophils, bind to cytoplasmic calmodulin, and induce Ca^{2+} influx, leading to neutrophil activation and immune system augmentation [276].

Granulysin is an effector molecule in the cytotoxic granules of cytotoxic T lymphocytes and natural killer (NK) cells. It can kill intracellular pathogens in infected cells in the presence of perforin and to induce a cytotoxic effect against tumor cells. Although perforin and granulysin can colocalize [277], it is unclear how they work together in bacterial killing. A recent study reveals that perforin can form pores that preferentially allow the entry of cationic molecules [278]. Thus, granulysin might have entered the cell via the perforin pores, thereby providing yet another mechanism for intracellular bacterial killing by forming a molecular pair.

6. Concluding Remarks and Potential Therapeutic Strategies

Human antimicrobial peptides and proteins occupy an important niche in the current research on human host defense and innate immunity [1–6,279]. Except for antimicrobial protein lysozyme, which was found in 1922, most of short cationic peptides were discovered after 1980 (Table 1). By the time this article was written, over 100 human AMPs have been identified and characterized. They were either isolated from human tissues or predicted from the human genome by bioinformatics. Although genomic prediction constitutes an invaluable method, isolation from natural sources remains important in determining the exact mature form of AMPs. The discovery story of LL-37 nicely illustrates this point (Section 2.3). These peptides have diverse amino acid sequences (Table 1) and physical properties (Table 2), leading to a panel of defense molecules with varying activities (Table 1). While psoriasin and KDAMP primarily inhibit the growth of Gram-negative bacteria, RegIIIα is mainly active against Gram-positive bacteria. In addition, histatins and drosomycin-like defensin are primarily fungicidal. Many human AMPs such as LL-37 and defensins are broad-spectrum peptides against pathogens.

Remarkably, human AMPs are able to hinder bacterial growth by interactions with different targets, ranging from surface molecules (e.g., cell walls), inner membranes, to intracellular molecules (Table 3). Some AMPs can interact with two or more molecules. For example, the binding of RegIIIα to peptidoglycans constitutes only the initial recognition step and subsequent pore formation in bacterial membranes could be the lethal step [246].

Table 3. Select human antimicrobial peptides and their proposed targets.

APD ID	AMP	Structure	Molecular target
181	HD-6	β	Aggregate on bacterial surface
283	hBD-3	αβ	Bacterial cell wall (lipid II)
176	HNP-1	β	Bacterial cell wall (lipid II)
2257	Lysozyme	α	Cell wall carbohydrate
2071	RegIIIα	αβ	Membrane pores
310	LL-37	α	Bacterial membranes and/or DNA
433	Dermcidin	α	Membranes ion channel
2017	hGAPDH(2-32)	Unknown	Intracellular targets of fungi
505	Histatin 5	α	Intracellular mitochondria
2352	Chromagranin A-derived peptides	Unknown	Cytoplasmic calmodulin of neutrophils
1161	Granulysin	α	Perforin generates a pore to allow granulysin to enter the cell and kill intracellular bacteria

For interactions with different molecules, human AMPs are capable of adopting a variety of 3D structures (Figures 1–4). It is clearly important to determine the structure to high quality so that the molecular basis of these interactions can be uncovered accurately (reviewed in ref. [52]). It is also important to correlate the structure with the active state of the peptide. In the case of dermcidin, which oligomerizes on bacterial surface, the helix-bundle structure determined by X-ray crystallography [216] should be more relevant. Likewise, the disulfide-bonded structure of HBD-1 does not explain peptide activity under reduced conditions [226]. Therefore, human AMPs are diverse in terms of amino acid sequence, 3D structure, activity, and mechanism of action.

Many human AMPs are currently under close examination for their functional roles as well as potential applications in detection and diagnosis of human diseases. The type and expression level of human AMPs, if accurately mapped, may have clinical relevance. A clear variation in the expression level of AMPs can serve as biomarkers for human diseases, such as eczema severity and cancer [280–283]. In addition, this remarkable array of molecules may be used for detection, imaging, and diagnosis of bacterial infection. An example of this application is based on the preferential association of Technetium-99m labeled ubiquicidin with bacteria, enabling the physician to differentiate infection from aseptic loosening of hip prostheses in 30 min with high accuracy [284–286].

The collection of human AMPs discussed herein also inspires us in developing novel therapeutics [287]. First, new antimicrobials may be developed using human AMPs as templates. The rationale is that AMPs have remained potent for millions of years and are thus less prone to microbial resistance [1–6]. In particular, peptides with different structural scaffolds may kill the same bacterium by different mechanisms (Table 3). Furthermore, the same peptide sequence can be tailored into various peptides that selectively target pathogens such as Gram-positive, Gram-negative bacteria, or viruses [83]. This is highly desirable for selective bacterial elimination without destroying the probiotic microbial flora. The success of this line depends on whether a selected template will achieve the desired potency *in vivo* against a target pathogen, low cytotoxicity to humans, stability to proteases, and cost-effective production [287]. One can also consider alternative peptide forms. For instance, a pro-drug can be used to reduce the cytotoxicity of AMPs if a mechanism can be found to release it when needed [288]. While portions of antimicrobial proteins are preferred to design novel antimicrobials [222,223,242,289], a whole protein may also be considered. Unlike short peptides, the folded structure of proteins confers stability to the action of proteases. However, the production of such a long polypeptide chain may require recombinant expression in bacteria or cell-free systems [199].

Second, new strategies are actively sought to bring the invading pathogens under control. It is appreciated that different receptors and signal pathways are activated in response to the invasion of different microbes [65]. Of outstanding interest is that non-pathogen factors can also induce AMP expression (Table 4). One of the earliest examples might be the light therapy invented by Niel Finsen [290]. The establishment of a link between light therapy, vitamin D and human cathelicidin LL-37 expression provides a completely different way for infection treatment. Instead of treating patients with traditional antibiotics, doctors may be able to use light or vitamin D [291,292]. Indeed using narrow-band UV B light, the level of vitamin D was increased in psoriasis patients (psoriasis is a common autoimmune disease on skin) [293]. In addition, other small molecules such as butyrate can induce LL-37 expression [294]. Components from Traditional Chinese Medicine may regulate the AMP expression as well [295]. These factors may induce the expression of a single peptide or multiple AMPs [296]. It is also possible that certain factors can work together to induce AMP expression. While cyclic AMP and butyrate synergistically stimulate the expression of chicken β-defensin 9 [297], 4-phenylbutyrate (PBA) and 1,25-dihydroxyvitamin D3 (or lactose) can induce AMP gene expression synergistically [294,298]. It appears that stimulation of LL-37 expression by histone deacetylase (HDAC) inhibitors is cell dependent. Trichostatin and sodium butyrate increased the peptide expression in human NCI-H292 airway epithelial cells but not in the primary cultures of normal nasal epithelial cells [299]. However, the induction of the human LL-37 expression may not be a general approach for bacterial clearance. During *Salmonella enterica* infection of human monocyte-derived macrophages, LL-37 is neither induced nor required for bacterial clearance [300].

Table 4. Some known factors that induce antimicrobial peptide expression

Factor	AMP induced	Cells	Ref
Bacteria/LPS	LL-37, HBD-2	keratinocytes	[296]
TNF-α	LL-37, HBD-2	keratinocytes	[286]
UV Light	LL-37, HBD-2, chemerin	keratinocytes	[286,301]
Vitamin D3	LL-37	neutrophil progenitors and EBV-transformed B cells	[302,303]
Lactose	LL-37	colonic epithelial cells T84, THP-1 monocytes and macrophages	[304]
Short-chain fatty acids	LL-37; pBD-2, pBD-3, pEP2C, and protegrins	human HT-29 colonic epithelial cells and U-937 monocytic cells;	[305,306]
Isoleucine	hBD-1; epithelial defensins	human colon cells, HCT-116; bovine kidney epithelial cells	[307–309]
Arginine	hBD-1	human colon cells, HCT-116	[307]
Ca^{2+}	hBD-2, hBD-3	human keratinocyte monolayers	[310]
Zn^{2+}	LL-37; pBD-1, pBD-2, pBD-3	Caco-2 cell; Intestinal epithelial cells	[311]
Butyrate	LL-37	colon, gastric and hepatocellular cells	[312]
Albumin	hBD-1	human colon cells, HCT-116	[307]
Cyclic AMP/Butyrate	Chicken β-defensin 9	macrophages and primary jejunal explants	[297]
Phenylbutyrate/ 1,25-dihydroxyvitamin D3	cathelicidins	immortalized human bronchial epithelial cell line VA10	[298]

Finally, immune modulation peptides may find therapeutic use because they do not act on microbes directly and thereby are less likely to induce antimicrobial resistance [4,5]. Immune modulation is activated via peptide binding to host cell receptors that initiate various signal transduction pathways. Recently, a natural peptide was found to have immune modulating activity but no antimicrobial activity [313]. Besides engineering peptides with distinct properties, there has been growing interest in elucidating the bacterial mechanisms in generating resistance to AMPs or by subverting host immune systems [314,315]. It can be anticipated that new therapeutic approaches will continue to emerge from our understanding of the host-pathogen interactions. All these strategies will facilitate the development of AMPs into novel antimicrobials to meet the challenge of antibiotics-resistant superbugs, RNA viral infections and difficult-to-treat cancers [287].

Acknowledgments: The author is grateful for the support of the fundings from the NIH (R56AI081975) and the state of Nebraska during this study.

References

1. Boman, H.G. Antibacterial peptides: Basic facts and emerging concepts. *J. Inter. Med.* **2003**, *254*, 197–215. [CrossRef]
2. Ganz, T.; Lehrer, R.I. Defensins. *Curr. Opin. Immunol.* **1994**, *6*, 584–589. [CrossRef]
3. Zasloff, M. Antimicrobial peptides of multicellullar organisms. *Nature* **2002**, *415*, 359–365. [CrossRef]
4. Hancock, R.E.W.; Sahl, H.G. Antimicrobial and host-defense peptides as new anti-infective therapeutic strategies. *Nat. Biotechnol.* **2006**, *24*, 1551–1557. [CrossRef]
5. Lai, Y.; Gallo, R.L. AMPed up immunity: How antimicrobial peptides have multiple roles in immune defense. *Trends Immunol.* **2009**, *30*, 131–141. [CrossRef]
6. Yount, N.Y.; Yeaman, M.R. Emerging themes and therapeutic prospects for anti-infective peptides. *Annu. Rev. Pharmacol. Toxicol.* **2012**, *52*, 337–360. [CrossRef]
7. Wang, Z.; Wang, G. APD: The antimicrobial peptide database. *Nucleic Acids Res.* **2004**, *32*, D590–D592. [CrossRef]
8. Wang, G.; Li, X.; Wang, Z. The updated antimicrobial peptide database and its application in peptide design. *Nucleic Acids Res.* **2009**, *37*, D933–D937. [CrossRef]
9. Marchini, G.; Lindow, S.; Brismar, H.; Ståbi, B.; Berggren, V.; Ulfgren, A.K.; Lonne-Rahm, S.; Agerberth, B.; Gudmundsson, G.H. The newborn infant is protected by an innate antimicrobial barrier: Peptide antibiotics are present in the skin and vernix caseosa. *Br. J. Dermatol.* **2002**, *147*, 1127–1134. [CrossRef]
10. Gschwandtner, M.; Zhong, S.; Tschachler, A.; Mlitz, V.; Karner, S.; Elbe-Bürger, A.; Mildner, M. Fetal Human Keratinocytes Produce Large Amounts of Antimicrobial Peptides: Involvement of Histone-Methylation Processes. *J. Invest. Dermatol.* **2014**. [CrossRef]
11. Wittersheim, M.; Cordes, J.; Meyer-Hoffert, U.; Harder, J.; Hedderich, J.; Gläser, R. Differential expression and *in vivo* secretion of the antimicrobial peptides psoriasin (S100A7), RNase 7, human beta-defensin-2 and -3 in healthy human skin. *Exp. Dermatol.* **2013**, *22*, 364–366. [CrossRef]
12. Gläser, R.; Meyer-Hoffert, U.; Harder, J.; Cordes, J.; Wittersheim, M.; Kobliakova, J.; Fölster-Holst, R.; Proksch, E.; Schröder, J.M.; Schwarz, T. The antimicrobial protein psoriasin (S100A7) is upregulated in atopic dermatitis and after experimental skin barrier disruption. *J. Invest. Dermatol.* **2009**, *129*, 641–649. [CrossRef]
13. McDermott, A.M. Antimicrobial compounds in tears. *Exp. Eye Res.* **2013**, *117*, 53–61. [CrossRef]
14. Underwood, M.; Bakaletz, L. Innate immunity and the role of defensins in otitis media. *Curr. Allergy Asthma Rep.* **2011**, *11*, 499–507. [CrossRef]
15. Sato, J.; Nishimura, M.; Yamazaki, M.; Yoshida, K.; Kurashige, Y.; Saitoh, M.; Abiko, Y. Expression profile of drosomycin-like defensin in oral epithelium and oral carcinoma cell lines. *Arch. Oral Biol.* **2013**, *58*, 279–285. [CrossRef]
16. Da Silva, B.R.; de Freitas, V.A.; Nascimento-Neto, L.G.; Carneiro, V.A.; Arruda, F.V.; de Aguiar, A.S.; Cavada, B.S.; Teixeira, E.H. Antimicrobial peptide control of pathogenic microorganisms of the oral cavity: A review of the literature. *Peptides* **2012**, *36*, 315–321. [CrossRef]
17. Tollner, T.L.; Bevins, C.L.; Cherr, G.N. Multifunctional glycoprotein DEFB126—A curious story of defensin-clad spermatozoa. *Nat. Rev. Urol.* **2012**, *9*, 365–375. [CrossRef]
18. Yu, H.; Dong, J.; Gu, Y.; Liu, H.; Xin, A.; Shi, H.; Sun, F.; Zhang, Y.; Lin, D.; Diao, H. The novel human β-defensin 114 regulates lipopolysaccharide (LPS)-mediated inflammation and protects sperm from motility loss. *J. Biol. Chem.* **2013**, *288*, 12270–12282.
19. Tollner, T.L.; Yudin, A.I.; Tarantal, A.F.; Treece, C.A.; Overstreet, J.W.; Cherr, G.N. Beta-defensin 126 on the surface of macaque sperm mediates attachment of sperm to oviductal epithelia. *Biol. Reprod.* **2008**, *78*, 400–412. [CrossRef]
20. Fleming, A. On a remarkable bacteriolytic element found in tissues and secretions. *Proc. R. Soc. B* **1922**, *93*, 306–317. [CrossRef]
21. Selsted, M.E.; Harwig, S.S.; Ganz, T.; Schilling, J.W.; Lehrer, R.I. Primary structures of three human neutrophil defensins. *J. Clin. Invest.* **1985**, *76*, 1436–1439. [CrossRef]

22. Oppenheim, F.G.; Xu, T.; McMillian, F.M.; Levitz, S.M.; Diamond, R.D.; Offner, G.D.; Troxler, R.F. Histatins, a novel family of histidine-rich proteins in human parotid secretion. Isolation, characterization, primary structure, and fungistatic effects on *Candida albicans*. *J. Biol. Chem.* **1988**, *263*, 7472–7477.
23. Wilde, C.G.; Griffith, J.E.; Marra, M.N.; Snable, J.L.; Scott, R.W. Purification and characterization of human neutrophil peptide 4, a novel member of the defensin family. *J. Biol. Chem.* **1989**, *264*, 11200–11203.
24. Hamann, K.J.; Gleich, G.J.; Checkel, J.L.; Loegering, D.A.; McCall, J.W.; Barker, R.L. *In vitro* killing of microfilariae of *Brugia pahangi* and *Brugia malayi* by eosinophil granule proteins. *J. Immunol.* **1990**, *144*, 3166–3173.
25. Jones, D.E.; Bevins, C.L. Paneth cells of the human small intestine express an antimicrobial peptide gene. *J. Biol. Chem.* **1992**, *267*, 23216–23225.
26. Jones, D.E.; Bevins, C.L. Defensin-6 mRNA in human Paneth cells: Implications for antimicrobial peptides in host defense of the human bowel. *FEBS Lett.* **1993**, *315*, 187–192. [CrossRef]
27. Bensch, K.W.; Raida, M.; Mägert, H.J.; Schulz-Knappe, P.; Forssmann, W.G. hBD-1: A novel beta-defensin from human plasma. *FEBS Lett.* **1995**, *368*, 331–335. [CrossRef]
28. Agerberth, B.; Gunne, H.; Odeberg, J.; Kogner, P.; Boman, H.G.; Gudmundsson, G.H. FALL-39, a putative human peptide antibiotic, is cysteine-free and expressed in bone marrow and testis. *Proc. Natl. Acad. Sci. USA* **1995**, *92*, 195–199. [CrossRef]
29. Larrick, J.W.; Hirata, M.; Balint, R.F.; Lee, J.; Zhong, J.; Wright, S.C. Human CAP18: A novel antimicrobial lipopolysaccharide-binding protein. *Infect. Immun.* **1995**, *63*, 1291–1297.
30. Cowland, J.B.; Johnsen, A.H.; Borregaard, N. hCAP-18, a cathelin/pro-bactenecin-like protein of human neutrophil specific granules. *FEBS Lett.* **1995**, *368*, 173–176. [CrossRef]
31. Harder, J.; Bartels, J.; Christophers, E.; Schröder, J.M. A peptide antibiotic from human skin. *Nature* **1997**, *387*, 861. [CrossRef]
32. Stenger, S.; Hanson, D.A.; Teitelbaum, R.; Dewan, P.; Niazi, K.R.; Froelich, C.J.; Ganz, T.; Thoma-Uszynski, S.; Melián, A.; Bogdan, C.; *et al.* An antimicrobial activity of cytolytic T cells mediated by granulysin. *Science* **1998**, *282*, 121–125. [CrossRef]
33. Hieshima, K.; Ohtani, H.; Shibano, M.; Izawa, D.; Nakayama, T.; Kawasaki, Y.; Shiba, F.; Shiota, M.; Katou, F.; Saito, T.; *et al.* CCL28 has dual roles in mucosal immunity as a chemokine with broad-spectrum antimicrobial activity. *J. Immunol.* **2003**, *170*, 1452–1461. [CrossRef]
34. Krijgsveld, J.; Zaat, S.A.; Meeldijk, J.; van Veelen, P.A.; Fang, G.; Poolman, B.; Brandt, E.; Ehlert, J.E.; Kuijpers, A.J.; Engbers, G.H.; *et al.* Thrombocidins, microbicidal proteins from human blood platelets, are C-terminal deletion products of CXC chemokines. *J. Biol. Chem.* **2000**, *275*, 20374–20381. [CrossRef]
35. Krause, A.; Neitz, S.; Mägert, H.J.; Schulz, A.; Forssmann, W.G.; Schulz-Knappe, P.; Adermann, K. LEAP-1, a novel highly disulfide-bonded human peptide, exhibits antimicrobial activity. *FEBS Lett.* **2000**, *480*, 147–150. [CrossRef]
36. Cutuli, M.; Cristiani, S.; Lipton, J.M.; Catania, A. Antimicrobial effects of alpha-MSH peptides. *J. Leukoc. Biol.* **2000**, *67*, 233–239.
37. Harder, J.; Bartels, J.; Christophers, E.; Schroeder, J.M. Isolation and characterization of human deta-defensin-3, a novel human inducible peptide antibiotic. *J. Biol. Chem.* **2001**, *276*, 5707–5713. [CrossRef]
38. García, J.R.; Krause, A.; Schulz, S.; Rodríguez-Jiménez, F.J.; Klüver, E.; Adermann, K.; Forssmann, U.; Frimpong-Boateng, A.; Bals, R.; Forssmann, W.G. Human beta-defensin 4: A novel inducible peptide with a specific salt-sensitive spectrum of antimicrobial activity. *FASEB J.* **2001**, *15*, 1819–1821.
39. Schittek, B.; Hipfel, R.; Sauer, B.; Bauer, J.; Kalbacher, H.; Stevanovic, S.; Schirle, M.; Schroeder, K.; Blin, N.; Meier, F.; *et al.* Dermcidin: A novel human antibiotic peptide secreted by sweat glands. *Nat. Immunol.* **2001**, *2*, 1133–1137. [CrossRef]
40. Harder, J.; Schroder, J.M. RNase 7, a novel innate immune defense antimicrobial protein of healthy human skin. *J. Biol. Chem.* **2002**, *277*, 46779–46784. [CrossRef]
41. Hooper, L.V.; Stappenbeck, T.S.; Hong, C.V.; Gordon, J.I. Angiogenins: A new class of microbicidal proteins involved in innate immunity. *Nat. Immunol.* **2003**, *4*, 269–273. [CrossRef]
42. Yang, D.; Chen, Q.; Hoover, D.M.; Staley, P.; Tucker, K.D.; Lubkowski, J.; Oppenheim, J.J. Many chemokines including CCL20/MIP-3alpha display antimicrobial activity. *J. Leukoc. Biol.* **2003**, *74*, 448–455. [CrossRef]
43. Gläser, R.; Harder, J.; Lange, H.; Bartels, J.; Christophers, E.; Schröder, J.M. Antimicrobial psoriasin (S100A7) protects human skin from *Escherichia coli* infection. *Nat. Immunol.* **2005**, *6*, 57–64. [CrossRef]

44. Cash, H.L.; Whitham, C.V.; Behrendt, C.L.; Hooper, L.V. Symbiotic bacteria direct expression of an intestinal bactericidal lectin. *Science* **2006**, *313*, 1126–1130. [CrossRef]
45. El Karim, I.A.; Linden, G.J.; Orr, D.F.; Lundy, F.T. Antimicrobial activity of neuropeptides against a range of micro-organisms from skin, oral, respiratory and gastrointestinal tract sites. *J. Neuroimmunol.* **2008**, *200*, 11–16. [CrossRef]
46. Simon, A.; Kullberg, B.J.; Tripet, B.; Boerman, O.C.; Zeeuwen, P.; van der Ven-Jongekrijg, J.; Verweij, P.; Schalkwijk, J.; Hodges, R.; van der Meer, J.W.; *et al.* Drosomycin-like defensin, a human homologue of Drosophila melanogaster drosomycin with antifungal activity. *Antimicrob. Agents Chemother.* **2008**, *52*, 1407–1412. [CrossRef]
47. Marischen, L.; Wesch, D.; Schröder, J.M.; Wiedow, O.; Kabelitz, D. Human $\gamma\delta$ T cells produce the protease inhibitor and antimicrobial peptide elafin. *Scand. J. Immunol.* **2009**, *70*, 547–552. [CrossRef]
48. Soscia, S.J.; Kirby, J.E.; Washicosky, K.J.; Tucker, S.M.; Ingelsson, M.; Hyman, B.; Burton, M.A.; Goldstein, L.E.; Duong, S.; Tanzi, R.E.; *et al.* The Alzheimer's disease-associated amyloid beta-protein is an antimicrobial peptide. *PLoS One* **2010**, *5*, e9505. [CrossRef]
49. Kulig, P.; Kantyka, T.; Zabel, B.A.; Banas, M.; Chyra, A.; Stefanska, A.; Tu, H.; Allen, S.J.; Handel, T.M.; Kozik, A.; *et al.* Regulation of chemerin chemoattractant and antibacterial activity by human cysteine cathepsins. *J. Immunol.* **2011**, *187*, 1403–1410. [CrossRef]
50. Wang, L.; Liu, Q.; Chen, J.C.; Cui, Y.X.; Zhou, B.; Chen, Y.X.; Zhao, Y.F.; Li, Y.M. Antimicrobial activity of human islet amyloid polypeptides: An insight into amyloid peptides' connection with antimicrobial peptides. *Biol. Chem.* **2012**, *393*, 641–646.
51. Tam, C.; Mun, J.J.; Evans, D.J.; Fleiszig, S.M. Cytokeratins mediate epithelial innate defense through their antimicrobial properties. *J. Clin. Invest.* **2012**, *122*, 3665–3677. [CrossRef]
52. Wang, G. Database-guided discovery of potent peptides to combat HIV-1 or superbugs. *Pharmaceuticals* **2013**, *6*, 728–758. [CrossRef]
53. Zhao, C.; Wang, I.; Lehrer, R.I. Widespread expression of beta-defensin hBD-1 in human secretory glands and epithelial cells. *FEBS Lett.* **1996**, *396*, 319–322. [CrossRef]
54. Ouellette, A.J.; Greco, R.M.; James, M.; Frederick, D.; Naftilan, J.; Fallon, J.T. Developmental regulation of cryptdin, a corticostatin/defensin precursor mRNA in mouse small intestinal crypt epithelium. *J. Cell Biol.* **1989**, *108*, 1687–1695. [CrossRef]
55. Ganz, T. Defensins in the urinary tract and other tissues. *J. Infect. Dis.* **2001**, *183* Suppl 1, S41–S42. [CrossRef]
56. Valore, E.V.; Park, C.H.; Quayle, A.J.; Wiles, K.R.; McCray, P.B., Jr.; Ganz, T. Human beta-defensin-1: An antimicrobial peptide of urogenital tissues. *J. Clin. Invest.* **1998**, *101*, 1633–1642. [CrossRef]
57. Goldman, M.J.; Anderson, G.M.; Stolzenberg, E.D.; Kari, U.P.; Zasloff, M.; Wilson, J.M. Human beta-defensin-1 is a salt-sensitive antibiotic in lung that is inactivated in cystic fibrosis. *Cell* **1997**, *88*, 553–560. [CrossRef]
58. Bals, R.; Wang, X.; Wu, Z.; Freeman, T.; Bafna, V.; Zasloff, M.; Wilson, J.M. Human beta-defensin 2 is a salt-sensitive peptide antibiotic expressed in human lung. *J. Clin. Invest.* **1998**, *102*, 874–880. [CrossRef]
59. Jia, H.P.; Schutte, B.C.; Schudy, A.; Linzmeier, R.; Guthmiller, J.M.; Johnson, G.K.; Tack, B.F.; Mitros, J.P.; Rosenthal, A.; Ganz, T.; *et al.* Discovery of new human beta-defensins using a genomics-based approach. *Gene* **2001**, *263*, 211–218. [CrossRef]
60. García, J.R.; Jaumann, F.; Schulz, S.; Krause, A.; Rodríguez-Jiménez, J.; Forssmann, U.; Adermann, K.; Klüver, E.; Vogelmeier, C.; Becker, D.; *et al.* Identification of a novel, multifunctional beta-defensin (human beta-defensin 3) with specific antimicrobial activity. Its interaction with plasma membranes of Xenopus oocytes and the induction of macrophage chemoattraction. *Cell Tissue Res.* **2001**, *306*, 257–264. [CrossRef]
61. Scheetz, T.; Bartlett, J.A.; Walters, J.D.; Schutte, B.C.; Casavant, T.L.; McCray, P.B., Jr. Genomics-based approaches to gene discovery in innate immunity. *Immunol. Rev.* **2002**, *190*, 137–145. [CrossRef]
62. Huang, L.; Leong, S.S.; Jiang, R. Soluble fusion expression and characterization of bioactive human beta-defensin 26 and 27. *Appl. Microbiol. Biotechnol.* **2009**, *84*, 301–308. [CrossRef]
63. Schulz, A.; Klüver, E.; Schulz-Maronde, S.; Adermann, K. Engineering disulfide bonds of the novel human beta-defensins hBD-27 and hBD-28: Differences in disulfide formation and biological activity among human beta-defensins. *Biopolymers* **2005**, *80*, 34–49. [CrossRef]
64. Xin, A.; Zhao, Y.; Yu, H.; Shi, H.; Liu, H.; Diao, H.; Zhang, Y. Soluble fusion expression, characterization and localization of human β-defensin 6. *Mol. Med. Rep.* **2014**, *9*, 149–155.

65. Lemaitre, B.; Reichhart, J.M.; Hoffmann, J.A. Drosophila host defense: Differential induction of antimicrobial peptide genes after infection by various classes of microorganisms. *Proc. Natl. Acad. Sci. USA* **1997**, *94*, 14614–14619. [CrossRef]
66. Selsted, M.E. Theta-defensins: cyclic antimicrobial peptides produced by binary ligation of truncated alpha-defensins. *Curr Protein Pept Sci.* **2004**, *5*, 365–371. [CrossRef]
67. Tang, Y.Q.; Yuan, J.; Osapay, G.; Osapay, K.; Tran, D.; Miller, C.J.; Ouellette, A.J.; Selsted, M.E. A cyclic antimicrobial peptide produced in primate leukocytes by the ligation of two truncated alpha-defensins. *Science* **1999**, *286*, 498–502. [CrossRef]
68. Cole, A.M.; Wang, W.; Waring, A.J.; Lehrer, R.I. Retrocyclins: Using past as prologue. *Curr. Protein Pept. Sci.* **2004**, *5*, 373–381. [CrossRef]
69. Yang, C.; Boone, L.; Nguyen, T.X.; Rudolph, D.; Limpakarnjanarat, K.; Mastro, T.D.; Tappero, J.; Cole, A.M.; Lal, R.B. Theta-Defensin pseudogenes in HIV-1-exposed, persistently seronegative female sex-workers from Thailand. *Infect Genet Evol.* **2005**, *5*, 11–15. [CrossRef]
70. Lehrer, R.I.; Cole, A.M.; Selsted, M.E. θ-Defensins: Cyclic peptides with endless potential. *J. Biol. Chem.* **2012**, *287*, 27014–27019. [CrossRef]
71. Troxler, R.F.; Offner, G.D.; Xu, T.; Vanderspek, J.C.; Oppenheim, F.G. Structural relationship between human salivary histatins. *J. Dent. Res.* **1990**, *69*, 2–6. [CrossRef]
72. Sabatini, L.M.; Azen, E.A. Histatins, a family of salivary histidine-rich proteins, are encoded by at least two loci (HIS1 and HIS2). *Biochem. Biophys. Res. Commun.* **1989**, *160*, 495–502. [CrossRef]
73. vanderSpek, J.C.; Wyandt, H.E.; Skare, J.C.; Milunsky, A.; Oppenheim, F.G.; Troxler, R.F. Localization of the genes for histatins to human chromosome 4q13 and tissue distribution of the mRNAs. *Am. J. Hum. Genet.* **1989**, *45*, 381–387.
74. Nizet, V.; Ohtake, T.; Lauth, X.; Trowbridge, J.; Rudisill, J.; Dorschner, R.A.; Pestonjamasp, V.; Piraino, J.; Huttner, K.; Gallo, R.L. Innate antimicrobial peptide protects the skin from invasive bacterial infection. *Nature* **2001**, *414*, 454–457. [CrossRef]
75. Braff, M.H.; Zaiou, M.; Fierer, J.; Nizet, V.; Gallo, R.L. Keratinocyte production of cathelicidin provides direct activity against bacterial skin pathogens. *Infect. Immun.* **2005**, *73*, 6771–6781. [CrossRef]
76. Lee, P.H.; Ohtake, T.; Zaiou, M.; Murakami, M.; Rudisill, J.A.; Lin, K.H.; Gallo, R.L. Expression of an additional cathelicidin antimicrobial peptide protects against bacterial skin infection. *Proc. Natl. Acad. Sci. USA* **2005**, *102*, 3750–3755.
77. Romeo, D.; Skerlavaj, B.; Bolognesi, M.; Gennaro, R. Structure and bactericidal activity of an antibiotic dodecapeptide purified from bovine neutrophils. *J. Biol. Chem.* **1988**, *263*, 9573–9575.
78. Zanetti, M. Cathelicidins, multifunctional peptides of the innate immunity. *J. Leukoc. Biol.* **2004**, *75*, 39–48. [CrossRef]
79. Gudmundsson, G.H.; Agerberth, B.; Odeberg, J.; Bergman, T.; Olsson, B.; Salcedo, R. The human gene FALL-39 and processing of the cathelin precursor to the antibacterial peptide LL-37 in granulocytes. *Eur. J. Biochem.* **1996**, *238*, 325–332.
80. Sørensen, O.E.; Gram, L.; Johnsen, A.H.; Andersson, E.; Bangsbøll, S.; Tjabringa, G.S.; Hiemstra, P.S.; Malm, J.; Egesten, A.; Borregaard, N. Processing of seminal plasma hCAP-18 to ALL-38 by gastricsin: A novel mechanism of generating antimicrobial peptides in vagina. *J. Biol. Chem.* **2003**, *278*, 28540–28546. [CrossRef]
81. Zhao, H.; Lee, W.H.; Shen, J.H.; Li, H.; Zhang, Y. Identification of novel semenogelin I-derived antimicrobial peptide from liquefied human seminal plasma. *Peptides* **2008**, *29*, 505–511. [CrossRef]
82. Yamasaki, K.; Schauber, J.; Coda, A.; Lin, H.; Dorschner, R.A.; Schechter, N.M.; Bonnart, C.; Descargues, P.; Hovnanian, A.; Gallo, R.L. Kallikrein-mediated proteolysis regulates the antimicrobial effects of cathelicidins in skin. *FASEB J.* **2006**, *20*, 2068–2080. [CrossRef]
83. Wang, G.; Mishra, B.; Epand, R.F.; Epand, R.M. High-quality 3D structures shine light on antibacterial, anti-biofilm and antiviral activities of human cathelicidin LL-37 and its fragments. *Biochim. Biophys. Acta* **2014**. [CrossRef]
84. Tailor, R.H.; Acland, D.P.; Attenborough, S.; Cammue, B.P.; Evans, I.J.; Osborn, R.W.; Ray, J.A.; Rees, S.B.; Broekaert, W.F. A novel family of small cysteine-rich antimicrobial peptides from seed of Impatiens balsamina is derived from a single precursor protein. *J. Biol. Chem.* **1997**, *272*, 24480–24487. [CrossRef]
85. Scocchi, M.; Bontempo, D.; Boscolo, S.; Tomasinsig, L.; Giulotto, E.; Zanetti, M. Novel cathelicidins in horse leukocytes. *FEBS Lett.* **1999**, *457*, 459–464. [CrossRef]

86. Anderson, R.C.; Yu, P.L. Isolation and characterisation of proline/arginine-rich cathelicidin peptides from ovine neutrophils. *Biochem. Biophys. Res. Commun.* **2003**, *312*, 1139–1146. [CrossRef]
87. Skerlavaj, B.; Benincasa, M.; Risso, A.; Zanetti, M.; Gennaro, R. SMAP-29: A potent antibacterial and antifungal peptide from sheep leukocytes. *FEBS Lett.* **1999**, *463*, 58–62. [CrossRef]
88. Castiglioni, B.; Scocchi, M.; Zanetti, M.; Ferretti, L. Six antimicrobial peptide genes of the cathelicidin family map to bovine chromosome 22q24 by fluorescence in situ hybridization. *Cytogenet. Cell Genet.* **1996**, *75*, 240–242. [CrossRef]
89. Murakami, M.; Ohtake, T.; Dorschner, R.A.; Schittek, B.; Garbe, C.; Gallo, R.L. Cathelicidin anti-microbial peptide expression in sweat, an innate defense system for the skin. *J. Invest. Dermatol.* **2002**, *119*, 1090–1095. [CrossRef]
90. Rieg, S.; Garbe, C.; Sauer, B.; Kalbacher, H.; Schittek, B. Dermcidinis constitutively produced by eccrine sweat glands and is not induced in epidermal cells under inflammatory skin conditions. *Br. J. Dermatol.* **2004**, *151*, 534–539. [CrossRef]
91. Rieg, S.; Saborowski, V.; Kern, W.V.; Jonas, D.; Bruckner-Tuderman, L.; Hofmann, S.C. Expression of the sweat-derived innate defence antimicrobial peptide dermcidin is not impaired in *Staphylococcus aureus* colonization or recurrent skin infections. *Clin. Exp. Dermatol.* **2013**. [CrossRef]
92. Schittek, B. The multiple facets of dermcidin in cell survival and host defense. *J. Innate Immun.* **2012**, *4*, 349–360.
93. Ghosh, R.; Maji, U.K.; Bhattacharya, R.; Sinha, A.K. The role of dermcidin isoform 2: A two-faceted atherosclerotic risk factor for coronary artery disease and the effect of acetyl salicylic acid on it. *Thrombosis* **2012**, *2012*, 987932.
94. Park, C.H.; Valore, E.V.; Waring, A.J.; Ganz, T. Hepcidin, a urinary antimicrobial peptide synthesized in the liver. *J. Biol. Chem.* **2001**, *276*, 7806–7801. [CrossRef]
95. Jordan, J.B.; Poppe, L.; Haniu, M.; Arvedson, T.; Syed, R.; Li, V.; Kohno, H.; Kim, H.; Schnier, P.D.; Harvey, T.S.; *et al.* Hepcidin revisited, disulfide connectivity, dynamics, and structure. *J. Biol. Chem.* **2009**, *284*, 24155–24167. [CrossRef]
96. Pigeon, C.; Ilyin, G.; Courselaud, B.; Leroyer, P.; Turlin, B.; Brissot, P.; Loréal, O. A new mouse liver-specific gene, encoding a protein homologous to human antimicrobial peptide hepcidin, is overexpressed during iron overload. *J. Biol. Chem.* **2001**, *276*, 7811–7819.
97. Roetto, A.; Papanikolaou, G.; Politou, M.; Alberti, F.; Girelli, D.; Christakis, J.; Loukopoulos, D.; Camaschella, C. Mutant antimicrobial peptide hepcidin is associated with severe juvenile hemochromatosis. *Nat. Genet.* **2003**, *33*, 21–22.
98. Krause, A.; Sillard, R.; Kleemeier, B.; Klüver, E.; Maronde, E.; Conejo-García, J.R.; Forssmann, W.G.; Schulz-Knappe, P.; Nehls, M.C.; Wattler, F.; *et al.* Isolation and biochemical characterization of LEAP-2, a novel blood peptide expressed in the liver. *Protein Sci.* **2003**, *12*, 143–152.
99. Park, C.B.; Kim, M.S.; Kim, S.C. A novel antimicrobial peptide from Bufo bufo gargarizans. *Biochem. Biophys. Res. Commun.* **1996**, *218*, 408–413. [CrossRef]
100. Minn, I.; Kim, H.S.; Kim, S.C. Antimicrobial peptides derived from pepsinogens in the stomach of the bullfrog, Rana catesbeiana. *Biochim. Biophys. Acta* **1998**, *1407*, 31–39. [CrossRef]
101. Cole, A.M.; Kim, Y.H.; Tahk, S.; Hong, T.; Weis, P.; Waring, A.J.; Ganz, T. Calcitermin, a novel antimicrobial peptide isolated from human airway secretions. *FEBS Lett.* **2001**, *504*, 5–10. [CrossRef]
102. Park, C.J.; Park, C.B.; Hong, S.S.; Lee, H.S.; Lee, S.Y.; Kim, S.C. Characterization and cDNA cloning of two glycine- and histidine-rich antimicrobial peptides from the roots of shepherd's purse, *Capsella. bursa*-pastoris. *Plant. Mol. Biol.* **2000**, *44*, 187–197. [CrossRef]
103. Chang, C.I.; Pleguezuelos, O.; Zhang, Y.A.; Zou, J.; Secombes, C.J. Identification of a novel cathelicidin gene in the rainbow trout, *Oncorhynchus. mykiss. Infect. Immun.* **2005**, *73*, 5053–5064. [CrossRef]
104. Bayer, A.; Freund, S.; Jung, G. Post-translational heterocyclic backbone modifications in the 43-peptide antibiotic microcin B17. Structure elucidation and NMR study of a ^{13}C,^{15}N-labelled gyrase inhibitor. *Eur. J. Biochem.* **1995**, *234*, 414–426.
105. Sousa1, J.C.; Berto1, R.F.; Gois, E.A.; Fontenele-Cardi, N.C.; Honório-Júnior, J.E.; Konno, K.; Richardson, M.; Rocha, M.F.; Camargo, A.A.; Pimenta, D.C.; *et al.* Leptoglycin: A new Glycine/Leucine-rich antimicrobial peptide isolated from the skin secretion of the South American frog *Leptodactylus. pentadactylus* (Leptodactylidae). *Toxicon* **2009**, *54*, 23–32. [CrossRef]

106. Couillault, C.; Pujol, N.; Reboul, J.; Sabatier, L.; Guichou, J.F.; Kohara, Y.; Ewbank, J.J. TLR-independent control of innate immunity in Caenorhabditis elegans by the TIR domain adaptor protein TIR-1, an ortholog of human SARM. *Nat. Immunol.* **2004**, *5*, 488–494. [CrossRef]
107. Hao, X.; Yang, H.; Wei, L.; Yang, S.; Zhu, W.; Ma, D.; Yu, H.; Lai, R. Amphibian cathelicidin fills the evolutionary gap of cathelicidin in vertebrate. *Amino Acids* **2012**, *43*, 677–685. [CrossRef]
108. Lorenzini, D.M.; da Silva, P.I., Jr.; Fogaça, A.C.; Bulet, P.; Daffre, S. Acanthoscurrin: A novel glycine-rich antimicrobial peptide constitutively expressed in the hemocytes of the spider *Acanthoscurria. gomesiana. Dev. Comp. Immunol.* **2003**, *27*, 781–791. [CrossRef]
109. Zeng, Y. Procambarin: A glycine-rich peptide found in the haemocytes of red swamp crayfish Procambarus clarkii and its response to white spot syndrome virus challenge. *Fish. Shellfish Immunol.* **2013**, *35*, 407–412. [CrossRef]
110. Lee, S.Y.; Moon, H.J.; Kurata, S.; Natori, S.; Lee, B.L. Purification and cDNA cloning of an antifungal protein from the hemolymph of *Holotrichia. diomphalia* larvae. *Biol. Pharm. Bull.* **1995**, *18*, 1049–1052. [CrossRef]
111. Hiemstra, P.S.; van den Barselaar, M.T.; Roest, M.; Nibbering, P.H.; van Furth, R. Ubiquicidin, a novel murine microbicidal protein present in the cytosolic fraction of macrophages. *J. Leukoc. Biol.* **1999**, *66*, 423–428.
112. Linde, C.M.; Grundström, S.; Nordling, E.; Refai, E.; Brennan, P.J.; Andersson, M. Conserved structure and function in the granulysin and NK-lysin peptide family. *Infect. Immun.* **2005**, *73*, 6332–6339. [CrossRef]
113. Drannik, A.G.; Nag, K.; Sallenave, J.M.; Rosenthal, K.L. *Antiviral activity of trappin-2 and elafin in vitro* and *in vivo* against genital herpes. *J. Virol.* **2013**, *87*, 7526–7538. [CrossRef]
114. Strub, J.M.; Garcia-Sablone, P.; Lonning, K.; Taupenot, L.; Hubert, P.; van Dorsselaer, A.; Aunis, D.; Metz-Boutigue, M.H. Processing of chromogranin B in bovine adrenal medulla. Identification of secretolytin, the endogenous C-terminal fragment of residues 614–626 with antibacterial activity. *Eur. J. Biochem.* **1995**, *229*, 356–368. [CrossRef]
115. Lugardon, K.; Raffner, R.; Goumon, Y.; Corti, A.; Delmas, A.; Bulet, P.; Aunis, D.; Metz-Boutigue, M.H. Antibacterial and antifungal activities of vasostatin-1, the N-terminal fragment of chromogranin A. *J. Biol. Chem.* **2000**, *275*, 10745–10753.
116. Briolat, J.; Wu, S.D.; Mahata, S.K.; Gonthier, B.; Bagnard, D.; Chasserot-Golaz, S.; Helle, K.B.; Aunis, D.; Metz-Boutigue, M.H. New antimicrobial activity for the catecholamine release-inhibitory peptide from chromogranin A. *Cell. Mol. Life Sci.* **2005**, *62*, 377–385. [CrossRef]
117. Goumon, Y.; Strub, J.M.; Moniatte, M.; Nullans, G.; Poteur, L.; Hubert, P.; van Dorsselaer, A.; Aunis, D.; Metz-Boutigue, M.H. The C-terminal bisphosphorylated proenkephalin-A-(209-237)-peptide from adrenal medullary chromaffin granules possesses antibacterial activity. *Eur. J. Biochem.* **1996**, *235*, 516–525.
118. Vindrola, O.; Padrós, M.R.; Sterin-Prync, A.; Ase, A.; Finkielman, S.; Nahmod, V. Proenkephalin system in human polymorphonuclear cells. Production and release of a novel 1.0-kD peptide derived from synenkephalin. *J. Clin. Invest.* **1990**, *86*, 531–537. [CrossRef]
119. Metz-Boutigue, M.H.; Goumon, Y.; Strub, J.M.; Lugardon, K.; Aunis, D. Antimicrobial chromogranins and proenkephalin-A-derived peptides. *Ann. N. Y. Acad. Sci.* **2003**, *992*, 168–178.
120. Shimizu, M.; Shigeri, Y.; Tatsu, Y.; Yoshikawa, S.; Yumoto, N. Enhancement of antimicrobial activity of neuropeptide Y by N-terminal truncation. *Antimicrob. Agents Chemother.* **1998**, *42*, 2745–2746.
121. Hansen, C.J.; Burnell, K.K.; Brogden, K.A. Antimicrobial activity of Substance P and Neuropeptide Y against laboratory strains of bacteria and oral microorganisms. *J. Neuroimmunol.* **2006**, *177*, 215–218. [CrossRef]
122. Allaker, R.P.; Zihni, C.; Kapas, S. An investigation into the antimicrobial effects of adrenomedullin on members of the skin, oral, respiratory tract and gut microflora. *FEMS Immunol. Med. Microbiol.* **1999**, *23*, 289–293. [CrossRef]
123. Chu, H.; Pazgier, M.; Jung, G.; Nuccio, S.P.; Castillo, P.A.; de Jong, M.F.; Winter, M.G.; Winter, S.E.; Wehkamp, J.; Shen, B.; *et al.* Human α-defensin 6 promotes mucosal innate immunity through self-assembled peptide nanonets. *Science* **2012**, *337*, 477–481. [CrossRef]
124. Wada, A.; Wong, P.F.; Hojo, H.; Hasegawa, M.; Ichinose, A.; Llanes, R.; Kubo, Y.; Senba, M.; Ichinose, Y. Alarin but not its alternative-splicing form, GALP (Galanin-like peptide) has antimicrobial activity. *Biochem. Biophys. Res. Commun.* **2013**, *434*, 223–227. [CrossRef]
125. Brogden, K.A.; Guthmiller, J.M.; Salzet, M.; Zasloff, M. The nervous system and innate immunity: The neuropeptide connection. *Nat. Immunol.* **2005**, *6*, 558–564.

126. Khemtémourian, L.; Killian, J.A.; Höppener, J.W.; Engel, M.F. Recent insights in islet amyloid polypeptide-induced membrane disruption and its role in beta-cell death in type 2 diabetes mellitus. *Exp. Diabetes Res.* **2008**, *2008*, 421287.
127. Shahnawaz, M.; Soto, C. Microcin amyloid fibrils A are reservoir of toxic oligomeric species. *J. Biol. Chem.* **2012**, *287*, 11665–11676. [CrossRef]
128. Domachowske, J.B.; Bonville, C.A.; Dyer, K.D.; Rosenberg, H.F. Evolution of antiviral activity in the ribonuclease A gene superfamily: Evidence for a specific interaction between eosinophil-derived neurotoxin (EDN/RNase 2) and respiratory syncytial virus. *Nucleic Acids Res.* **1998**, *26*, 5327–5332. [CrossRef]
129. Pulido, D.; Torrent, M.; Andreu, D.; Nogués, M.V.; Boix, E. Two human host defense ribonucleases against mycobacteria, the eosinophil cationic protein (RNase 3) and RNase 7. *Antimicrob. Agents Chemother.* **2013**, *57*, 3797–3805. [CrossRef]
130. Huang, Y.C.; Lin, Y.M.; Chang, T.W.; Wu, S.J.; Lee, Y.S.; Chang, M.D.; Chen, C.; Wu, S.H.; Liao, Y.D. The flexible and clustered lysine residues of human ribonuclease 7 are critical for membrane permeability and antimicrobial activity. *J. Biol. Chem.* **2007**, *282*, 4626–4633. [CrossRef]
131. Spencer, J.D.; Schwaderer, A.L.; Dirosario, J.D.; McHugh, K.M.; McGillivary, G.; Justice, S.S.; Carpenter, A.R.; Baker, P.B.; Harder, J.; Hains, D.S. Ribonuclease 7 is a potent antimicrobial peptide within the human urinary tract. *Kidney Int.* **2011**, *80*, 174–180. [CrossRef]
132. Spencer, J.D.; Schwaderer, A.L.; Wang, H.; Bartz, J.; Kline, J.; Eichler, T.; DeSouza, K.R.; Sims-Lucas, S.; Baker, P.; Hains, D.S. Ribonuclease 7, an antimicrobial peptide upregulated during infection, contributes to microbial defense of the human urinary tract. *Kidney Int.* **2013**, *83*, 615–625.
133. Nielsen, K.L.; Dynesen, P.; Larsen, P.; Jakobsen, L.; Andersen, P.S.; Frimodt-Møller, N. Role of urinary cathelicidin LL-37 and human β-defensin 1 in uncomplicated *Escherichia coli* urinary tractinfections. *Infect Immun.* **2014**, *82*, 1572–1578. [CrossRef]
134. Chromek, M.; Slamová, Z.; Bergman, P.; Kovács, L.; Podracká, L.; Ehrén, I.; Hökfelt, T.; Gudmundsson, G.H.; Gallo, R.L.; Agerberth, B.; *et al.* The antimicrobial peptide cathelicidin protects the urinary tract against invasive bacterial infection. *Nat. Med.* **2006**, *12*, 636–641. [CrossRef]
135. Becknell, B.; Spencer, J.D.; Carpenter, A.R.; Chen, X.; Singh, A.; Ploeger, S.; Kline, J.; Ellsworth, P.; Li, B.; Proksch, E.; *et al.* Expression and antimicrobial function of beta-defensin 1 in the lower urinary tract. *PLoS One.* **2013**, *8*, e77714.
136. Wiedłocha, A. Following angiogenin during angiogenesis: A journey from the cell surface to the nucleolus. *Arch. Immunol. Ther. Exp. (Warsz)* **1999**, *47*, 299–305.
137. Avdeeva, S.V.; Chernukha, M.U.; Shaginyan, I.A.; Tarantul, V.Z.; Naroditsky, B.S. Human angiogenin lacks specific antimicrobial activity. *Curr. Microbiol.* **2006**, *53*, 477–478. [CrossRef]
138. Rudolph, B.; Podschun, R.; Sahly, H.; Schubert, S.; Schröder, J.M.; Harder, J. Identification of RNase 8 as a novel human antimicrobial protein. *Antimicrob. Agents Chemother.* **2006**, *50*, 3194–3196. [CrossRef]
139. Boix, E.; Torrent, M.; Sánchez, D.; Nogués, M.V. The antipathogen activities of eosinophil cationic protein. *Curr. Pharm. Biotechnol.* **2008**, *9*, 141–152. [CrossRef]
140. Hoffmann, H.J.; Olsen, E.; Etzerodt, M.; Madsen, P.; Thøgersen, H.C.; Kruse, T.; Celis, J.E. Psoriasin binds calcium and is upregulated by calcium to levels that resemble those observed in normal skin. *J. Invest. Dermatol.* **1994**, *103*, 370–375.
141. Porre, S.; Heinonen, S.; Mäntyjärvi, R.; Rytkönen-Nissinen, M.; Perola, O.; Rautiainen, J.; Virtanen, T. Psoriasin, a calcium-binding protein with chemotactic properties is present in the third trimester amniotic fluid. *Mol. Hum. Reprod.* **2005**, *11*, 87–92. [CrossRef]
142. Ostergaard, M.; Rasmussen, H.H.; Nielsen, H.V.; Vorum, H.; Orntoft, T.F.; Wolf, H.; Celis, J.E. Proteome profiling of bladder squamous cell carcinomas: Identification of markers that define their degree of differentiation. *Cancer Res.* **1997**, *57*, 4111–4117.
143. Narushima, Y.; Unno, M.; Nakagawara, K.; Mori, M.; Miyashita, H.; Suzuki, Y.; Noguchi, N.; Takasawa, S.; Kumagai, T.; Yonekura, H.; *et al.* Structure, chromosomal localization and expression of mouse genes encoding type III Reg, RegIII α, RegIII β, RegIII γ. *Gene* **1997**, *185*, 159–168. [CrossRef]
144. Feng, Y.; Huang, N.; Wu, Q.; Wang, B. HMGN2: A novel antimicrobial effector molecule of human mononuclear leukocytes? *J. Leukoc. Biol.* **2005**, *78*, 1136–1141. [CrossRef]

145. Domachowske, J.B.; Dyer, K.D.; Bonville, C.A.; Rosenberg, H.F. Recombinant human eosinophil-derived neurotoxin/RNase 2 functions as an effective antiviral agent against respiratory syncytial virus. *J. Infect. Dis.* **1998**, *177*, 1458–64. [CrossRef]
146. Domachowske, J.B.; Dyer, K.D.; Adams, A.G.; Leto, T.L.; Rosenberg, H.F. Eosinophil cationic protein/RNase 3 is another RNase A-family ribonuclease with direct antiviral activity. *Nucleic Acids Res.* **1998**, *26*, 3358–63. [CrossRef]
147. Shugars, D.C. Endogenous mucosal antiviral factors of the oral cavity. *J. Infect. Dis.* **1999**, *179*, S431–S435. [CrossRef]
148. Wang, W.; Owen, S.M.; Rudolph, D.L.; Cole, A.M.; Hong, T.; Waring, A.J.; Lal, R.B.; Lehrer, R.I. Activity of alpha- and theta-defensins against primary isolates of HIV-1. *J. Immunol.* **2004**, *173*, 515–520. [CrossRef]
149. Dugan, A.S.; Maginnis, M.S.; Jordan, J.A.; Gasparovic, M.L.; Manley, K.; Page, R.; Williams, G.; Porter, E.; O'Hara, B.A.; Atwood, W.J. Human alpha-defensins inhibit BK virus infection by aggregating virions and blocking binding to host cells. *J. Biol. Chem.* **2008**, *283*, 31125–31132. [CrossRef]
150. Quiñones-Mateu, M.E.; Lederman, M.M.; Feng, Z.; Chakraborty, B.; Weber, J.; Rangel, H.R.; Marotta, M.L.; Mirza, M.; Jiang, B.; Kiser, P.; *et al.* Human epithelial beta-defensins 2 and 3 inhibit HIV-1 replication. *AIDS* **2003**, *17*, F39–F48.
151. Bergman, P.; Walter-Jallow, L.; Broliden, K.; Agerberth, B.; Söderlund, J. The antimicrobial peptide LL-37 inhibits HIV-1 replication. *Curr. HIV Res.* **2007**, *5*, 410–415. [CrossRef]
152. Wang, G.; Watson, K.M.; Buckheit, R.W., Jr. Anti-human immunodeficiency virus type 1 activities of antimicrobial peptides derived from human and bovine cathelicidins. *Antimicrob. Agents Chemother.* **2008**, *52*, 3438–3440. [CrossRef]
153. Groot, F.; Sanders, R.W.; ter Brake, O.; Nazmi, K.; Veerman, E.C.; Bolscher, J.G.; Berkhout, B. Histatin 5-derived peptide with improved fungicidal properties enhances human immunodeficiency virus type 1 replication by promoting viral entry. *J. Virol.* **2006**, *80*, 9236–9243. [CrossRef]
154. Wang, G. Natural antimicrobial peptides as promising anti-HIV candidates. *Curr. Topics Peptide Protein Res.* **2012**, *13*, 93–110.
155. López-García, B.; Lee, P.H.; Yamasaki, K.; Gallo, R.L. Anti-fungal activity of cathelicidins and their potential role in Candida albicans skin infection. *J. Invest. Dermatol.* **2005**, *125*, 108–115. [CrossRef]
156. Den Hertog, A.L.; van Marle, J.; Veerman, E.C.; Valentijn-Benz, M.; Nazmi, K.; Kalay, H.; Grün, C.H.; Van't Hof, W.; Bolscher, J.G.; Nieuw Amerongen, A.V. The human cathelicidin peptide LL-37 and truncated variants induce segregation of lipids and proteins in the plasma membrane of *Candida albicans*. *Biol. Chem.* **2006**, *387*, 1495–1502.
157. Dabirian, S.; Taslimi, Y.; Zahedifard, F.; Gholami, E.; Doustdari, F.; Motamedirad, M.; Khatami, S.; Azadmanesh, K.; Nylen, S.; Rafati, S. Human neutrophil peptide-1 (HNP-1): A new anti-leishmanial drug candidate. *PLoS Negl. Trop. Dis.* **2013**, *7*, e2491. [CrossRef]
158. Söbirk, S.K.; Mörgelin, M.; Egesten, A.; Bates, P.; Shannon, O.; Collin, M. Human chemokines as antimicrobial peptides with direct parasiticidal effect on Leishmania mexicana *in vitro*. *PLoS One* **2013**, *8*, e58129.
159. Rico-Mata, R.; De Leon-Rodriguez, L.M.; Avila, E.E. Effect of antimicrobial peptides derived from human cathelicidin LL-37 on Entamoeba histolytica trophozoites. *Exp. Parasitol.* **2013**, *133*, 300–306. [CrossRef]
160. Love, M.S.; Millholland, M.G.; Mishra, S.; Kulkarni, S.; Freeman, K.B.; Pan, W.; Kavash, R.W.; Costanzo, M.J.; Jo, H.; Daly, T.M.; *et al.* Platelet factor 4 activity against P. falciparum and its translation to nonpeptidic mimics as antimalarials. *Cell Host Microbe.* **2012**, *12*, 815–823. [CrossRef]
161. Baker, M.A.; Maloy, W.L.; Zasloff, M.; Jacob, L.S. Anticancer efficacy of Magainin2 and analogue peptides. *Cancer Res.* **1993**, *53*, 3052–3057.
162. Winder, D.; Günzburg, W.H.; Erfle, V.; Salmons, B. Expression of antimicrobial peptides has an antitumour effect in human cells. *Biochem. Biophys. Res. Commun.* **1998**, *242*, 608–612. [CrossRef]
163. Lichtenstein, A.; Ganz, T.; Selsted, M.E.; Lehrer, R.I. *In vitro* tumor cell cytolysis mediated by peptide defensins of human and rabbit granulocytes. *Blood* **1986**, *68*, 1407–1410.
164. Gaspar, D.; Veiga, A.S.; Castanho, M.A. From antimicrobial to anticancer peptides. A review. *Front. Microbiol.* **2013**, *4*, 294.
165. Riedl, S.; Zweytick, D.; Lohner, K. Membrane-active host defense peptides—Challenges and perspectives for the development of novel anticancer drugs. *Chem. Phys. Lipids* **2011**, *164*, 766–781. [CrossRef]

166. Hoskin, D.W.; Ramamoorthy, A. Studies on anticancer activities of antimicrobial peptides. *Biochim. Biophys. Acta* **2008**, *1778*, 357–375.
167. Kishi, A.; Takamori, Y.; Ogawa, K.; Takano, S.; Tomita, S.; Tanigawa, M.; Niman, M.; Kishida, T.; Fujita, S. Differential expression of granulysin and perforin by NK cells in cancer patients and correlation of impaired granulysin expression with progression of cancer. *Cancer Immunol. Immunother.* **2002**, *50*, 604–614. [CrossRef]
168. Sekiguchi, N.; Asano, N.; Ito, T.; Momose, K.; Momose, M.; Ishida, F. Elevated serum granulysin and its clinical relevance in mature NK-cell neoplasms. *Int. J. Hematol.* **2012**, *96*, 461–468. [CrossRef]
169. Xu, N.; Wang, Y.S.; Pan, W.B.; Xiao, B.; Wen, Y.J.; Chen, X.C.; Chen, L.J.; Deng, H.X.; You, J.; Kan, B.; *et al.* Human alpha-defensin-1 inhibits growth of human lung adenocarcinoma xenograft in nude mice. *Mol. Cancer Ther.* **2008**, *7*, 1588–1597. [CrossRef]
170. Mizukawa, N.; Sugiyama, K.; Fukunaga, J.; Ueno, T.; Mishima, K.; Takagi, S.; Sugahara, T. Defensin-1, a peptide detected in the saliva of oral squamous cell carcinoma patients. *Anticancer Res.* **1998**, *18*, 4645–4649.
171. Müller, C.A.; Markovic-Lipkovski, J.; Klatt, T.; Gamper, J.; Schwarz, G.; Beck, H.; Deeg, M.; Kalbacher, H.; Widmann, S.; Wessels, J.T.; *et al.* Human alpha-defensins HNPs-1, -2, and -3 in renal cell carcinoma: Influences on tumor cell proliferation. *Am. J. Pathol.* **2002**, *160*, 1311–1324. [CrossRef]
172. Sun, C.Q.; Arnold, R.; Fernandez-Golarz, C.; Parrish, A.B.; Almekinder, T.; He, J.; Ho, S.M.; Svoboda, P.; Pohl, J.; Marshall, F.F.; *et al.* Human beta-defensin-1, a potential chromosome 8p tumor suppressor: Control of transcription and induction of apoptosis in renal cell carcinoma. *Cancer Res.* **2006**, *66*, 8542–8549.
173. Bullard, R.S.; Gibson, W.; Bose, S.K.; Belgrave, J.K.; Eaddy, A.C.; Wright, C.J.; Hazen-Martin, D.J.; Lage, J.M.; Keane, T.E.; Ganz, T.A.; *et al.* Functional analysis of the host defense peptide Human Beta Defensin-1: New insight into its potential role in cancer. *Mol. Immunol.* **2008**, *45*, 839–848. [CrossRef]
174. Winter, J.; Pantelis, A.; Reich, R.; Martini, M.; Kraus, D.; Jepsen, S.; Allam, J.P.; Novak, N.; Wenghoefer, M. Human beta-defensin-1, -2, and -3 exhibit opposite effects on oral squamous cell carcinoma cell proliferation. *Cancer Invest.* **2011**, *29*, 196–201.
175. Wu, W.K.; Wang, G.; Coffelt, S.B.; Betancourt, A.M.; Lee, C.W.; Fan, D.; Wu, K.; Yu, J.; Sung, J.J.; Cho, C.H. Emerging roles of the host defense peptide LL-37 in human cancer and its potential therapeutic applications. *Int. J. Cancer.* **2010**, *127*, 1741–1747. [CrossRef]
176. van den Broek, I.; Sparidans, R.W.; Engwegen, J.Y.; Cats, A.; Depla, A.C.; Schellens, J.H.; Beijnen, J.H. Evaluation of human neutrophil peptide-1, -2 and -3 as serum markers for colorectal cancer. *Cancer Biomark.* **2010**, *7*, 109–115.
177. Albrethsen, J.; Bøgebo, R.; Gammeltoft, S.; Olsen, J.; Winther, B.; Raskov, H. Upregulated expression of human neutrophil peptides 1, 2 and 3 (HNP 1–3) in colon cancer serum and tumours: A biomarker study. *BMC Cancer* **2005**, *5*, 8. [CrossRef]
178. Albrethsen, J.; Møller, C.H.; Olsen, J.; Raskov, H.; Gammeltoft, S. Human neutrophil peptides 1, 2 and 3 are biochemical markers for metastatic colorectal cancer. *Eur. J. Cancer* **2006**, *42*, 3057–3064. [CrossRef]
179. Li, X.; Li, Y.; Han, H.; Miller, D.W.; Wang, G. Solution structures of human LL-37 fragments and NMR-based identification of a minimal membrane-targeting antimicrobial and anticancer region. *J. Am. Chem. Soc.* **2006**, *128*, 5776–5785. [CrossRef]
180. Ren, S.X.; Shen, J.; Cheng, A.S.; Lu, L.; Chan, R.L.; Li, Z.J.; Wang, X.J.; Wong, C.C.; Zhang, L.; Ng, S.S.; *et al.* FK-16 derived from the anticancer peptide LL-37 induces caspase-independent apoptosis and autophagic cell death in colon cancer cells. *PLoS One* **2013**, *8*, e63641. [CrossRef]
181. Zhou, J.; Shi, J.; Hou, J.; Cao, F.; Zhang, Y.; Rasmussen, J.T.; Heegaard, C.W.; Gilbert, G.E. Phosphatidylserine exposure and procoagulant activity in acute promyelocytic leukemia. *J. Thromb. Haemost.* **2010**, *8*, 773–782. [CrossRef]
182. Wang, G. Structures of human host defense cathelicidin LL-37 and its smallest antimicrobial peptide KR-12 in lipid micelles. *J. Biol. Chem.* **2008**, *283*, 32637–32643.
183. Svensson, D.; Westman, J.; Wickström, C.; Jönsson, D.; Herwald, H.; Nilsson, B.O. Human endogenous peptide p33 inhibits detrimental effects of LL-37 on osteoblast viability. *J. Periodontal Res.* **2014**. [CrossRef]
184. Hiemstra, T.F.; Charles, P.D.; Gracia, T.; Hester, S.S.; Gatto, L.; Al-Lamki, R.; Floto, R.A.; Su, Y.; Skepper, J.N.; Lilley, K.S.; *et al.* Human Urinary Exosomes as Innate Immune Effectors. *J. Am. Soc. Nephrol.* **2014**, in press.
185. Yung, S.C.; Murphy, P.M. Antimicrobial chemokines. *Front Immunol.* **2012**, *3*, 276.

186. Yang, D.; Chen, Q.; Schmidt, A.P.; Anderson, G.M.; Wang, J.M.; Wooters, J.; Oppenheim, J.J.; Chertov, O. LL-37, the neutrophil granule- and epithelial cell-derived cathelicidin, utilizes formyl peptide receptor-like 1 (FPRL1) as a receptor to chemoattract human peripheral blood neutrophils, monocytes, and T cells. *J. Exp. Med.* **2000**, *192*, 1069–1074. [CrossRef]
187. Ciornei, C.D.; Tapper, H.; Bjartell, A.; Sternby, N.H.; Bodelsson, M. Human antimicrobial peptide LL-37 is present in atherosclerotic plaques and induces death of vascular smooth muscle cells: A laboratory study. *BMC Cardiovasc. Disord.* **2006**, *6*, 49. [CrossRef]
188. Barlow, P.G.; Li, Y.; Wilkinson, T.S.; Bowdish, D.M.; Lau, Y.E.; Cosseau, C.; Haslett, C.; Simpson, A.J.; Hancock, R.E.; Davidson, D.J. The human cationic host defense peptide LL-37 mediates contrasting effects on apoptotic pathways in different primary cells of the innate immune system. *J. Leukoc. Biol.* **2006**, *80*, 509–520. [CrossRef]
189. Aarbiou, J.; Tjabringa, G.S.; Verhoosel, R.M.; Ninaber, D.K.; White, S.R.; Peltenburg, L.T.; Rabe, K.F.; Hiemstra, P.S. Mechanisms of cell death induced by the neutrophil antimicrobial peptides alpha-defensins and LL-37. *Inflamm. Res.* **2006**, *55*, 119–127. [CrossRef]
190. Okumura, K.; Itoh, A.; Isogai, E.; Hirose, K.; Hosokawa, Y.; Abiko, Y.; Shibata, T.; Hirata, M.; Isogai, H. C-terminal domain of human CAP18 antimicrobial peptide induces apoptosis in oral squamous cell carcinoma SAS-H1 cells. *Cancer Lett.* **2004**, *212*, 185–194. [CrossRef]
191. Ciornei, C.D.; Egesten, A.; Bodelsson, M. Effects of human cathelicidin antimicrobial peptide LL-37 on lipopolysaccharide-induced nitric oxide release from rat aorta *in vitro*. *Acta Anaesthesiol. Scand.* **2003**, *47*, 213–220. [CrossRef]
192. Chamorro, C.I.; Weber, G.; Grönberg, A.; Pivarcsi, A.; Ståhle, M. The human antimicrobial peptide LL-37 suppresses apoptosis *in* keratinocytes. *J. Invest. Dermatol.* **2009**, *129*, 937–944. [CrossRef]
193. Nagaoka, I.; Tamura, H.; Hirata, M. An antimicrobial cathelicidin peptide, human CAP18/LL-37, suppresses neutrophil apoptosis via the activation of formyl-peptide receptor-like 1 and P2X7. *J. Immunol.* **2006**, *176*, 3044–3052. [CrossRef]
194. Lee, W.Y.; Savage, J.R.; Zhang, J.; Jia, W.; Oottamasathien, S.; Prestwich, G.D. Prevention of anti-microbial peptide LL-37-induced apoptosis and ATP release in the urinary bladder by a modified glycosaminoglycan. *PLoS One* **2013**, *8*, e77854.
195. Suzuki, K.; Murakami, T.; Kuwahara-Arai, K.; Tamura, H.; Hiramatsu, K.; Nagaoka, I. Human anti-microbial cathelicidin peptide LL-37 suppresses the LPS-induced apoptosis of endothelial cells. *Int. Immunol.* **2011**, *23*, 185–193. [CrossRef]
196. Ren, S.X.; Cheng, A.S.; To, K.F.; Tong, J.H.; Li, M.S.; Shen, J.; Wong, C.C.; Zhang, L.; Chan, R.L.; Wang, X.J.; *et al.* Host immune defense peptide LL-37 activates caspase-independent apoptosis and suppresses colon cancer. *Cancer Res.* **2012**, *72*, 6512–6523. [CrossRef]
197. Oudhoff, M.J.; Blaauboer, M.E.; Nazmi, K.; Scheres, N.; Bolscher, J.G.; Veerman, E.C. The role of salivary histatin and the human cathelicidin LL-37 in wound healing and innate immunity. *Biol. Chem.* **2010**, *391*, 541–548.
198. Wang, G. NMR of membrane-associated peptides and proteins. *Curr. Protein Pept. Sci.* **2008**, *9*, 50–69. [CrossRef]
199. Wang, G. NMR of membrane proteins. In "Advances in Protein and Peptide Sciences" (edited by Dunn BM). *Bentham Sci.* **2013**, *1*, 128–188.
200. Nguyen, L.T.; Haney, E.F.; Vogel, H.J. The expanding scope of antimicrobial peptide structures and their modes of action. *Trends Biotechnol.* **2011**, *29*, 464–472. [CrossRef]
201. Wang, G.; Li, X.; Zasloff, M. A Database View of Natural Antimicrobial Peptides: Nomenclature, Classification and Amino acid Sequence Analysis. In *Antimicrobial Peptides: Discovery, Design and Novel Therapeutic Strategies*; Wang, G., Ed.; CABI: Wallingford, UK, 2010; pp. 1–21.
202. Rose, P.W.; Bi, C.; Bluhm, W.F.; Christie, C.H.; Dimitropoulos, D.; Dutta, S.; Green, R.K.; Goodsell, D.S.; Prlic, A.; Quesada, M.; *et al.* The RCSB Protein Data Bank: New resources for research and education. *Nucleic Acids Res.* **2013**, *41*, D475–D482. [CrossRef]
203. Xu, T.; Levitz, S.M.; Diamond, R.D.; Oppenheim, F.G. Anticandidal activity of major human salivary histatins. *Infect. Immun.* **1991**, *59*, 2549–2554.
204. Raj, P.A.; Edgerton, M.; Levine, M.J. Salivary histatin 5: Dependence of sequence, chain length, and helical conformation for candidacidal activity. *J. Biol. Chem.* **1990**, *265*, 3898–3905.

205. Rothstein, D.M.; Spacciapoli, P.; Tran, L.T.; Xu, T.; Roberts, F.D.; Dalla Serra, M.; Buxton, D.K.; Oppenheim, F.G.; Friden, P. Anticandida activity is retained in P-113, a 12-amino-acid fragment of histatin 5. *Antimicrob. Agents Chemother.* **2001**, *45*, 1367–1373. [CrossRef]
206. Zuo, Y.; Xu, T.; Troxler, R.F.; Li, J.; Driscoll, J.; Oppenheim, F.G. Recombinant histatins: Functional domain duplication enhances candidacidal activity. *Gene* **1995**, *161*, 87–91. [CrossRef]
207. Situ, H.; Tsai, H.; Bobek, L.A. Construction and characterization of human salivary histatin-5 multimers. *J. Dent. Res.* **1999**, *78*, 690–698. [CrossRef]
208. Situ, H.; Balasubramanian, S.V.; Bobek, L.A. Role of alpha-helical conformation of histatin-5 in candidacidal activity examined by proline variants. *Biochim. Biophys. Acta* **2000**, *1475*, 377–382. [CrossRef]
209. Melino, S.; Rufini, S.; Sette, M.; Morero, R.; Grottesi, A.; Paci, M.; Petruzzelli, R. Zn^{2+} ions selectively induce antimicrobial salivary peptide histatin-5 to fuse negatively charged vesicles. Identification and characterization of a zinc-binding motif present in the functional domain. *Biochemistry* **1999**, *38*, 9626–9633. [CrossRef]
210. Rydengård, V.; Andersson Nordahl, E.; Schmidtchen, A. Zinc potentiates the antibacterial effects of histidine-rich peptides against *Enterococcus faecalis*. *FEBS J.* **2006**, *273*, 2399–2406. [CrossRef]
211. Melino, S.; Gallo, M.; Trotta, E.; Mondello, F.; Paci, M.; Petruzzelli, R. Metal-binding and nuclease activity of an antimicrobial peptide analogue of the salivary histatin 5. *Biochemistry* **2006**, *45*, 15373–15383. [CrossRef]
212. Wang, G. Structural studies of antimicrobial peptides provide insight into their mechanisms of action. In *Antimicrobial Peptides: Discovery, Design and Novel Therapeutic Strategies*; Wang, G., Ed.; CABI: Wallingford, UK, 2010; pp. 141–168.
213. Xhindoli, D.; Pacor, S.; Guida, F.; Antcheva, N.; Tossi, A. Native oligomerization determines the mode of action and biological activities of human cathelicidin LL-37. *Biochem. J.* **2014**, *457*, 263–275. [CrossRef]
214. Wang, G.; Elliott, M.; Cogen, A.L.; Ezell, E.L.; Gallo, R.L.; Hancock, R.E.W. Structure, dynamics, antimicrobial and immune modulatory activities of human LL-23 and its single residue variants mutated based on homologous primate cathelicidins. *Biochemistry* **2012**, *51*, 653–664. [CrossRef]
215. Paulmann, M.; Arnold, T.; Linke, D.; Özdirekcan, S.; Kopp, A.; Gutsmann, T.; Kalbacher, H.; Wanke, I.; Schuenemann, V.J.; Habeck, M.; *et al.* Structure-activity analysis of the dermcidin-derived peptide DCD-1L, an anionic antimicrobial peptide present in human sweat. *J. Biol. Chem.* **2012**, *287*, 8434–8443. [CrossRef]
216. Song, C.; Weichbrodt, C.; Salnikov, E.S.; Dynowski, M.; Forsberg, B.O.; Bechinger, B.; Steinem, C.; de Groot, B.L.; Zachariae, U.; Zeth, K. Crystal structure and functional mechanism of a human antimicrobial membrane channel. *Proc. Natl. Acad. Sci. USA* **2013**, *110*, 4586–4591. [CrossRef]
217. Jung, H.H.; Yang, S.T.; Sim, J.Y.; Lee, S.; Lee, J.Y.; Kim, H.H.; Shin, S.Y.; Kim, J.I. Analysis of the solution structure of the human antibiotic peptide dermcidin and its interaction with phospholipid vesicles. *BMB Rep.* **2010**, *43*, 362–368. [CrossRef]
218. Koradi, R.; Billeter, M.; Wüthrich, K. MOLMOL: A program for display and analysis of macromolecular structures. *J. Mol. Graph.* **1996**, *14*, 51–55. [CrossRef]
219. Anderson, D.H.; Sawaya, M.R.; Cascio, D.; Ernst, W.; Modlin, R.; Krensky, A.; Eisenberg, D. Granulysin crystal structure and a structure-derived lytic mechanism. *J. Mol. Biol.* **2003**, *325*, 355–365.
220. Peña, S.V.; Krensky, A.M. Granulysin, a new human cytolytic granule-associated protein with possible involvement in cell-mediated cytotoxicity. *Semin. Immunol.* **1997**, *9*, 117–125. [CrossRef]
221. Bruhn, H. A short guided tour through functional and structural features of saposin-like proteins. *Biochem. J.* **2005**, *389*, (Pt 2). 249–257.
222. da Silva, A.P.; Unks, D.; Lyu, S.C.; Ma, J.; Zbozien-Pacamaj, R.; Chen, X.; Krensky, A.M.; Clayberger, C. *In vitro* and *in vivo* antimicrobial activity of granulysin-derived peptides against Vibrio cholerae. *J. Antimicrob Chemother.* **2008**, *61*, 1103–1109. [CrossRef]
223. McInturff, J.E.; Wang, S.J.; Machleidt, T.; Lin, T.R.; Oren, A.; Hertz, C.J.; Krutzik, S.R.; Hart, S.; Zeh, K.; Anderson, D.H.; *et al.* Granulysin-derived peptides demonstrate antimicrobial and anti-inflammatory effects against *Propionibacterium. acnes*. *J. Invest. Dermatol.* **2005**, *125*, 256–263.
224. Ericksen, B.; Wu, Z.; Lu, W.; Lehrer, R.I. Antibacterial activity and specificity of the six human α-defensins. *Antimicrob. Agents Chemother.* **2005**, *49*, 269–275. [CrossRef]
225. Schibli, D.J.; Hunter, H.N.; Aseyev, V.; Starner, T.D.; Wiencek, J.M.; McCray PB, Jr.; Tack, B.F.; Vogel, H.J. The solution structures of the human beta-defensins lead to a better understanding of the potent bactericidal activity of HBD3 against *Staphylococcus aureus*. *J. Biol. Chem.* **2002**, *277*, 8279–8289. [CrossRef]

226. Schroeder, B.O.; Wu, Z.; Nuding, S.; Groscurth, S.; Marcinowski, M.; Beisner, J.; Buchner, J.; Schaller, M.; Stange, E.F.; Wehkamp, J. Reduction of disulphide bonds unmasks potent antimicrobial activity of human β-defensin 1. *Nature* **2011**, *469*, 419–423. [CrossRef]
227. Keizer, D.W.; Crump, M.P.; Lee, T.W.; Slupsky, C.M.; Clark-Lewis, I.; Sykes, B.D. Human CC chemokine I-309, structural consequences of the additional disulfide bond. *Biochemistry* **2000**, *39*, 6053–6059. [CrossRef]
228. Blaszczyk, J.; Coillie, E.V.; Proost, P.; Damme, J.V.; Opdenakker, G.; Bujacz, G.D.; Wang, J.M.; Ji, X. Complete crystal structure of monocyte chemotactic protein-2, a CC chemokine that interacts with multiple receptors. *Biochemistry* **2000**, *39*, 14075–14081.
229. Crump, M.P.; Rajarathnam, K.; Kim, K.S.; Clark-Lewis, I.; Sykes, B.D. Solution structure of eotaxin, a chemokine that selectively recruits eosinophils in allergic inflammation. *J. Biol. Chem.* **1998**, *273*, 22471–22479.
230. Love, M.; Sandberg, J.L.; Ziarek, J.J.; Gerarden, K.P.; Rode, R.R.; Jensen, D.R.; McCaslin, D.R.; Peterson, F.C.; Veldkamp, C.T. Solution structure of CCL21 and identification of a putative CCR7 binding site. *Biochemistry* **2012**, *51*, 733–735.
231. Jansma, A.L.; Kirkpatrick, J.P.; Hsu, A.R.; Handel, T.M.; Nietlispach, D. NMR analysis of the structure, dynamics, and unique oligomerization properties of the chemokine CCL27. *J. Biol. Chem.* **2010**, *285*, 14424–14437.
232. Veldkamp, C.T.; Ziarek, J.J.; Su, J.; Basnet, H.; Lennertz, R.; Weiner, J.J.; Peterson, F.C.; Baker, J.E.; Volkman, B.F. Monomeric structure of the cardioprotective chemokine SDF-1/CXCL12. *Protein Sci.* **2009**, *18*, 1359–1369.
233. Hoover, D.M.; Boulegue, C.; Yang, D.; Oppenheim, J.J.; Tucker, K.; Lu, W.; Lubkowski, J. The structure of human macrophage inflammatory protein-3alpha/CCL20. Linking antimicrobial and CC chemokine receptor-6-binding activities with human beta-defensins. *J. Biol. Chem.* **2002**, *277*, 37647–37654.
234. Barinka, C.; Prahl, A.; Lubkowski, J. Structure of human monocyte chemoattractant protein 4 (MCP-4/CCL13). *Acta. Crystallogr. D Biol. Crystallogr.* **2008**, *64*, (Pt 3). 273–278. [CrossRef]
235. Kim, K.S.; Clark-Lewis, I.; Sykes, B.D. Solution structure of GRO/melanoma growth stimulatory activity determined by ^{1}H-NMR spectroscopy. *J. Biol. Chem.* **1994**, *269*, 32909–32915.
236. Swaminathan, G.J.; Holloway, D.E.; Colvin, R.A.; Campanella, G.K.; Papageorgiou, A.C.; Luster, A.D.; Acharya, K.R. Crystal structures of oligomeric forms of the IP-10/CXCL-10 chemokine. *Structure* **2003**, *11*, 521–532. [CrossRef]
237. Yung, S.C.; Parenti, D.; Murphy, P.M. Host chemokines bind to *Staphylococcus aureus* and stimulate protein A release. *J. Biol. Chem.* **2011**, *286*, 5069–5077. [CrossRef]
238. Nguyen, L.T.; Kwakman, P.H.; Chan, D.I.; Liu, Z.; de Boer, L.; Zaat, S.A.; Vogel, H.J. Exploring platelet chemokine antimicrobial activity: Nuclear magnetic resonance backbone dynamics of NAP-2 and TC-1. *Antimicrob. Agents Chemother.* **2011**, *55*, 2074–2083. [CrossRef]
239. Wang, G.; Epand, R.F.; Mishra, B.; Lushnikova, T.; Thomas, V.C.; Bayles, K.W.; Epand, R.M. Decoding the functional roles of cationic side chains of the major antimicrobial region of human cathelicidin LL-37. *Antimicrob. Agents Chemother.* **2012**, *56*, 845–856. [CrossRef]
240. Lequin, O.; Thüring, H.; Robin, M.; Lallemand, J.Y. Three-dimensional solution structure of human angiogenin determined by ^{1}H,^{15}N-NMR spectroscopy–characterization of histidine protonation states and pKa values. *Eur. J. Biochem.* **1997**, *250*, 712–726.
241. Wang, H.; Schwaderer, A.L.; Kline, J.; Spencer, J.D.; Kline, D.; Hains, D.S. Contribution of structural domains to the activity of ribonuclease 7 against uropathogenic bacteria. *Antimicrob. Agents Chemother.* **2013**, *57*, 766–774. [CrossRef]
242. Torrent, M.; Pulido, D.; Valle, J.; Nogués, M.V.; Andreu, D.; Boix, E. Ribonucleases as a host-defence family: Evidence of evolutionarily conserved antimicrobial activity at the N-terminus. *Biochem. J.* **2013**, *456*, 99–108. [CrossRef]
243. Boix, E.; Salazar, V.A.; Torrent, M.; Pulido, D.; Nogués, M.V.; Moussaoui, M. Structural determinants of the eosinophil cationic protein antimicrobial activity. *Biol. Chem.* **2012**, *393*, 801–815.
244. Spencer, J.D.; Schwaderer, A.L.; Eichler, T.; Wang, H.; Kline, J.; Justice, S.S.; Cohen, D.M.; Hains, D.S. An endogenous ribonuclease inhibitor regulates the antimicrobial activity of ribonuclease 7 in the human urinary tract. *Kidney Int.* **2013**, *85*, 1179–1191.
245. Lehotzky, R.E.; Partch, C.L.; Mukherjee, S.; Cash, H.L.; Goldman, W.E.; Gardner, K.H.; Hooper, L.V. Molecular basis for peptidoglycan recognition by a bactericidal lectin. *Proc. Natl. Acad. Sci. USA* **2010**, *107*, 7722–7727.

246. Mukherjee, S.; Zheng, H.; Derebe, M.G.; Callenberg, K.M.; Partch, C.L.; Rollins, D.; Propheter, D.C.; Rizo, J.; Grabe, M.; Jiang, Q.X.; *et al.* Antibacterial membrane attack by a pore-forming intestinal C-type lectin. *Nature* **2013**, *505*, 103–107. [CrossRef]
247. De Leeuw, E.; Li, C.; Zeng, P.; Li, C.; Diepeveen-de Buin, M.; Lu, W.Y.; Breukink, E.; Lu, W. Functional interaction of human neutrophil peptide-1 with the cell wall precursor lipid II. *FEBS Lett.* **2010**, *584*, 1543–1548. [CrossRef]
248. Böhling, A.; Hagge, S.O.; Roes, S.; Podschun, R.; Sahly, H.; Harder, J.; Schröder, J.M.; Grötzinger, J.; Seydel, U.; Gutsmann, T. Lipid-specific membrane activity of human beta-defensin-3. *Biochemistry* **2006**, *45*, 5663–5670. [CrossRef]
249. Sass, V.; Schneider, T.; Wilmes, M.; Körner, C.; Tossi, A.; Novikova, N.; Shamova, O.; Sahl, H.G. Human beta-defensin 3 inhibits cell wall biosynthesis in Staphylococci. *Infect. Immun.* **2010**, *78*, 2793–2800. [CrossRef]
250. Schmitt, P.; Wilmes, M.; Pugnière, M.; Aumelas, A.; Bachère, E.; Sahl, H.G.; Schneider, T.; Destoumieux-Garzón, D. Insight into invertebrate defensin mechanism of action: Oyster defensins inhibit peptidoglycan biosynthesis by binding to lipid II. *Biol. Chem.* **2010**, *285*, 29208–29216. [CrossRef]
251. Bierbaum, G.; Sahl, H.G. Lantibiotics: Mode of action, biosynthesis and bioengineering. *Curr. Pharm. Biotechnol.* **2009**, *10*, 2–18. [CrossRef]
252. Schneider, T.; Kruse, T.; Wimmer, R.; Wiedemann, I.; Sass, V.; Pag, U.; Jansen, A.; Nielsen, A.K.; Mygind, P.H.; Raventós, D.S.; *et al.* Plectasin, a fungal defensin, targets the bacterial cell wall precursor Lipid II. *Science* **2010**, *328*, 1168–1172. [CrossRef]
253. Derouaux, A.; Turk, S.; Olrichs, N.K.; Gobec, S.; Breukink, E.; Amoroso, A.; Offant, J.; Bostock, J.; Mariner, K.; Chopra, I.; *et al.* Small molecule inhibitors of peptidoglycan synthesis targeting the lipid II precursor. *Biochem. Pharmacol.* **2011**, *81*, 1098–1105. [CrossRef]
254. Varney, K.M.; Bonvin, A.M.; Pazgier, M.; Malin, J.; Yu, W.; Ateh, E.; Oashi, T.; Lu, W.; Huang, J.; Diepeveen-de Buin, M.; *et al.* Turning Defense into Offense: Defensin Mimetics as Novel Antibiotics Targeting Lipid II. *PLoS Pathog.* **2013**, *9*, e1003732. [CrossRef]
255. Poon, I.K.h.; Baxter, A.A.; Lay, F.T.; Mills, G.D.; Adda, C.G.; Payne, J.A.; Phan, T.K.; Ryan, G.F.; White, J.A.; Veneer, P.K.; *et al.* Phosphoinositide-mediated oligomerization of a defensin induces cell lysis. *Elife* **2014**, *3*, e01808. [CrossRef]
256. Silva, P.M.; Gonçalves, S.; Santos, N.C. Defensins: Antifungal lessons from eukaryotes. *Front. Microbiol.* **2014**, *5*, 97.
257. Sagaram, U.S.; El-Mounadi, K.; Buchko, G.W.; Berg, H.R.; Kaur, J.; Pandurangi, R.S.; Smith, T.J.; Shah, D.M. Structural and functional studies of a phosphatidic acid-binding antifungal plant defensin MtDef4: identification of an RGFRRR motif governing fungal cell entry. *PLoS One.* **2013**, *8*, e82485. [CrossRef]
258. Miki, T.; Holst, O.; Hardt, W.D. The bactericidal activity of the C-type lectin RegIIIβ against Gram-negative bacteria involves binding to lipid A. *J. Biol. Chem.* **2012**, *287*, 34844–34855. [CrossRef]
259. Formanek, H. A three dimensional model of the digestion of peptidoglycan by lysozyme. *Biophys. Struct. Mech.* **1977**, *4*, 1–14. [CrossRef]
260. Ma, G.; Greenwell-Wild, T.; Lei, K.; Jin, W.; Swisher, J.; Hardegen, N.; Wild, C.T.; Wahl, S.M. Secretory leukocyte protease inhibitor binds to annexin II, a cofactor for macrophage HIV-1 infection. *J. Exp. Med.* **2004**, *200*, 1337–1346. [CrossRef]
261. Oren, Z.; Lerman, J.C.; Gudmundsson, G.H.; Agerberth, B.; Shai, Y. Structure and organization of the human antimicrobial peptide LL-37 in phospholipid membranes: Relevance to the molecular basis for its non-cell-selective activity. *Biochem. J.* **1999**, *341*, (Pt. 3). 501–513.
262. Lee, C.C.; Sun, Y.; Qian, S.; Huang, H.W. Transmembrane pores formed by human antimicrobial peptide LL-37. *Biophys. J.* **2011**, *100*, 1688–1696. [CrossRef]
263. Maisetta, G.; Vitali, A.; Scorciapino, M.A.; Rinaldi, A.C.; Petruzzelli, R.; Brancatisano, F.L.; Esin, S.; Stringaro, A.; Colone, M.; Luzi, C.; *et al.* pH-dependent disruption of *Escherichia coli* ATCC 25922 and model membranes by the human antimicrobial peptides hepcidin 20 and 25. *FEBS J.* **2013**, *280*, 2842–2854. [CrossRef]
264. Natividad, J.M.; Hayes, C.L.; Motta, J.P.; Jury, J.; Galipeau, H.J.; Philip, V.; Garcia-Rodenas, C.L.; Kiyama, H.; Bercik, P.; Verdu, E.F. Differential Induction of Antimicrobial REGIII by the Intestinal Microbiota and Bifidobacterium breve NCC2950. *Appl. Environ. Microbiol.* **2013**, *79*, 7745–7754. [CrossRef]

265. Parker, M.W.; Feil, S.C. Pore-forming protein toxins: From structure to function. *Prog. Biophys. Mol. Biol.* **2005**, *88*, 91–142. [CrossRef]
266. Birck, C.; Damian, L.; Marty-Detraves, C.; Lougarre, A.; Schulze-Briese, C.; Koehl, P.; Fournier, D.; Paquereau, L.; Samama, J.P. A new lectin family with structure similarity to actinoporins revealed by the crystal structure of Xerocomus chrysenteron lectin XCL. *J. Mol. Biol.* **2004**, *344*, 1409–1420. [CrossRef]
267. Mechaly, A.E.; Bellomio, A.; Gil-Cartón, D.; Morante, K.; Valle, M.; González-Mañas, J.M.; Guérin, D.M. Structural insights into the oligomerization and architecture of eukaryotic membrane pore-forming toxins. *Structure* **2011**, *19*, 181–191. [CrossRef]
268. Miller, K.W.; Evans, R.J.; Eisenberg, S.P.; Thompson, R.C. Secretory leukocyte protease inhibitor binding to mRNA and DNA as a possible cause of toxicity to Escherichia coli. *J. Bacteriol.* **1989**, *171*, 2166–2172.
269. den Hertog, A.L.; van Marle, J.; van Veen, H.A.; Van't Hof, W.; Bolscher, J.G.; Veerman, E.C.; Nieuw Amerongen, A.V. Candidacidal effects of two antimicrobial peptides: Histatin 5 causes small membrane defects, but LL-37 causes massive disruption of the cell membrane. *Biochem. J.* **2005**, *388*, 689–695. [CrossRef]
270. Gyurko, C.; Lendenmann, U.; Troxler, R.F.; Oppenheim, F.G. *Candida albicans* mutants deficient in respiration are resistant to the small cationic salivary antimicrobial peptide histatin 5. *Antimicrob. Agents Chemother.* **2000**, *44*, 348–354. [CrossRef]
271. Gyurko, C.; Lendenmann, U.; Helmerhorst, E.J.; Troxler, R.F.; Oppenheim, F.G. Killing of *Candida albicans* by histatin 5: Cellular uptake and energy requirement. *Antonie. Van Leeuwenhoek.* **2001**, *79*, 297–309. [CrossRef]
272. Li, X.S.; Sun, J.N.; Okamoto-Shibayama, K.; Edgerton, M. *Candida albicans* cell wall ssa proteins bind and facilitate import of salivary histatin 5 required for toxicity. *J. Biol. Chem.* **2006**, *281*, 22453–22463.
273. Helmerhorst, E.J.; Breeuwer, P.; Van't Hof, W.; Walgreen-Weterings, E.; Amerongen, A.V.; Abee, T. The cellular target of histatin 5 on *Candida albicans* is the energized mitochondrion. *J. Biol. Chem.* **1999**, *274*, 7286–7291.
274. Vylkova, S.; Jang, W.S.; Li, W.; Nayyar, N.; Edgerton, M. Histatin 5 initiates osmotic stress response in *Candida albicans* via activation of the Hog1 mitogen-activated protein kinase pathway. *Eukaryot. Cell* **2007**, *6*, 1876–1888. [CrossRef]
275. Wagener, J.; Schneider, J.J.; Baxmann, S.; Kalbacher, H.; Borelli, C.; Nuding, S.; Küchler, R.; Wehkamp, J.; Kaeser, M.D.; Mailänder-Sanchez, D.; *et al.* A peptide derived from the highly conserved protein Glyceraldehyde-3-phosphate dehydrogenase (GAPDH) is involved in tissue protection by different antifungal strategies and epithelial immunomodulation. *J. Invest. Dermatol.* **2013**, *133*, 144–153. [CrossRef]
276. Aslam, R.; Atindehou, M.; Lavaux, T.; Haïkel, Y.; Schneider, F.; Metz-Boutigue, M.H. Chromogranin A-derived peptides are involved in innate immunity. *Curr. Med. Chem.* **2012**, *19*, 4115–4123. [CrossRef]
277. Ochoa, M.T.; Stenger, S.; Sieling, P.A.; Thoma-Uszynski, S.; Sabet, S.; Cho, S.; Krensky, A.M.; Rollinghoff, M.; Nunes Sarno, E.; Burdick, A.E.; *et al.* T-cell release of granulysin contributes to host defense in leprosy. *Nat. Med.* **2001**, *7*, 174–179. [CrossRef]
278. Stewart, S.E.; Kondos, S.C.; Matthews, A.Y.; D'Angelo, M.E.; Dunstone, M.A.; Whisstock, J.C.; Trapani, J.A.; Bird, P.I. The Perforin Pore Facilitates the Delivery of Cationic Cargos. *J. Biol. Chem.* **2014**, *289*, 9172–9181. [CrossRef]
279. Diamond, G.; Beckloff, N.; Weinberg, A.; Kisich, K.O. The roles of antimicrobial peptides in innate host defense. *Curr. Pharm Des.* **2009**, *15*, 2377–2392. [CrossRef]
280. Leung, T.F.; Ching, K.W.; Kong, A.P.; Wong, G.W.; Chan, J.C.; Hon, K.L. Circulating LL-37 is a biomarker for eczema severity in children. *J. Eur. Acad. Dermatol. Venereol.* **2012**, *26*, 518–522. [CrossRef]
281. Weber, G.; Chamorro, C.I.; Granath, F.; Liljegren, A.; Zreika, S.; Saidak, Z.; Sandstedt, B.; Rotstein, S.; Mentaverri, R.; Sánchez, F.; *et al.* Human antimicrobial protein hCAP18/LL-37 promotes a metastatic phenotype in breast cancer. *Breast Cancer Res.* **2009**, *11*, R6. [CrossRef]
282. Cheng, W.L.; Wang, C.S.; Huang, Y.H.; Liang, Y.; Lin, P.Y.; Hsueh, C.; Wu, Y.C.; Chen, W.J.; Yu, C.J.; Lin, S.R.; *et al.* Overexpression of a secretory leukocyte protease inhibitor in human gastric cancer. *Int. J. Cancer* **2008**, *123*, 1787–1796. [CrossRef]
283. Emson, C.L.; Fitzmaurice, S.; Lindwall, G.; Li, K.W.; Hellerstein, M.K.; Maibach, H.I.; Liao, W.; Turner, S.M. A pilot study demonstrating a non-invasive method for the measurement of protein turnover in skin disorders: Application to psoriasis. *Clin. Transl. Med.* **2013**, *2*, 12. [CrossRef]

284. Welling, M.M.; Paulusma-Annema, A.; Balter, H.S.; Pauwels, E.K.; Nibbering, P.H. Technetium-99m labeled antimicrobial peptides discriminate between bacterial infections and sterile inflammations. *Eur. J. Nucl. Med.* **2000**, *27*, 292–301. [CrossRef]
285. Saeed, S.; Zafar, J.; Khan, B.; Akhtar, A.; Qurieshi, S.; Fatima, S.; Ahmad, N.; Irfanullah, J. Utility of ^{99}mTc-labelled antimicrobial peptide ubiquicidin (29–41) in the diagnosis of diabetic foot infection. *Eur. J. Nucl. Med. Mol. Imaging* **2013**, *40*, 737–743. [CrossRef]
286. Aryana, K.; Hootkani, A.; Sadeghi, R.; Davoudi, Y.; Naderinasab, M.; Erfani, M.; Ayati, N. (99m)Tc-labeled ubiquicidin scintigraphy: A promising method in hip prosthesis infection diagnosis. *Nuklearmedizin* **2012**, *51*, 133–139. [CrossRef]
287. Wang, G. *Antimicrobial Peptides: Discovery, Design and Novel Therapeutic Strategies*; CABI: Wallingford, UK, 2010.
288. Forde, E.; Humphreys, H.; Greene, C.M.; Fitzgerald-Hughes, D.; Devocelle, M. The potential of host defence peptide prodrugs as neutrophil elastase-dependent anti-infective agents for cystic fibrosis. *Antimicrob. Agents. Chemother.* **2013**, *58*, 978–985.
289. Reynolds, N.L.; de Cecco, M.; Taylor, K.; Stanton, C.; Kilanowski, F.; Kalapothakis, J.; Seo, E.; Uhrin, D.; Campopiano, D.; Govan, J.; *et al.* Peptide fragments of a beta-defensin derivative with potent bactericidal activity. *Antimicrob. Agents Chemother.* **2010**, *54*, 1922–1929. [CrossRef]
290. Roelandts, R. The history of phototherapy: Something new under the sun? *J. Am. Acad. Dermatol.* **2002**, *46*, 926–930. [CrossRef]
291. Wang, T.T.; Nestel, F.P.; Bourdeau, V.; Nagai, Y.; Wang, Q.; Liao, J.; Tavera-Mendoza, L.; Lin, R.; Hanrahan, J.W.; Mader, S.; *et al.* Cutting edge: 1,25-dihydroxyvitamin D3 is a direct inducer of antimicrobial peptide gene expression. *J. Immunol.* **2004**, *173*, 2909–2912. [CrossRef]
292. Gombart, A.F.; Borregaard, N.; Koeffler, H.P. Human cathelicidin antimicrobial peptide (CAMP) gene is a direct target of the vitamin D receptor and is strongly up-regulated in myeloid cells by 1,25-dihydroxyvitamin D3. *FASEB J.* **2005**, *19*, 1067–1077. [CrossRef]
293. Ala-Houhala, M.J.; Karppinen, T.; Vähävihu, K.; Kautiainen, H.; Dombrowski, Y.; Snellman, E.; Schauber, J.; Reunala, T. Narrow-band Ultraviolet B Treatment Boosts Serum 25-hydroxyvitamin D in Patients with Psoriasis on Oral Vitamin D Supplementation. *Acta Derm. Venereol.* **2014**, *94*, 146–151.
294. Steinmann, J.; Halldórsson, S.; Agerberth, B.; Gudmundsson, G.H. Phenylbutyrate (PBA) induces antimicrobial peptide expression. *Antimicrob. Agents Chemother.* **2009**, *53*, 5127–5133. [CrossRef]
295. Gan, Y.; Cui, X.; Ma, T.; Liu, Y.; Li, A.; Huang, M. Paeoniflorin Upregulates β-Defensin-2 Expression in Human Bronchial Epithelial Cell Through the p38 MAPK, ERK, and NF-κB Signaling Pathways. *Inflammation.* **2014**, in press.
296. Kim, B.J.; Rho, Y.K.; Lee, H.I.; Jeong, M.S.; Li, K.; Seo, S.J.; Kim, M.N.; Hong, C.K. The effect of calcipotriol on the expression of human beta defensin-2 and LL-37 in cultured human keratinocytes. *Clin. Dev. Immunol.* **2009**, *2009*, 645898.
297. Sunkara, L.T.; Zeng, X.; Curtis, A.R.; Zhang, G. Cyclic AMP synergizes with butyrate in promoting β-defensin9 expression in chickens. *Mol. Immunol.* **2014**, *57*, 171–180. [CrossRef]
298. Cederlund, A.; Nylén, F.; Miraglia, E.; Bergman, P.; Gudmundsson, G.H.; Agerberth, B. Label-Free Quantitative Mass Spectrometry Reveals Novel Pathways Involved in LL-37 Expression. *J. Innate Immun.* **2014**, *6*, 365–376.
299. Liu, Q.; Liu, J.; Roschmann, K.I.; van Egmond, D.; Golebski, K.; Fokkens, W.J.; Wang, D.; van Drunen, C.M. Histone deacetylase inhibitors up-regulate LL-37 expression independent of toll-like receptor mediated signalling in airway epithelial cells. *J. Inflamm. (Lond)* **2013**, *10*, 15. [CrossRef]
300. Strandberg, K.L.; Richards, S.M.; Gunn, J.S. Cathelicidin antimicrobial peptide expression is not induced or required for bacterial clearance during *salmonella enterica* infection of human monocyte-derived macrophages. *Infect. Immun.* **2012**, *80*, 3930–3938. [CrossRef]
301. Yin, Q.; Xu, X.; Lin, Y.; Lv, J.; Zhao, L.; He, R. Ultraviolet B irradiation induces skin accumulation of plasmacytoid dendritic cells: A possible role for chemerin. *Autoimmunity.* **2013**, *47*, 185–192.
302. Karlsson, J.; Carlsson, G.; Larne, O.; Andersson, M.; Pütsep, K. Vitamin D3 induces pro-LL-37 expression in myeloid precursors from patients with severe congenital neutropenia. *J. Leukoc. Biol.* **2008**, *84*, 1279–1286. [CrossRef]

303. Martineau, A.R.; Wilkinson, K.A.; Newton, S.M.; Floto, R.A.; Norman, A.W.; Skolimowska, K.; Davidson, R.N.; Sørensen, O.E.; Kampmann, B.; Griffiths, C.J.; *et al.* IFN-gamma- and TNF-independent vitamin D-inducible human suppression of mycobacteria: The role of cathelicidin LL-37. *J. Immunol.* **2007**, *178*, 7190–7198. [CrossRef]

304. Cederlund, A.; Kai-Larsen, Y.; Printz, G.; Yoshio, H.; Alvelius, G.; Lagercrantz, H.; Strömberg, R.; Jörnvall, H.; Gudmundsson, G.H.; Agerberth, B. Lactose in human breast milk an inducer of innate immunity with implications for a role in intestinal homeostasis. *PLoS One* **2013**, *8*, e53876.

305. Jiang, W.; Sunkara, L.T.; Zeng, X.; Deng, Z.; Myers, S.M.; Zhang, G. Differential regulation of human cathelicidin LL-37 by free fatty acids and their analogs. *Peptides* **2013**, *50C*, 129–138.

306. Zeng, X.; Sunkara, L.T.; Jiang, W.; Bible, M.; Carter, S.; Ma, X.; Qiao, S.; Zhang, G. Inductionof porcine host defense peptidegene expression by short-chain fatty acids and their analogs. *PLoS One* **2013**, *8*, e72922.

307. Sherman, H.; Chapnik, N.; Froy, O. Albumin and amino acids upregulate the expression of human beta-defensin 1. *Mol. Immunol.* **2006**, *43*, 1617–1623. [CrossRef]

308. Fehlbaum, P.; Rao, M.; Zasloff, M.; Anderson, G.M. An essential amino acid induces epithelial beta-defensin expression. *Proc. Natl. Acad. Sci. USA* **2000**, *97*, 12723–12728. [CrossRef]

309. Rivas-Santiago, C.E.; Rivas-Santiago, B.; León, D.A.; Castañeda-Delgado, J.; Hernández Pando, R. Induction of β-defensins by l-isoleucine as novel immunotherapy in experimental murine tuberculosis. *Clin. Exp. Immunol.* **2011**, *164*, 80–89. [CrossRef]

310. Pernet, I.; Reymermier, C.; Guezennec, A.; Branka, J.E.; Guesnet, J.; Perrier, E.; Dezutter-Dambuyant, C.; Schmitt, D.; Viac, J. Calcium triggers beta-defensin (hBD-2 and hBD-3) and chemokine macrophage inflammatory protein-3 alpha (MIP-3alpha/CCL20) expression in monolayers of activated human keratinocytes. *Exp. Dermatol.* **2003**, *12*, 755–760. [CrossRef]

311. Talukder, P.; Satho, T.; Irie, K.; Sharmin, T.; Hamady, D.; Nakashima, Y.; Kashige, N.; Miake, F. Trace metal zinc stimulates secretion of antimicrobial peptide LL-37 from Caco-2 cells through ERK and p38 MAP kinase. *Int. Immunopharmacol.* **2011**, *11*, 141–144. [CrossRef]

312. Schauber, J.; Iffland, K.; Frisch, S.; Kudlich, T.; Schmausser, B.; Eck, M.; Menzel, T.; Gostner, A.; Lührs, H.; Scheppach, W. Histone-deacetylase inhibitors induce the cathelicidin LL-37 in gastrointestinal cells. *Mol. Immunol.* **2004**, *41*, 847–854. [CrossRef]

313. Thivierge, K.; Cotton, S.; Schaefer, D.A.; Riggs, M.W.; To, J.; Lund, M.E.; Robinson, M.W.; Dalton, J.P.; Donnelly, S.M. Cathelicidin-like helminth defence molecules (HDMs): Absence of cytotoxic, anti-microbial and anti-protozoan activities imply a specific adaptation to immune modulation. *PLoS Negl. Trop. Dis.* **2013**, *7*, e2307.

314. Yeaman, M.R.; Yount, N.Y. Mechanisms of antimicrobial peptide action and resistance. *Pharmacol. Rev.* **2003**, *55*, 27–55. [CrossRef]

315. Peschel, A. How do bacteria resist human antimicrobial peptides? *Trends Microbiol.* **2002**, *10*, 179–186. [CrossRef]

6

Development and Characterization of a Semi-Solid Dosage Form of Meglumine Antimoniate for Topical Treatment of Cutaneous Leishmaniasis

Diana Berenguer [1], Lilian Sosa [2], Magdalena Alcover [1], Marcella Sessa [2], Lyda Halbaut [2], Carme Guillén [1], Roser Fisa [1], Ana Cristina Calpena-Campmany [2] and Cristina Riera [1,*]

1 Department of Biology, Health and Environment, Laboratory of Parasitology, Faculty of Pharmacy and Food Sciences, University of Barcelona, 08028 Barcelona, Spain; berenguer.diana@gmail.com (D.B.); mmagdalenaalcoveramengual@ub.edu (M.A.); carmeguillen@ub.edu (C.G.); rfisa@ub.edu (R.F.)

2 Department of Pharmaceutical Technology and Physicochemistry, Faculty of Pharmacy and Food Sciences, University of Barcelona, 08028 Barcelona, Spain; liliansosa2012@gmail.com (L.S.); marcellass93@gmail.com (M.S.); halbaut@ub.edu (L.H.); anacalpena@ub.edu (A.C.C.-C.)

* Correspondence: mcriera@ub.edu;

Abstract: Cutaneous leishmaniasis (CL) is treated with painful intralesional injections of meglumine antimoniate (MA). With the aim of developing an alternative topical treatment for CL, a gel-based formulation with 30% MA was prepared and its physicochemical properties, stability and rheological behavior were studied. The following were assessed: drug release on propylene hydrophilic membranes ex vivo human skin permeation, tolerance in healthy volunteers, cytotoxicity in three cell lines and anti-leishmanial activity against *Leishmania infantum* promastigotes and amastigotes. The MA gel formulation was found to have suitable pH, and good spreadability and stability. Low quantities of pentavalent antimony (Sb^V) were observed in release and permeation tests, whereas retention was high in both non-damaged and damaged skin (71,043.69 ± 10,641.57 and 10,728 ± 2254.61 μg/g/cm^2 of Sb^V, respectively). The formulation did not have a toxic effect on the cell lines, and presented lower Sb^V IC_{50} values against amastigotes (15.76 ± 4.81 μg/mL) in comparison with the MA solution. The high amount of drug retained in the skin and the Sb^V IC_{50} values obtained suggest that this semi-solid dosage form has potential as an alternative treatment of CL.

Keywords: *Leishmania infantum*; cutaneous leishmaniasis; meglumine antimoniate; Sepigel 305®; topical treatment

---

1. Introduction

Leishmaniasis is caused by protozoan parasites, including more than 20 *Leishmania* species, and is transmitted through the bites of infected female phlebotomine sandflies. It is a neglected tropical disease that is prevalent in low-income countries [1] and is endemic in 98 countries with tropical, temperate and mild temperate climates, with an estimated 12 million people infected by the disease. There are three types of leishmaniasis: cutaneous (CL), mucocutaneous (MCL) and visceral (VL). The most common form of the disease worldwide is CL, with 0.6–1 million new cases estimated to occur annually [2]. In the Mediterranean area, *Leishmania infantum* is the main species responsible for CL and VL [3]. Depending on the *Leishmania* species involved, manifestations of CL range from self-resolving ulcerative lesions, which may take up to two years to heal, to painful open wounds that leave permanent scars or even disseminate and affect other areas of the body [4].

Treatments proposed for CL depend on the infecting species, patient immunity, as well as the number, sizes and location of lesions, but none of them are universally effective [5]. CL cases presenting small and localized lesions are usually treated with pentavalent antimony salts, sodium stibogluconate or meglumine antimoniate (MA). These first-line drugs are administered by intralesional infiltrations requiring multiple injections that cause acute pain to the extent that patients are often unable to complete the treatment [6]. As it is a common mistake when talking about MA treatments for leishmaniasis to confuse the therapeutic dose that refers to MA with the amount of pentavalent antimony (Sb^V), henceforth we will refer all the concentrations to the amount of Sb^V since it is the main active ingredient.

Consequently, efforts have been made to develop alternative drugs and forms of administration.

According to the World Health Organization (WHO), topical and local therapies with less systemic toxicity (thermotherapy, cryotherapy, paromomycin ointment, local infiltration with antimonials) are good treatment options for patients with a low number of small lesions [7].

Topical treatments have many advantages: they are easy to administer, do not require hospitalization or other infrastructure, favor patient commitment, are low cost and have fewer toxic side effects [8–10].

A widely used treatment is the application of 15% paromomycin ointments in association with 12% methylbenzethonium chloride twice a day for 20 days, although results are variable, and patients experience significant irritation, inflammation, pain and pigmentation [11,12]. Cure rates of around 80% have been obtained in some clinical trials [13,14], whereas others report lower efficiency [15]. Liposomes and a nanogel formulation containing paromomycin have also been developed [6,16,17].

Alternatively, topical conjugates with amphotericin B were reported to penetrate the skin in a murine model [18]. However, the cure rates in a phase II study with topical 3% amphotericin B cream for uncomplicated CL were low and its clinical development as a therapeutic option was discontinued [19].

Clinical trials have also been performed with a topical formulation of miltefosine, but no efficacy against CL has been proven [10] despite experimental trials in mice reporting a reduction in lesion size and full recovery, albeit with relapse [20].

Regarding antimonials, there are few data available on semi-solid dosage forms for topical administration. The development and characterization of liposomes loading sodium stibogluconate and MA has been described [21–23].

Sepigel 305®, a product used in gels and gel-creams, consists of a gelling agent (polyacrylamide), a non-ionic emulsifier (polyoxyethylene 7 lauryl ether) and a fatty oil (isoparaffin). Simple gel formulations containing Sepigel 305® have medium to high viscosity [24], a degree of cooling power, evanescent properties and optimal dermocosmetic qualities. They also allow the incorporation of both hydrophilic and lipophilic substances, and previous studies on different drugs have reported that formulations containing this polymer have good stability [24–26].

In this context, the use of hydrogels could be a promising strategy to deliver MA for the management and healing of CL. The aim of the present study was therefore to design and develop a gel-based formulation containing MA for CL treatment. Physico-chemical parameters were monitored to determine stability over time. Human skin permeation and retention ex vivo and tolerance in vivo were tested to optimize a new dosage system of the drug with fewer side effects. Cytotoxic effects and leishmanicidal activity in vitro were assayed in promastigotes and intracellular amastigotes of *L. infantum*.

2. Materials and Methods

2.1. Materials

Meglumine antimoniate was obtained from Acros Organics (Thermo Fisher Scientific, Waltham, MA, USA). Gentamicin was acquired from Sigma-Aldrich (Darmstadt, Germany), and Sepigel 305® from Acofarma (Barcelona, Spain). Distilled water utilized in the experiments was obtained from a Mili-Q® Plus System (Millipore Co., Burlington, MA, USA).

2.2. Preparation of the Gel

Briefly, a gel-based formulation containing 30% of MA (with 31.6% Sb^V *w/w*) was prepared. MA was dissolved in water with 0.5% of gentamicin. Sepigel 305® was added under continuous stirring to obtain the gel formulation at a concentration of 4.5%.

2.3. Physicochemical Characterization of the MA Gel

2.3.1. Morphological Analysis

To analyze its morphology, the MA gel was dried over a period of 7 days using a vacuum desiccator. Once totally dried, 0.1 g was coated with carbon as a conductive agent. The internal structure of the gel was examined by scanning electron microscopy (SEM) using a JEOL J-7100FE (Peabody, MA, USA).

2.3.2. Swelling and Degradation Tests

A gravimetric method was used to obtain the swelling ratio (SR) and to test degradation, which was represented as the percentage of weight loss (WL). Dried and fresh MA gel were used to carry out the swelling and degradation tests, respectively. In both experiments the MA gel was incubated in PBS (pH = 5.5) at 32 °C for 20 min. Samples ($n = 6$) were removed and weighed after blotting the surface water at predetermined time intervals of 3 min. The SR was calculated using the following equation and expressed by kinetic modeling:

$$SR = \frac{Ws - Wd}{Wd} \quad (1)$$

where Ws is the weight of the swollen MA gel at 3 min intervals for 20 min and Wd is the weight of dried gel.

WL was calculated following the equation and expressed by kinetic modeling:

$$WL\ (\%) = \frac{Wi - Wd}{Wi} \times 100 \quad (2)$$

where Wi is the initial weight of the MA gel and Wd is the gel weight each 3 min.

2.3.3. Water Loss Due to Drying

Water loss was evaluated by weighing 1 g of fresh MA gel, which was placed in a vacuum desiccator for 7 days until the weight was constant.

2.3.4. Porosity Study

The porosity percentage (P) was calculated by a solvent displacement method, which consisted of immersing the previously dried MA gel in absolute ethanol for 2 min and then weighing it after the excess ethanol on the surface was blotted. The porosity percentage was calculated using the following equation:

$$P\ (\%) = \frac{W2 - W1}{\rho \times V} \times 100 \quad (3)$$

where $W1$ represents the weight of the dried MA gel, $W2$ stands for the weight of the MA gel after being immersed in ethanol, ρ is the density of absolute ethanol and V is the volume of the gel.

2.4. Stability Studies

The MA gel was stored at room temperature (RT), 4 °C and 37 °C. The pH values of the formulation were measured with universal test paper (Filter-Lab®) by direct spread of the samples ($n = 3$). Appearance was visually inspected, and pH was measured after 30 days and after 6 months.

Sb^V was quantified by ICP-OES (Inductively coupled plasma-optical emission spectrometry, Perkin Elmer Elan 6000, Waltham, MA, USA) after previous treatment of the samples with HNO_3 and

H_2O_2 in a microwave digester at 220 °C for 72 h. The drug content was evaluated at the beginning and end of the 6-month experiment.

2.5. Rheological Studies

The rheological measurements were performed in duplicate 24 h after gel preparation using a rotational rheometer (Thermo Scientific HaakeRheostress 1, Thermo Fischer Scientific, Karlsruhe, Germany) equipped with a cone plate set-up (0.105 mm gap between cone and plate) with a fixed lower plate and a mobile upper cone Haake C60/2° Ti (60 mm diameter, 2° angle). The rheometer was connected to a temperature control ThermoHaake Phoenix II + Haake C25P (Thermo Fischer Scientific, Waltham, MA, USA) and a computer provided with the HaakeRheowin® Job Manager v. 4.0 (Thermo Fischer Scientific, Waltham, MA, USA) to carry out the tests and HaakeRheowin® Data Manager v.4.0 (Thermo Fischer Scientific) to carry out the analyses of the obtained data. Viscosity curves ($\eta = f(\dot{\gamma})$) and flow curves ($\tau = f(\dot{\gamma})$) were recorded at 25 °C. The shear rate ramp program included: a ramp-up period from 0 to 50 s^{-1} for 3 min; constant shear rate period of 50 s^{-1} for 1 min; and a ramp-down period from 50 to 0 s^{-1} for 3 min. The data from the flow curves ($\tau = f(\dot{\gamma})$) were fitted to different mathematical models equations: Newton, Bingham, Ostwald-de-Waele, Herschel-Bulkley, Casson and Cross [27]. Best fit of mathematical models was based on the correlation coefficient value (r). The viscosity mean value (Pa·s) was determined from the constant share section at 50 s^{-1}.

2.6. Spreadability Test

The spreadability of MA gel and MA solution was determined in triplicate as follows: 0.5 g of formulation and 150 μL of MA solution were placed within 1 cm diameter circles previously marked on a glass plate, and also on a plastic plate. A series of weights (5, 10, 20, 50 and 100 g) were successively added and allowed to rest for 2 min each at RT. The diameters (cm^2) of the circle spreads were measured and recorded as comparative values.

2.7. In Vitro Release Studies

Vertical Franz diffusion cells (FDC 400; Crown Glass, Somerville, NJ, USA) were used to assay the MA release with hydrophilic polypropylene membranes (GH Polypro, Life Sciences). The receptor medium was water at 32 ± 0.5 °C under stirring at 600 rpm in sink conditions. The experiment was performed with a diffusion area of 0.64 cm^2. Small quantities of MA gels (0.3 g) or MA solution (300 μL) were added to the donor compartment. At the end of the study at 55 h, the amount of Sb^V in the receptor compartment was analyzed by ICP-OES (Perkin Elmer Elan 6000). Results were reported as the mean ± SD of five replicates.

2.8. Ex Vivo Permeation Studies

Ex vivo permeation tests were performed as described in Section 2.7 using damaged and non-damaged human skin samples with a thickness of 400 μm from a single donor. The skin was damaged using the tape stripping technique, which involves repeated application of adhesive tapes to the skin surface to remove stratum corneum layers. For the assay, adhesive tapes were applied to the skin 7 times to damage the skin but not remove it completely. Then 0.3 g of MA gel was placed in the donor compartment. After 27 h the quantity of Sb^V was determined by ICP-OES in five replicates.

To determine the amount of drug retained in the epidermal tegument, the skin membranes were detached from the Franz cells, cleaned with gauze soaked in 0.05% sodium dodecylsulphate solution and washed in distilled water. The area of permeation was then cut and weighed. Finally, the Sb^V retained was extracted in an ultrasound bath with water for 30 min. The resulting solutions were measured by ICP-OES for quantification.

The Plastic Surgery Department of Barcelona-SCIAS Hospital (Barcelona, Spain) provided the human skin from the abdominal region of a healthy woman, and the Bioethics Committee of the same hospital approved the experimental protocol (reference number: BEC/001/16; date: 15 January 2016).

Written informed consent forms were provided. Human skin was dermatomed (GA630 dermatome, Aesculap, Tuttlingen, Germany) into pieces with a thickness of 400 μm [28]. The integrity of skin samples was assessed in triplicate by measuring the trans-epidermal water loss (TEWL) values using a DermaLab® module (Cortex Technology, Hadsund, Denmark).

2.9. *In Vivo Tolerance Study*

Ten female volunteers with healthy skin between 25 and 35 years old participated in the study. The study was approved by the Ethics Committee of the University of Barcelona (reference number: IRB00003099; date: 20 March 2018) following the guidelines of the Declaration of Helsinki [29] and all volunteers signed written informed consent forms. Skin-care cosmetics were not permitted on the test areas for two days prior to the study. Volunteers stayed in the test room for at least 30 min prior to the measurements. Measurements were performed before applying the gel (to establish the baseline readings) and 15 min, 1 h and 2 h after the application of 0.5 g on the flexor side of the left forearm.

Trans epidermal water loss (TEWL), referring to the total amount of water vapor lost through the skin was measured by a Tewameter® TM 300 (Courage-Khazaka electronic GmbH, Cologne, Germany). The stratum corneum hydration (SCH) was determined using a Corneometer® CM 825 (Courage-Khazaka electronic GmbH). Measurements were performed according to international guidelines [30].

2.10. *Parasite Strains and Cultures*

The *Leishmania infantum* strain MHOM/ES/2016/CATB101 isolated from an individual with CL from Mallorca (Spain) was used. Promastigotes were cultured at 26 °C in Schneider insect medium, pH 7.0, with 20% heat-inactivated fetal calf serum, 25 μg/mL gentamicin solution (Sigma G-1397, St. Louis, MO, USA), and 1% penicillin (100 U/mL)-streptomycin (100 mg/mL) solution (Sigma P4333).

2.11. *In Vitro Cytotoxicity Assay*

In order to study the cytotoxicity of the MA gel and the gel excipients, 5×10^4 cells/mL of the cell lines RAW 264.7, J774A.1 and HaCaT were cultured in 96-well plates (Costar 3595). Serial dilutions of the gel in RPMI-1640 medium with 10% heat-inactivated fetal calf serum and 1% penicillin (100 U/mL)-streptomycin (100 mg/mL) were added. After 24 h of incubation at 37 °C in a 5% CO_2 atmosphere, WST-1 reagent (Roche Diagnostics GmbH, Mannheim, Germany) was added to each well and the plate was incubated in the same conditions for 4 h. The absorbance of the samples was measured at 450 nm using a spectrophotometer (Multiskan EX, Thermo Electron Corporation, Shanghai, China). The concentration inhibiting 50% of cell viability (CC_{50}) was determined by linear regression analysis and experiments were performed in triplicate [31].

2.12. *In Vitro Anti-Leishmanial Activity against Promastigotes*

The activity of MA gel, gel alone and MA solution was studied on promastigotes in microtiter plates (Costar 3595). Serial dilutions of the gel in Schneider medium were seeded, and then 10^6 promastigotes/mL in their logarithmic growth phase were added to each well and incubated at 26 °C for 48 h. Growth was measured through acid phosphatase and the optical density was determined at 405 nm with a spectrophotometer (Multiskan EX, Thermo Electron Corporation). The concentration inhibiting 50% of parasite growth (IC_{50}) was determined by linear regression analysis of the minimum squares of parasitic growth versus the logarithm of the drug concentration with 95% confidence interval. Experiments were performed in triplicate [32].

2.13. *In Vitro Anti-Leishmanial Activity against Intracellular Amastigotes*

J774A.1 cells at a concentration of 5×10^4 cells/mL were cultured in an eight LabTek chamber slide system (Nunc®). After 24 h, late stationary phase promastigotes from a 5-day culture in RPMI-1640 complete medium with 10% heat-inactivated fetal calf serum and 1% penicillin (100 U/mL)-streptomycin (100 mg/mL) were added at a concentration of 5×10^5 cells/mL and incubated for 24 h at 37 °C in 5% CO_2 atmosphere. Free promastigotes were removed by washing. RPMI-1640 complete medium with serial dilutions of the gel was added to each well and incubated at 37 °C in 5% CO_2 atmosphere for 48 h. Infected cells were washed and slides were stained with Giemsa. Drug activity was evaluated by counting the number of infected cells by examining 300 macrophages in triplicate [33].

2.14. Statistical Analysis

Experimental data obtained were analyzed by one-way parametric analysis of variance (ANOVA), followed by a multiple comparison Tukey test. A $p < 0.05$ indicated the differences were statistically significant. Prism® V. 5 (GraphPad Software Inc., San Diego, CA, USA) was used for calculations.

3. Results

3.1. Physicochemical Characterization of the MA Gel

As shown in Figure 1A,B, SEM revealed a laminar disposition in the gel formulation. The layers were regularly organized and a porous structure was evident.

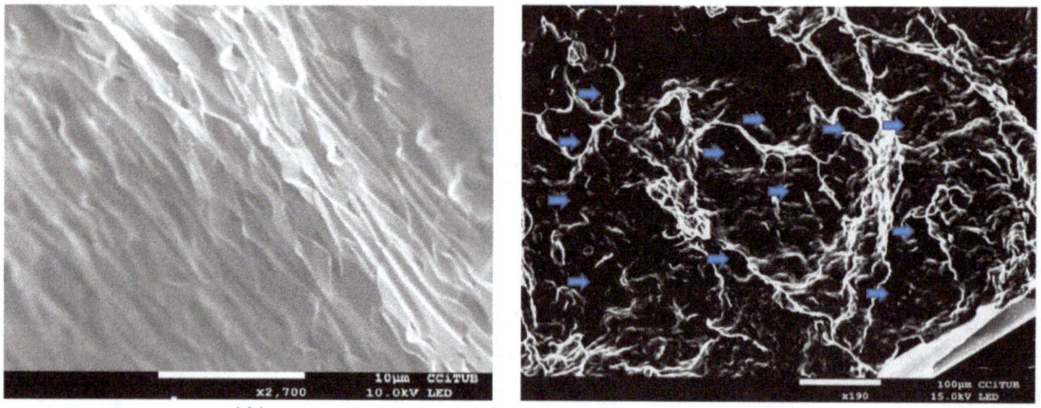

(A) (B)

Figure 1. SEM images of the meglumine antimoniate (MA) gel, (**A**) laminar disposition (2700×) and (**B**) porous structure (190×).

The swelling process of MA gel followed a hyperbolic model, which was represented by the kinetic constants $k = 0.64\ min^{-1}$ ($r^2 = 0.9986$) (Figure 2A). The degradation of MA gel was completed in 15 min and followed a one phase exponential model with a kinetic constant $k = 0.01\ min^{-1}$ ($r^2 = 0.9995$) (Figure 2B), and the P percentage of MA gel was ~89.37 ± 0.15%.

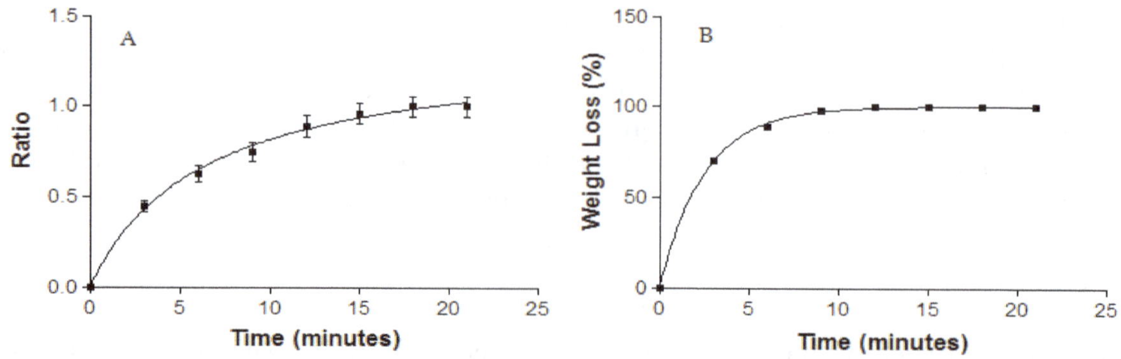

Figure 2. (**A**) Swelling ratio and (**B**) percentage of weight loss in the degradation of MA gel.

After 7 days of drying the gel, the sample showed 22 ± 2.13% loss of water content.

3.2. Drug Quantification and Stability Studies

Determination of the drug content revealed 72.7% entrapment efficiency of Sb^V in the gel formulation. The concentration of Sb^V in the reference solution and in the gel over time is summarized in Table 1. The Sb^V content of the gel samples at the tested temperatures did not present statistical differences ($p > 0.05$) after 6 months (Figure 3).

Table 1. Concentration of Sb^V and SD in the reference solution and MA gel samples at the beginning of the experiment and 6 months later at different storage temperatures (t_0 = initial time; t_{180} = after 6 months).

Formulations	Sb^V (µg/mL) ± SD			
	t_0	t_{180} RT	t_{180} 37 °C	t_{180} 4 °C
MA solution	79,659.92 ± 1023.45			
MA gel	57,936.62 ± 894.92	57,436.62 ± 854.92	58,575.93 ± 654.07	59,255.83 ± 524.49

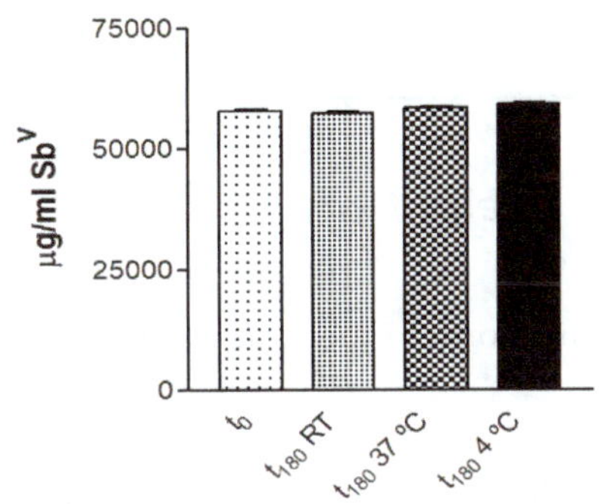

Figure 3. Concentration of Sb^V in the gel at different storage temperatures at the beginning of the experiment and 6 months later.

The MA gel had a pH value of 5–6 at the beginning and end of the experiment.

When freshly prepared, the gel formulation was a semi-transparent white with homogeneous appearance without precipitates. After 30 days at RT and 4 °C, the formulation had the same appearance as at the beginning of the experiment, whereas at 37 °C it turned yellow. After 6 months at 4 °C it looked the same as at the beginning of the experiment, while at RT it was a semi-transparent light yellow and at 37 °C a semi-transparent dark yellow.

3.3. Rheological Studies

The MA gel formulation exhibited pseudoplastic behavior (Cross model; $r^2 = 0.9997$) (Figure 4A). Viscosity at 50 s^{-1} was 677.8 ± 1.76 mPa·s, and it was non-thixotropic. The MA solution showed Newtonian behavior (Newton model; $r^2 = 0.9967$) (Figure 4B) and viscosity at 50 s^{-1} was 2.67 ± 0.06 mPa·s.

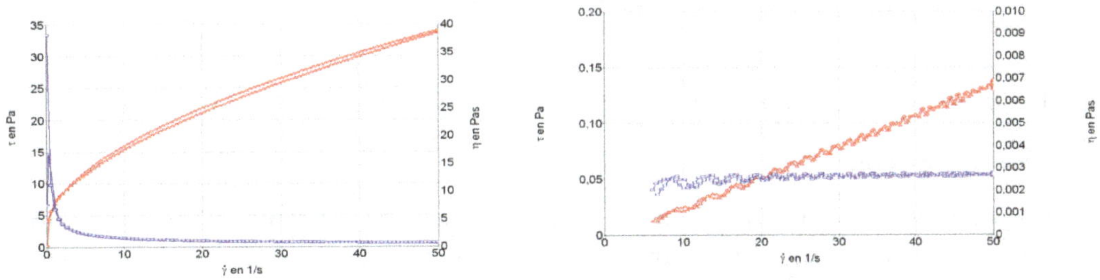

(A) (B)

Figure 4. Rheological behavior of (**A**) MA gel and (**B**) MA solution.

3.4. Spreadability Test

The equation that best fitted the spreadability behavior of the MA gel and solution followed a first-order kinetic model [$S = S_{max} \times (1 - \exp(-k \times W))$], where S is the extension surface (cm^2), S_{max} is the maximum extension surface (cm^2), k is the kinetic constant (g^{-1}) and W is the weight added (g). The resulting graphics and equations are shown in Figure 5. Spreadability of the MA gel increased as more weight was applied, until a maximum value was reached.

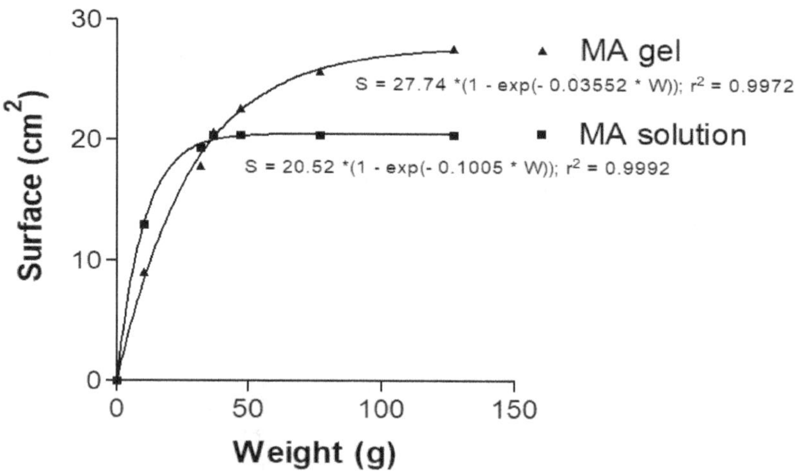

Figure 5. Spreadability graphic and first-order kinetic model equations for the MA gel and MA solution.

3.5. In Vitro Release Studies

After 55 h the amount of Sb^V released in the receptor compartment through the hydrophilic polypropylene membranes was 13,646.53 ± 960.63 μg/cm^2 of Sb^V for MA solution and 9081.13 ± 1446.20 μg/cm^2 of Sb^V for the gel, corresponding to a release of 32.3 ± 3.56% and 21.5 ± 3.43%, respectively, from the total amount seeded. The differences ($p < 0.01$) between the Sb^V released from the solution and the gel are statistically significant (Figure 6).

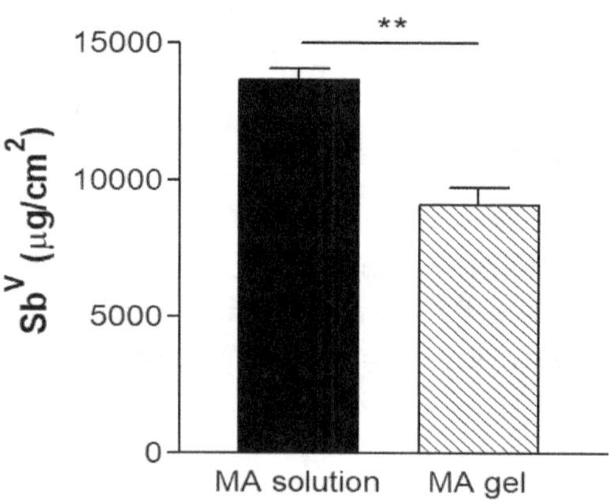

Figure 6. Flux of Sb^V released after 55 h through hydrophilic polypropylene membranes (** $p < 0.01$).

3.6. Ex Vivo Permeation Studies

Table 2 summarizes the amount of Sb^V permeated (μg/cm^2) through the skin and the amount retained (μg/g/cm^2). In both permeation and retention assays, higher Sb^V values were obtained for non-damaged than damaged skin when testing the reference solution and the MA gel. The percentage of Sb^V in the reference solution and MA gel that permeated through the healthy skin was 7.03 ± 1.23% and 2.89 ± 0.83%, and through the damaged skin 0.29 ± 0.51% and 1.84 ± 0.65%, respectively.

Table 2. Sb^V permeation across the skin barrier and Sb^V retained after 27 h in damaged and non-damaged skin.

Assay	MA Solution		MA Gel	
	Non-Damaged Skin	Damaged Skin	Non-Damaged Skin	Damaged Skin
Permeation (µg/cm^2) ± SD	2966.50 ± 562.37	121.00 ± 59.45	1217.53 ± 279.41	774.81 ± 179.63
Retention in skin (µg/g/cm^2) ± SD	51,672.84 ± 8964.28	2057.47 ± 381.67	71,043.69 ± 10,641.57	10,728.23 ± 2254.61

3.7. *In Vivo Tolerance Study*

The results for the TEWL and SCH are shown in Figure 7. The MA solution decreased the TEWL with statistically significant differences for all of the experiment times (Figure 7A). The MA gel increased the TEWL after 15 min, and basal values were almost recovered after 1 h, with statistically significant differences between 15 min and 60 min, and between 15 min and 120 min (Figure 7C). As the graph shows, significant differences in SCH values were found when comparing baseline values with all the experiment times for both formulations, revealing the dehydration of the stratum corneum and its slow gradual recovery (Figure 7B,D).

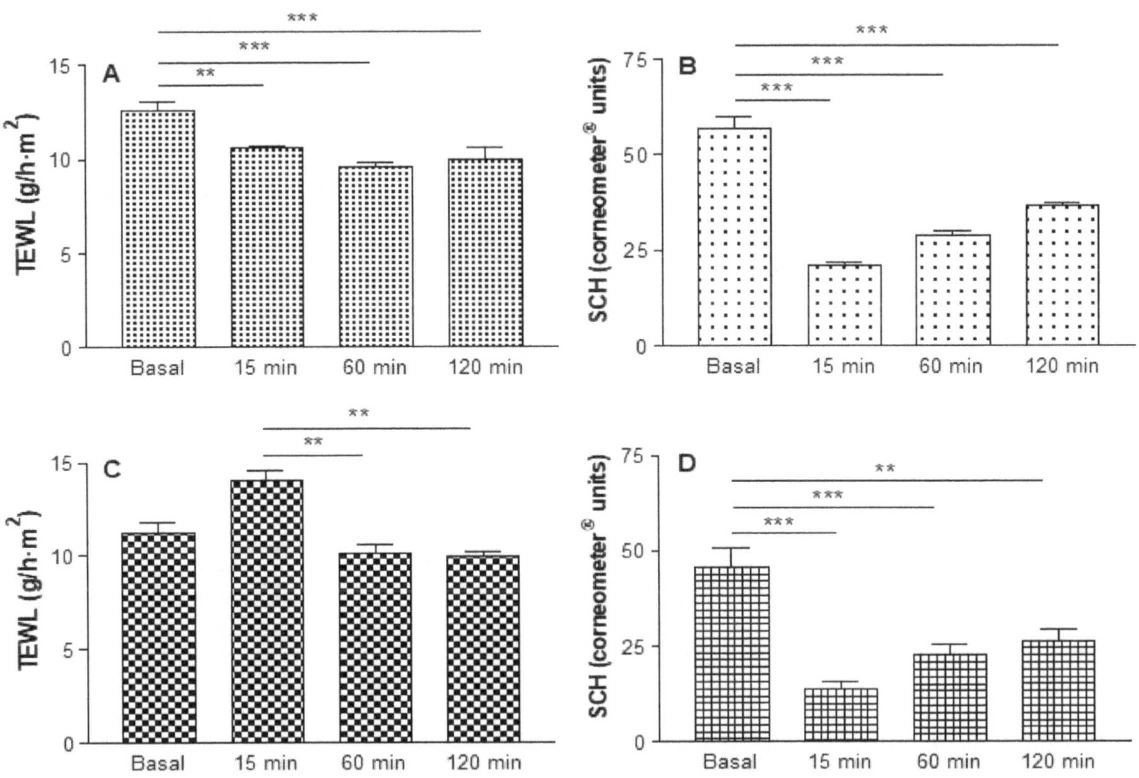

Figure 7. Measurements of biomechanical parameters of skin for 2 h after application of the gel and solution. (**A**) Change in trans-epidermal water loss (TEWL) and (**B**) Stratum corneum hydration (SCH) values after application of MA solution. (**C**) Change in TEWL and (**D**) SCH values after application of MA gel (** $p < 0.01$; *** $p < 0.001$).

3.8. *In Vitro Cytotoxicity Assay*

Figures 8 and 9 show the cytotoxic effects on the cell lines assayed. No cytotoxicity was observed in the keratinocyte cell line HaCaT at the ranges of dilution tested. The gel formulation with and without MA showed cytotoxicity in the RAW264.7 and J774A.1 cell lines only at the highest concentrations of the gelling excipients and Sb^V assayed. The CC_{50} of the MA gel and the gel alone are summarized in Tables 3 and 4.

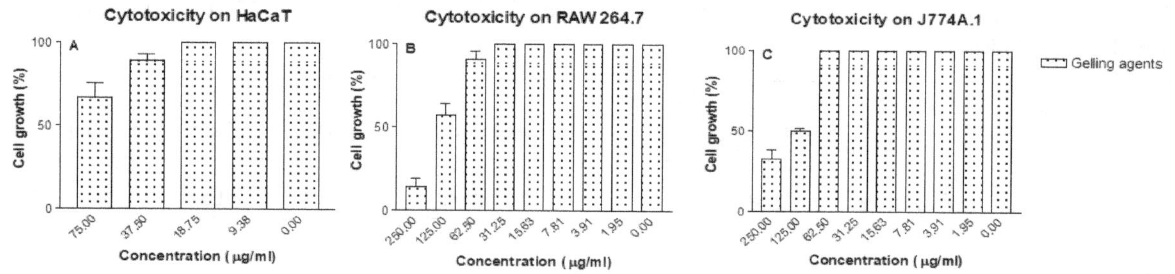

Figure 8. Cytotoxicity of the gelling excipients in cell lines (**A**) HaCaT, (**B**) RAW 264.7 and (**C**) J774A.1.

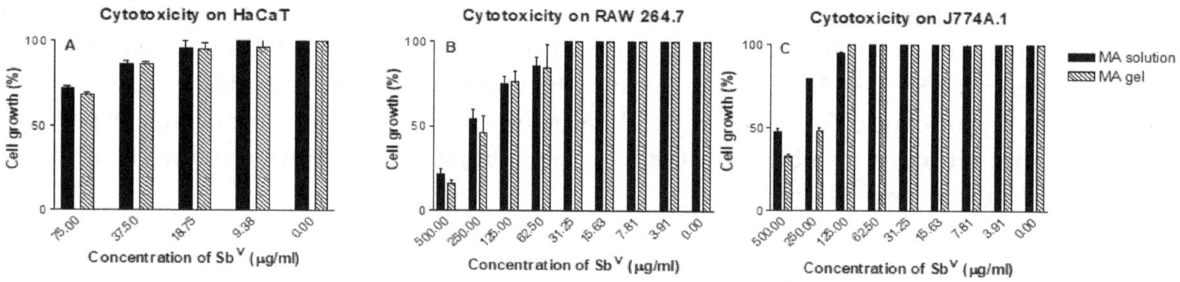

Figure 9. Cytotoxicity of MA solution and MA gel in cell lines (**A**) HaCaT, (**B**) RAW 264.7 and (**C**) J774A.1.

Table 3. In vitro activity against promastigotes and amastigotes, and cytotoxicity of the reference MA solution and the MA gel and selectivity index (SI).

Formulations (µg/mL Sb^V)	IC_{50} (µg/mL Sb^V ± SD)		SI		CC_{50} (µg/mL Sb^V ± SD)	
	Promastigotes	Amastigotes	SI_{RAW}	SI_{J774}	RAW 264.7	J774A.1
MA solution	>750 (* na)	57.35 ± 2.76	6.66	6.37	381.76 ± 94.74	365.14 ± 165.26
MA gel	633.15 ± 43.26 (* na)	15.76 ± 4.81	14.19	14.03	223.66 ± 46.82	221.05 ± 65.41

* na: not active.

Table 4. In vitro activity against promastigotes and amastigotes, and cytotoxicity of the gel alone and selectivity index (SI).

Excipients	IC_{50} (µg/mL ± SD)		SI		CC_{50} (µg/mL ± SD)	
	Promastigotes	Amastigotes	SI_{RAW}	SI_{J774}	RAW 264.7	J774A.1
Gelling agents (375–0.37 µg/mL)	>375	20.39 ± 5.43	6.57	6.13	134.00 ± 42.57	125.00 ± 20.80

3.9. Anti-Leishmanial In Vitro Activity against Promastigotes

The effects of the MA solution and MA gel are summarized in Table 3, and Table 4 shows the effect of the gel without the drug. Neither the MA gel nor the gel alone were able to inhibit the growth of *L. infantum* promastigotes, with Sb^V IC_{50} values of 633.15 ± 43.26 µg/mL (0.70% of gel) for the MA gel and IC_{50} values greater than 375 µg/mL (0.71% of gel) for the gel alone.

3.10. Anti-Leishmanial In Vitro Activity against Intracellular Amastigotes

The activity of the MA solution and MA gel is summarized in Table 3. In the amastigote assay the MA gel presented lower Sb^V IC_{50} values (15.76 ± 4.81 µg/mL) in comparison with the MA solution (57.35 ± 2.76 µg/mL). As shown in Table 4, the gelling excipients showed some activity against the amastigotes of *L. infantum*. Figure 10 shows the images of control infected macrophages and infected macrophages treated with MA gel.

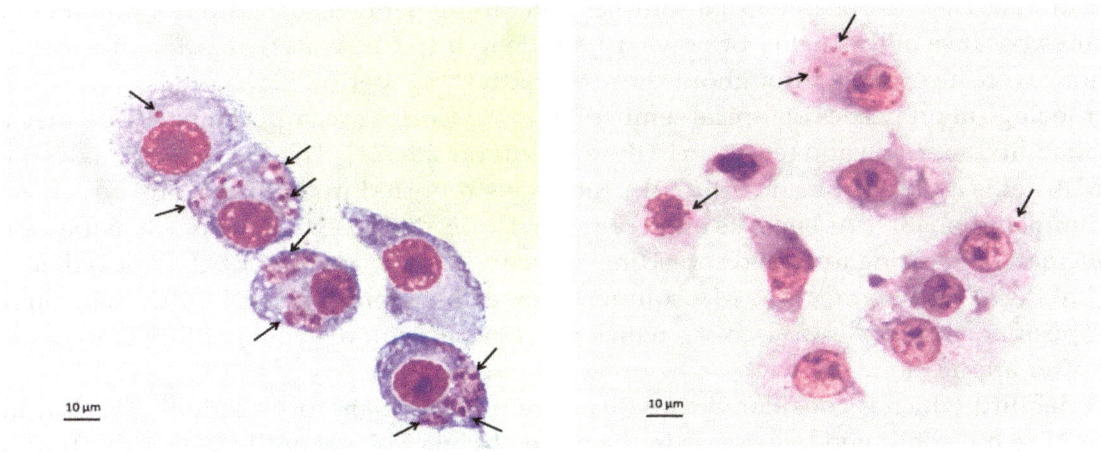

Figure 10. Effect of the MA gel on the infection of J774A.1 macrophages with *L. infantum*. (**A**) Infected and untreated control cultures. (**B**) Cultures treated with 15.63 µg/mL of Sb^V of the MA gel. Amastigotes are indicated by arrows.

4. Discussion

The development of an effective topical treatment for CL is an interesting but difficult challenge. One of the main problems in topical administration is that *Leishmania* amastigotes are localized within dermal macrophages, in the papillary dermis beneath the epidermis [34]. Thus, after the drug is released from the vehicle, it must cross the stratum corneum in the skin barrier and reach the macrophages to deliver the pharmacological action.

In this study, we developed a Sepigel 305®-based formulation for the dermal delivery of MA with qualities that could enhance the activity of MA against CL with minimal side effects.

The water content in the MA gel formulation represented almost a quarter of its composition. Degradation was constant over time, indicating it did not depend on the remaining polymer concentration, and the process was completed in 15 min. The very high porosity percentage of the MA gel was corroborated by SEM images, which also revealed a regular laminar disposition in the superficial structure of the gel layers. The porous structure, similar to that described by Dong et al. (2015) [35], allows the drug to be released when applied on membranes or skin.

The pH plays an important role in the stability of gels as well as in skin tolerability, and should be between 5 and 6 for skin formulations [26]. The tested formulation maintained a pH of 5–6 throughout the experiment, indicating biocompatibility for skin applications, with minimal risk of irritation or bacterial or fungal infection [36]. Anchisi et al. (2001) studied the stability of a wide range of formulations containing the same gel base over 6 months, and observed minimal changes in the pH [24].

At the beginning of the experiment the quantity of Sb^V found in the gel was 57,936.62 µg/mL, 27.3% less than in the reference solution consisting of MA in water. This reduction may be explained by incomplete digestion during the analytical procedure, considering the high quantity of organic material, which may mask the actual amount of Sb^V. The stability test indicated that the amount of Sb^V in the gels remained constant for 6 months at all the tested storage temperatures, although the organoleptic characteristics varied. Samples stored at 4 °C retained the same visual properties throughout the 6 months (a homogeneous semi-transparent white appearance), whereas samples stored at RT turned pale yellow in the third month, and at 37 °C they turned yellow after the first month. This change in color may be due to meglumine oxidation with increasing temperature. Gel homogeneity was observed in all samples, without any biphasic formation.

When comparing different topical formulations, Bilia et al. (2006) found the best long-term stability with polyacrylamide, C13-14 isoparaffin and laureth-7 [25]. Similar results were reported by

Anchisi et al. (2001), who observed that samples containing Sepigel 305® did not polymerize at high temperatures because of the ability of polyacrylamide to trap free water; organoleptic features of the formulations were also stable throughout the six-month study period [24].

The rheological properties of topical semi-solid dosage forms are important because they influence skin spreadability, adhesion and retention in the application site [21]. The rheological analysis indicated that the MA gel is a pseudoplastic fluid, like most gels reported in the literature, which is ideal for topical administration [37]. As such, its main characteristic is decreased viscosity when the deformation speed is increased, resulting in a good spreading capacity. The pseudoplastic behavior is determined by the cross linking of the polymer. The MA solution showed Newtonian behavior due to its predominant water composition and very low viscosity, which makes it difficult to avoid spilling or to maintain skin adhesion after application.

Spreadability, which is considered a quality parameter for skin formulations, was lost in the MA solution at 37 g, but continued to increase in the more viscous MA gel until 127 g, indicating its ease of application (see rheograms in Figure 4A,B).

The profile of drug release from the delivery vehicle can be useful for predicting in vivo behavior of the product. At 55 h, drug release from the formulation was incomplete: only 32.3 ± 3.56% of Sb^V from the MA solution and 21.5 ± 3.43% from the MA gel had been released. This was probably due to the large amount of sample located in the donor compartment, the slow release of the drug from the gel, and the chemical binding of the meglumine.

In addition, the permeation study performed with damaged and healthy human skin showed very low amounts of Sb^V in the receptor compartment at 27 h for both the MA solution and MA gel. The percentage of permeation was higher through healthy skin than damaged skin with both vehicles. In the retention study, the drug in the skin was determined in terms of μg of Sb^V per g and cm^2 of skin. Higher Sb^V retention values were obtained for the MA gel when the skin was undamaged, probably due to better functioning and ability to absorb more drug. The same behavior was observed for the MA solution, although a lower amount of Sb^V was detected. Similar results were obtained by Dar et al. (2018), who tested nano-deformable liposomes with sodium stibogluconate and the same liposomes in a Carbopol gel on rat skin, and observed a low percentage of Sb^V permeated into the receptor compartment and a high percentage was retained in the skin [21]. Other studies with liposomes encapsulating MA, MA combined with oleic acid and MA plus stearylamine also showed low permeation of Sb^V across the skin barrier and high retention in mouse skin [22,23]. Bilia et al. (2006) found the highest amounts of sesquiterpenes retained in stripped skin when using a mixture of polyacrylamide, C13-14 isoparaffin and laureth-7 and other excipients, since the level of lipophilicity enhanced the permeation compared with other topical delivery systems [25].

Most substances penetrate the skin through the transepidermic route, mainly across the spaces between cells [38]. The level of penetration depends essentially on two coefficients: that of the vehicle-skin partition and the diffusion. Small molecules are able to cross the skin more easily [39], while highly lipophilic molecules can be retained in the stratum corneum [40]. The drug of our formulation may cross the skin through the intercellular route, as MA is a small molecule (MW: 365.98 g/mol), thereby allowing proper diffusion despite its hydrophilicity. In the permeation experiments, we found lower Sb^V values in the damaged skin than when it was not. This indicates that stratum corneum plays an important role as a drug reservoir that allows a slow release, as we could detect Sb^V in the receptor compartment. Regarding the new formulation, the low permeation of Sb^V to the receptor compartment through the skin barrier, and retention of sufficient quantities of Sb^V in the damaged skin after 27 h suggests the drug could remain in the skin layers where leishmania parasites are located.

In relation to biomechanical properties, the MA solution maintained TEWL values below 12 $g/h{\cdot}m^2$, which is considered normal, and the integrity of the stratum corneum was not affected. The slight decreasing pattern observed could be due to an occlusive effect of the solution. The solution also caused a loss of water in the skin but with a tendency to recover after 1 h. When applying the MA gel, an increase in water loss from the stratum corneum was observed 15 min after the application, pointing to an alteration in the constitution of the skin. However, within one hour the basal values were recovered, which indicated the alterations were reversible. When using gels containing polymers with a high capacity to capture water, the skin hydration is strongly affected and water is lost from the stratum corneum. In the current study, this effect was marked at 15 min, followed by a slow gradual recuperation of hydration over the next 2 h. The application of the MA gel did not induce any visual skin irritation and was well tolerated by all the individuals participating in the study, none of whom reported pain or any inconveniences from its administration.

At the highest concentrations tested, the gel formulation with or without MA showed cytotoxicity effects on the RAW 264.7 and J774A.1 cell lines. Cytotoxicity in the macrophage cell lines was similar for all the compounds tested, indicating a similar resistance to the excipients and the MA in the formulation.

The in vitro anti-leishmanial activity on intracellular amastigotes showed the MA gel inhibited amastigote survival to a greater extent than the MA solution. Analysis of the selectivity index (SI) showed higher SI values for the MA gel formulation than for the MA solution, which indicated that the gel was less toxic and with higher activity against the parasite.

Interestingly, the amount of Sb^V retained in damaged and undamaged skin was greater when the gel formulation was applied compared to the solution, which makes it more advantageous for therapeutic application. These skin retention values, as well as the IC_{50} results against amastigotes (Table 3) and considering the density of the hydrated skin (0.964 g/mL) [41], indicate that the new MA gel formulation could provide high local amounts of Sb^V, even in damaged skin, and may exert an efficient action against CL. Future experiments in an animal model need to be performed to confirm our preliminary results and determine the efficacy in vivo.

5. Conclusions

We have developed an easy to prepare topical MA gel-based formulation, an administration route that avoids injections and has higher patient acceptance and tolerability. It was shown to be stable for at least 6 months and has optimal properties for use in CL treatment: a biocompatible pH, easy spreadability and no skin irritant effects.

Experiments showed low permeation of the Sb^V through the skin, which would represent a low concentration of the drug in blood, and high retention in the skin layers. Thus, the gel formulation almost completely avoids the toxic side effects of Sb^V and could supply a therapeutic level of MA at the local site for an extended period.

Low cytotoxicity in the keratinocyte cell line and the two macrophages cell lines was observed. The study of anti-leishmanial activity in intracellular amastigotes treated with the MA gel showed a reduction of the IC_{50} in comparison to the reference solution. These preliminary results indicate the MA formulation could be a promising alternative for CL treatment, although further studies are required to establish a proper dosage schedule in vivo.

Author Contributions: D.B. carried out and analyzed the experiments and wrote the original draft of the manuscript. L.S. conceptualized the idea, carried out the swelling, degradation and porosity tests, and edited the manuscript. M.A. and C.G. collaborated in the preparation of the parasitology experiments. M.S. carried out and analyzed the experiments. L.H. directed the rheological tests. R.F. reviewed the manuscript. A.C.C.-C. conceptualized the idea of the investigation and validated and supervised the biopharmaceutical results. C.R. conceptualized the idea, validated and supervised the parasitology experiments, reviewed and edited the manuscript.

Acknowledgments: The authors would like to thank the University of Barcelona for the financial support to cover the cost of open access publication. We appreciate the help of Silvia Tebar for the preparation of culture mediums. We would like to thank the group of Josefa Badia, and specially Rodrigo Vera for helping us with the assay on keratinocyte cell line. We value the contribution of Joan Garcias for his expertise in dermatology. Additionally, thanks to Lucy Brzoska for the revision of the use of the English language.

References

1. Weng, H.B.; Chen, H.X.; Wang, M.W. Innovation in neglected tropical disease drug discovery and development. *Infect. Dis. Poverty* **2018**, *7*, 67–76. [CrossRef] [PubMed]
2. Alvar, J.; Vélez, I.D.; Bern, C.; Herrero, M.; Desjeux, P.; Cano, J.; Janin, J.; den Boer, M.; WHO Leishmaniasis Control Team. Leishmaniasis worldwide and global estimates of its incidence. *PLoS ONE* **2012**, *7*, e35671. [CrossRef] [PubMed]
3. Alcover, M.M.; Rocamora, V.; Guillén, M.C.; Berenguer, D.; Cuadrado, M.; Riera, C.; Fisa, R. Case Report: Diffuse Cutaneous Leishmaniasis by *Leishmania infantum* in a Patient Undergoing Immunosuppressive Therapy: Risk Status in an Endemic Mediterranean Area. *Am. J. Trop. Med. Hyg.* **2018**, *98*, 1313–1316. [CrossRef] [PubMed]
4. Rajni, E.; Ghiya, B.C.; Singh, S.; Shankar, P.; Swami, T.; Jadon, D.S.; Negi, S.R.; Malik, M.; Khatri, P.K. Cutaneous leishmaniasis in Bikaner, India: Clinicoepidemiological profile; parasite identification using conventional, molecular methods and CL Detect^{TM} rapid test, a new Food and Drug Administration-approved test. *Trop. Parasitol.* **2019**, *9*, 115–123. [CrossRef] [PubMed]
5. Olliaro, P.; Vaillant, M.; Arana, B.; Grogl, M.; Modabber, F.; Magill, A.; Lapujade, O.; Buffet, P.; Alvar, J. Methodology of Clinical Trials Aimed at Assessing Interventions for Cutaneous Leishmaniasis. *PLoS Negl. Trop. Dis.* **2013**, *7*, e2130. [CrossRef] [PubMed]
6. Jaafari, M.R.; Bavarsad, N.; Fazly-Bazzaz, B.S.; Samiei, A.; Soroush, D.; Ghorbani, S.; Lotfi-Heravi, M.M.; Khamesipour, A. Effect of Topical Liposomes Containing Paromomycin Sulfate in the Course of *Leishmania major* Infection in Susceptible BALB/c Mice. *Antimicrob. Agents Chemother.* **2009**, *53*, 2259–2265. [CrossRef]
7. Royal Society of Chemistry. Available online: https://doi.org/10.1039/9781788010177-00001 (accessed on 9 October 2019).
8. Trinconi, C.T.; Reimao, J.Q.; Bonano, V.I.; Espada, C.R.; Miguel, D.C.; Yokoyama-Yasunaka, J.K.U.; Uliana, S.R.B. Topical tamoxifen in the therapy of cutaneous leishmaniasis. *Parasitology* **2018**, *145*, 490–496. [CrossRef]
9. Alexandrino-Junior, F.; Silva, K.G.H.E.; Freire, M.C.L.C.; Lione, V.O.F.; Cardoso, E.A.; Marcelina, H.R.; Genre, J.; Oliveira, A.G.; Egito, E.S.T.D. A Functional Wound Dressing as a Potential Treatment for Cutaneous Leishmaniasis. *Pharmaceutics* **2019**, *11*, 200. [CrossRef]
10. Garnier, T.; Croft, S.L. Topical treatment for cutaneous leishmaniasis. *Curr. Opin. Investig. Drugs* **2002**, *3*, 538–544.
11. Zur, E. Topical Treatment of Cutaneous Leishmaniasis in Israel, Part 1. *Int. J. Pharm. Compd.* **2019**, *23*, 200–207.
12. El-On, J.; Livshin, R.; Even-Paz, Z.; Hamburger, D.; Weinrauch, L. Topical treatment of cutaneous leishmaniasis. *J. Investig. Dermatol.* **1986**, *87*, 284–288. [CrossRef] [PubMed]
13. Ben Salah, A.; Ben Messaoud, N.; Guedri, E.; Zaatour, A.; Ben Alaya, N.; Bettaieb, J.; Gharbi, A.; Belhadj Hamida, N.; Boukthir, A.; Chlif, S.; et al. Topical paromomycin with or without gentamicin for cutaneous leishmaniasis. *N. Engl. J. Med.* **2013**, *368*, 524–532. [CrossRef] [PubMed]
14. Sosa, N.; Pascale, J.M.; Jiménez, A.I.; Norwood, J.A.; Kreishman-Detrick, M.; Weina, P.J.; Lawrence, K.; McCarthy, W.F.; Adams, R.C.; Scott, C.; et al. Topical paromomycin for New World cutaneous leishmaniasis. *PLoS Negl. Trop. Dis.* **2019**, *13*, e0007253. [CrossRef] [PubMed]
15. Soto, J.; Fuya, P.; Herrera, R.; Berman, J. Topical paromomycin/methylbenzethonium chloride plus parenteral meglumine antimoniate as treatment for American cutaneous leishmaniasis: Controlled study. *Clin. Infect. Dis.* **1998**, *26*, 56–58. [CrossRef]
16. Carneiro, G.; Santos, D.C.; Oliveira, M.C.; Fernandes, A.P.; Ferreira, L.S.; Ramaldes, G.A.; Nunan, E.A.; Ferreira, L.A. Topical delivery and in vivo antileishmanial activity of paromomycin-loaded liposomes for treatment of cutaneous leishmaniasis. *J. Liposome Res.* **2010**, *20*, 16–23. [CrossRef]
17. Brugués, A.P.; Naveros, B.C.; Calpena Campmany, A.C.; Pastor, P.H.; Saladrigas, R.F.; Lizandra, C.R. Developing cutaneous applications of paromomycin entrapped in stimuli-sensitive block copolymer nanogel dispersions. *Nanomedicine (Lond.)* **2015**, *10*, 227–240. [CrossRef]
18. Frankenburg, S.; Glick, D.; Klaus, S.; Barenholz, Y. Efficacious topical treatment for murine cutaneous leishmaniasis with ethanolic formulations of amphoteicin B. *Antimicrob. Agents Chemother.* **1998**, *42*, 3092–3096. [CrossRef]

19. López, L.; Vélez, I.; Asela, C.; Cruz, C.; Alves, F.; Robledo, S.; Arana, B. A phase II study to evaluate the safety and efficacy of topical 3% amphotericin B cream (Anfoleish) for the treatment of uncomplicated cutaneous leishmaniasis in Colombia. *PLoS Negl. Trop. Dis.* **2018**, *12*, e0006653. [CrossRef]
20. Schmidt-Ott, R.; Klenner, T.; Overath, P.; Aebischer, T. Topical treatment with hexadecylphosphocholine (Miltex) efficiently reduces parasite burden in experimental cutaneous leishmaniasis. *Trans. R. Soc. Trop. Med. Hyg.* **1999**, *93*, 85–90. [CrossRef]
21. Dar, M.J.; Din, F.U.; Khan, G.M. Sodium stibogluconate loaded nano-deformable liposomes for topical treatment of leishmaniasis: Macrophage as a target cell. *Drug Deliv.* **2018**, *25*, 1595–1606. [CrossRef]
22. Moosavian Kalat, S.A.; Khamesipour, A.; Bavarsad, N.; Fallah, M.; Khashayarmanesh, Z.; Feizi, E.; Neghabi, K.; Abbasi, A.; Jaafari, M.R. Use of topical liposomes containing meglumine antimoniate (Glucantime) for the treatment of L. major lesion in BALB/c mice. *Exp. Parasitol.* **2014**, *143*, 5–10. [CrossRef] [PubMed]
23. Moosavian, S.A.; Fallah, M.; Jaafari, M.R. The activity of encapsulated meglumine antimoniate in stearylamine-bearing liposomes against cutaneous leishmaniasis in BALB/c mice. *Exp. Parasitol.* **2019**, *200*, 30–35. [CrossRef] [PubMed]
24. Anchisi, C.; Maccioni, A.M.; Sinico, C.; Valenti, D. Stability studies of new cosmetic formulations with vegetable extracts as functional agents. *Farmaco* **2001**, *56*, 427–431. [CrossRef]
25. Bilia, A.R.; Bergonzi, M.C.; Mazzi, G.; Vincieri, F.F. Development and stability of semisolid preparations based on a supercritical CO2 Arnica extract. *J. Pharm. Biomed. Anal.* **2006**, *41*, 449–454. [CrossRef] [PubMed]
26. Risaliti, L.; Piazzini, V.; Di Marzo, M.G.; Brunetti, L.; Cecchi, R.; Lencioni, P.; Bilia, A.R.; Bergonzi, M.C. Topical formulations of delta-aminolevulinic acid for the treatment of actinic keratosis: Characterization and efficacy evaluation. *Eur. J. Pharm. Sci.* **2018**, *115*, 345–351. [CrossRef] [PubMed]
27. Suñer, J.; Calpena, A.C.; Clares, B.; Cañadas, C.; Halbaut, L. Development of Clotrimazole Multiple W/O/W Emulsions as Vehicles for Drug Delivery: Effects of Additives on Emulsion Stability. *AAPS Pharm. Sci. Tech.* **2017**, *18*, 539–550. [CrossRef]
28. Council regulation (EC) no 440/2008 Test guideline for skin absorption: In vitro method (B45). *J. Eur. Union* **2008**, *142*, 438–443.
29. World medical association declaration of Helsinki: Ethical Principles for Medical Research Involving Human Subjects. *JAMA* **2013**, *310*, 2191–2194. [CrossRef]
30. Du Plessis, J.; Stefaniak, A.; Eloff, F.; John, S.; Agner, T.; Chou, T.C.; Nixon, R.; Steiner, M.; Franken, A.; Kudla, I.; et al. International guidelines for the in vivo assessment of skin properties in non-clinical settings: Part 2. Transepidermal water loss and skin hydration. *Skin. Res. Technol.* **2013**, *19*, 265–278. [CrossRef]
31. Pujol, A.; Urbán, P.; Riera, C.; Fisa, R.; Molina, I.; Salvador, F.; Estelrich, J.; Fernández-Busquets, X. Application of Quantum Dots to the Study of Liposome Targeting in Leishmaniasis and Malaria. *Int. J. Theoret. Appiel. Nanotech.* **2014**, *2*, 1–8. [CrossRef]
32. Carrió, J.; de Colmenares, M.; Riera, C.; Gállego, M.; Arboix, M.; Portús, M. Leishmania infantum: Stage-specific activity of pentavalent antimony related with the assay conditions. *Exp. Parasitol.* **2000**, *95*, 209–214. [CrossRef] [PubMed]
33. Carrió, J.; Riera, C.; Gállego, M.; Portús, M. In vitro activity of pentavalent antimony derivates on promastigotes and intracellular amastigotes of Leishmania infantum strains from humans and dogs in Spain. *Acta Trop.* **2001**, *79*, 179–183. [CrossRef]
34. Handler, M.Z.; Patel, P.A.; Kapila, R.; Al-Qubati, Y.; Schwarts, R.A. Cutaneous and mucocutaneous leishmaniasis: Differential diagnosis, diagnosis, histopathology, and management. *J. Am. Acad Dermatol.* **2015**, *73*, 911–926. [CrossRef] [PubMed]
35. Dong, L.; Liu, C.; Cun, D.; Fang, L. The effect of rheological behavior and microstructure of the emulgels on the release and permeation profiles of Terpinen-4-ol. *Eur. J. Pharm. Sci.* **2015**, *78*, 140–150. [CrossRef]
36. Sosa, L.; Calpena, A.C.; Silva-Abreu, M.; Espinoza, L.C.; Rincón, M.; Bozal, N.; Domenech, O.; Rodríguez-Lagunas, M.J.; Clares, B. Thermoreversible Gel-Loaded Amphotericin B for the treatment of Dermal and Vaginal Candidiasis. *Pharmaceutics* **2019**, *11*, 312. [CrossRef]
37. Kaur, L.; Jain, S.K.; Singh, K. Vitamin E TPGS based nanogel for the skin targeting of high molecular weight anti-fungal drug: Development and *in vitro* and *in vivo* assessment. *RSC Adv.* **2015**, *5*, 53671–53686. [CrossRef]
38. Elias, P.M. Epidermal lipids, barrier function, and desquamation. *J. Investig. Dermatol.* **1983**, *80*, 44–49. [CrossRef]

39. Marzulli, F.N.; Callahan, J.F.; Brown, D.W. Chemical structure and skin penetrating capacity of a short series of organic phosphates and phosphoric acid. *J. Investig. Dermatol.* **1965**, *44*, 339–344. [CrossRef]
40. Anderson, B.D.; Raykar, P.V. Solute structure-permeability relationships in human stratum corneum. *J. Investig. Dermatol.* **1989**, *93*, 280–286. [CrossRef]
41. Rins, M.; Diez, I.; Calpena, A.C.; Obach, R. Skin density in the hairless rat. Evidence of regional differences. *Eur. J. Drug Metab. Pharmacokinet.* **1991**, *3*, 456–457.

7

A Recombinant Enolase-Montanide™ PetGel A Vaccine Promotes a Protective Th1 Immune Response against a Highly Virulent *Sporothrix schenckii* by Toluene Exposure

Damiana Téllez-Martínez, Deivys Leandro Portuondo, Maria Luiza Loesch, Alexander Batista-Duharte * and Iracilda Zeppone Carlos *

Department of Clinical Analysis, School of Pharmaceutical Sciences, São Paulo State University (UNESP), Araraquara 14800-903, SP, Brazil; damianatellezm@gmail.com (D.T.-M.); deivysleandro@gmail.com (D.L.P.); ma_luizaloesch@hotmail.com (M.L.L.)

* Correspondence: batistaduhartea@gmail.com or batistaduhartea@fcfar.unesp.br (A.B.-D.); carlosiz@fcfar.unesp.br (I.Z.C.)

Abstract: The effect of vaccination in fungal strains that suffered changes in their virulence by exposure to environmental contaminants is largely known. Growing reports of resistance to antifungal drugs and the emergence of new highly virulent strains, possibly acquired in the environment, prompt the design of new vaccines able to prevent and combat emerging mycotic diseases. In this study, we evaluated the protective capacity of an enolase-based vaccine and Montanide PetGel A (PGA) as an adjuvant against *S. schenckii* with increased virulence by exposure to toluene. The adjuvanted vaccine induced a strong specific Th1 response and protective immunity against a challenge with either wildtype or toluene-adapted *S. schenckii* in Balb/c mice. This study highlights the role of the adjuvant PGA driving the quality of the anti-sporothrix immunity and the key component in the vaccine efficacy.

Keywords: vaccine; adjuvants; *Sporothrix schenckii*; toluene; virulence; enolase; Montanide PetGel A

---

1. Introduction

Sporotrichosis is an emergent subcutaneous mycosis in tropical and subtropical regions, caused by several pathogenic species of the genus *Sporothrix*; that include *Sporothrix brasiliensis*, *S. schenckii sensu stricto*, *Sporothrix globosa*, and *Sporothrix luriei* [1]. Classically, infection is acquired after traumatic inoculation of contaminated soil, plants, and organic matter into skin or mucosa or, more rarely, by inhalation of conidia. Over the last years, cat–human zoonotic transmission of sporotrichosis caused by *S. brasiliensis* has become a health problem in Brazil [2]. The disease can manifest as fixed cutaneous and regional lymphocutaneous forms in immunocompetent individuals, and disseminated forms, mainly reported in immunocompromised patients [3].

Ecological determinants of the genus *Sporothrix* remain poorly understood [4,5]. However, experimental evidence suggests that environmental contaminants can modify the fungal virulence by reducing the host immunity [6] or modifying the fungal biology [4,7]. Previous studies showed that fungal exposure to toluene, a common soil contaminant that shares the same environmental niche of *S. schenckii*, is able to increase the *S. schenckii* virulence [7]. Ongoing studies are evaluating the role of chemical contamination and other environmental factors in sporotrichosis outbreaks.

Conventional treatment of sporotrichosis requires long periods of antifungal drug administration often accompanied by adverse effects and fungal resistance, principally during the treatment of disseminated sporotrichosis [8]. These problems have stimulated the search for new strategies for sporotrichosis management, including anti-sporothrix vaccination that has been proposed as a feasible way for both therapeutic and prophylactic purposes [9,10]. However, the development of antifungal vaccines has not been as successful as antiviral and antibacterial vaccines due to, among other things, a general under-appreciation for the impact of fungal diseases and the high cost of preclinical and clinical studies [11]. Another challenge has been the use of immunological adjuvants with an adequate safety and efficacy profile [12]. Aluminium-derived adjuvants have been used in human and veterinary vaccines for more than eight decades in licensed vaccines [13,14]. However, they have not been successful in preventing intracellular infection due to a weak capacity to induce cell-mediated immunity when used along with small immunogenic antigens [13]. Moreover, there are reports of tumors in the inoculation site in felines vaccinated with alum-based vaccines and a possible causal association between chronic inflammation induced by alum and these tumors has been suggested [15].

Current advances in the understanding of antifungal immune response support rational use of more effective adjuvants, such as pattern recognition receptors (PRR) agonists, inhibitors of regulatory T cells, and others [12,16,17], to achieve effective immune responses against specific fungi.

For several decades, biodegradable natural and synthetic polymers have been used for antigen delivery and as immunological adjuvants. Due to their biocompatibility, biodegradability, easy production and low toxicity polymers are attractive candidates for substituting conventional adjuvants [18]. MontanideTM PetGel A (PGA), is a polymer-based adjuvant composed of highly stable dispersion of microspherical particles of sodium polyacrylate in water (Figure 1A, Table 1). This polymeric technology has already been used in several vaccine models, including pet vaccines, with a promising safety and efficacy profile [19].

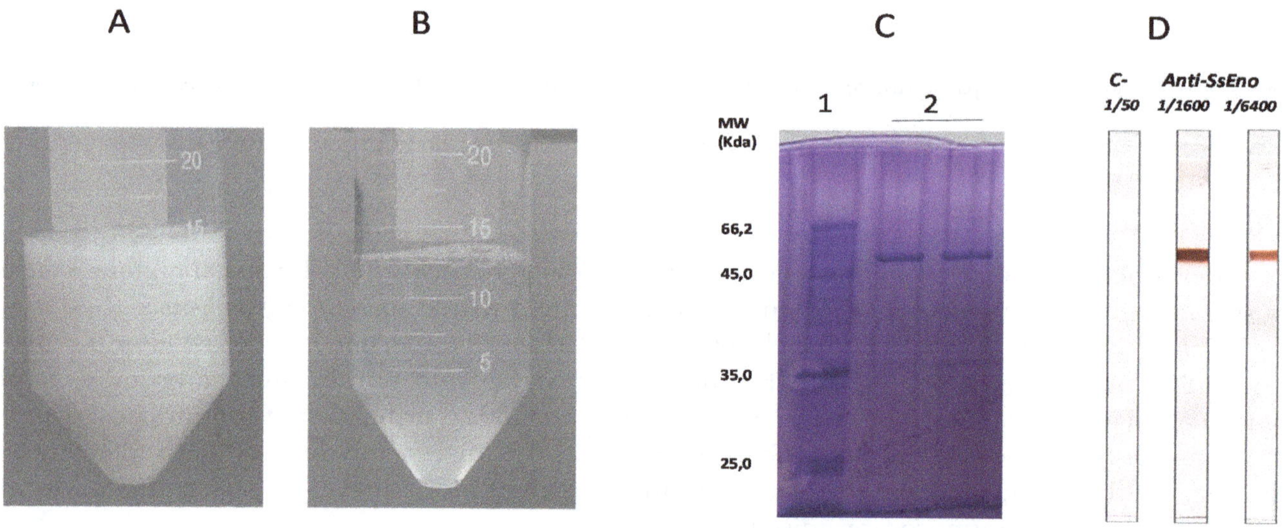

Figure 1. External aspect of (**A**) Montanide^{TM} PetGel (PGA) and (**B**) PGA+rSsEno vaccine formulation. (**C**) SDS-PAGE showing the expression and purification of *rSsEno*. C1. Molecular pattern, C2. rSsEno band stained with Coomassie blue with the expected 47 kDa molecular mass (in duplicate). (**D**) Immunoblotting analysis of rSsEno with a pooled anti-*rSsEno* serum from Balb/c mice immunized with Freund's adjuvant/rSsEno (Either 1/1600 or 1/6400 dilutions of serum were used). A pooled serum from non-immunized mice (dilution 1/50) was used as negative control (C−) to identify non-specific binding.

Table 1. General properties of Montanide™ GEL adjuvants.

	Description
Composition	Gel particles of sodium polyacrylate in water.
Particle size	90% of the particles are smaller than 1.2 μm in diameter.
Stability	Highly stable at room temperature.
Mechanisms of action	Depot effect with slow release of antigens, due to polymer adsorption properties. Improves the recruitment and activation of the innate immune system cells and inducement of specific immune response.
Vaccine preparation	Montanide™ GEL adjuvants are ready-to-use adjuvants that can be combined with a wide range of antigens by gentle mixing.
Routes of administration	Parenteral and mucosal administration.
Uses	Montanide™ GEL adjuvants are recommended for a wide variety of livestock species and for pets and horses. They can be formulated with a wide range of antigens.
Safety	Montanide™ adjuvants and their components have been considered as safe by the Committee for Veterinary Medical Products (CVMP) for use in immunological products. They are included in Part I of the Annex of the European Council Regulation n° 37/2010/EU as substances needing no further MRL studies, in the Out of Scope list (EMACVMP-519714-2009), and included in already registered veterinary commercial products.

Recently, our group evaluated a cell-wall protein extracted from *S. schenckii* (SsCWPs) in an experimental vaccine formulated with Aluminum hydroxide (AH) gel [20]. Immunized mice developed a specific immune response characterized by a balanced Th1/Th2/Th17 response and the production of protective antibody response. In a more recent study, the AH-based vaccine was compared with other experimental vaccine candidate containing SsCWPs and PGA. Both formulations induced a protective immune response in mice. However, AH stimulated the development of granulomas in the inoculation site while PGA-based vaccine exhibited a Th1 protective response and better local tolerance than AH-based vaccine in vaccinated mice [21]. In other recent study, we evaluated the immunogenic and protective effect of enolase, one of the main antigens that were found in SsCWPs, against *S. brasilensis*, the most virulent species of the genus *Sporothrix* [22]. The recombinant enolase of *S. schenckii* (SsEno) was formulated with PGA and after three subcutaneous administrations in mice, a significant specific immune response was observed. Furthermore, a reduction in mortality (over 90%) was observed after 45 days of an intravenous challenge with viable yeast, compared with non-vaccinated mice.

Until now, there are no studies on the effects of vaccination on fungal strains whose virulence changed due to exposure to environmental contaminants. In the current context of growing reports of fungal resistance to antifungal drugs and the emergence of new highly virulent strains, possibly acquired in the environment, these assessments can provide important information on the ability of new vaccines to prevent and combat emerging mycotic diseases.

In this study, we evaluated the protective capacity of an enolase-based vaccine formulated with PGA as an adjuvant, against *S. schenckii* with increased virulence by experimental exposure to toluene [7].

2. Materials and Methods

2.1. Animals

Male Balb/c mice (five to seven weeks old) were purchased from "Centro Multidisciplinar para Investigação Biológica na Área da Ciência de Animais de Laboratório" (CEMIB), Universidade de Campinas (UNICAMP), São Paulo, Brasil. Mice were housed in microisolator cages in a controlled ambient and receiving water and food ad libitum. The study was carried out in accordance with the Guide for the Care and Use of Laboratory Animals of the National Institutes of Health. The experiments were approved by the Ethics Committee for Animal Use in Research of Araraquara's School of Pharmaceutical Sciences from UNESP (Protocol CEUA/FCF/CAr: 19/2018).

2.2. Microorganisms and Preparations

The *S. schenckii sensu stricto* strain ATCC 16345 (here named as *S. schenckii*) used in this work was kindly provided by the Oswaldo Cruz Foundation (Rio de Janeiro, Brazil). The mycelial phase was maintained at room temperature in Mycosel (BD Biosciences) agar. A piece of a well-defined colony was grown in 100 mL of Sabouraud dextrose broth (SDB) (Difco, Detroit, MI, USA) for four days in a rotary shaker (130 rpm and 30 °C). The conidia were separated from the hyphae by filtration with sterile gauze using a Buchner funnel. Them conidia were counted and suspended in phosphate-buffered saline (PBS) at 1×10^7/mL.

2.3. S. schenckii Growth in Toluene

Fungal cultures were performed in 125-mL Erlenmeyer flasks containing 50 mL of Sabouraud dextrose broth (SDB) and sealed with Teflon Mininert valves (SUPELCO, 24 mm, (Merck KGaA Darmstadt, Germany) to prevent evaporation of the solvent. SDB was supplemented with toluene 0.1% (v/v). An aliquot of 1×10^7 conidia was inoculated and incubated during five days on a rotary shaker (30 °C and 130 rpm). Control cultures without toluene were included. Fungal viability was determined at fifth day by counting colony forming units (CFU) on Sabouraud dextrose agar (SDA) plates [7].

2.4. Expression and Purification of Recombinant S. schenckii Enolase (rSsEno)

The detailed procedures were previously described [22]. Briefly, the gene that encodes *S. schenckii* enolase with molecular mass 47 kDa and 438 amino acids (access code: ERS97971.1, GenBank database) was synthesized by Epoch Life Science Inc. (Missouri, TX, USA). The enolase gen was subcloned into the pET28a plasmid and optimized for production in *Escherichia coli* (pET28a::SsEno). *E. coli* DH5α was used for the propagation of pET28a::SsEno on lysogeny broth (LB) agar medium containing 30 µg/mL of kanamycin. For recombinant protein expression, *E. coli* BL21 cells cotransformed with pET28a::SsEno were grown at 37 °C in LB medium with kanamycin until they reached an OD600 in the range of 0.5–0.7. The expression of rSsEno was induced by 0.2 mmol/L of isopropyl β-D-1-thiogalactopyranoside (IPTG) at 30 °C for 4 h. The cells were centrifuged (20 min at 8000 rpm), and the pellet was resuspended in buffer A (NaPO4 20 mM, NaCl 500 mM and imidazole 20 mM, pH 7,4) containing 5 U of DNAse (Promega, Madison, WI, USA) and 30 µg/mL lysozyme (Merck KGaA Darmstadt, Germany) for 30 min on ice. The cell homogenate was sonicated, filtrated and then centrifuged at 19,000 rpm for 20 min at 4 °C. The supernatant containing rSsEno was filtered (0.45 µm nitrocellulose membrane, Millipore and initially purified by Ni^{2+}-affinity chromatography in buffer A. The rSsEno eluted in buffer B ($NaPO_4$ 20 mM, NaCl 500 mM, and imidazole 500 mM, pH 7.4) was subjected to size exclusion chromatography (SEC) with a Superdex 200 pg 16/60 column (GE Healthcare Life Sciences, Chicago, IL, USA) in Tris-HCl 25 mM, NaCl 100 mM and β-mercaptoethanol 2 mM at pH 7.5, and the eluted protein was concentrated using the Amicon® Ultra 15 mL 3k device (Millipore, Burlington, MA, USA) after being dialyzed for 24 h at 4 °C against phosphate buffer saline. The rSsEno concentration was measured by the Pierce BCA assay (Thermo Scientific, Waltham, MA, USA), and the efficacy of the expression and purification processes was assessed by 12% SDS-polyacrylamide gel electrophoresis (SDS-PAGE) and immunoblotting using anti-rSsEno serum.

2.5. Adjuvants and Vaccine Formulation

The vaccine formulation was prepared by mixing 100 µg of rSsEno with 5% PGA adjuvant kindly provided by Seppic (Paris, France) (Figure 1B). Other formulations composed by either PGA or rSsEno alone were used as control.

2.6. *Immunization Schedule*

Balb/c mice ($n = 5$) received subcutaneous (s.c.) vaccination (on days 0 for priming and 14 for booster) in the back of the neck, with 100 µL of one of the following formulations: PGA+rSsEno, 100 µg rSsEno or PBS alone as a negative control. One week after the booster, mice were euthanized in CO_2 chamber and bled by heart puncture to obtain serum, which was aliquoted and stored at −20 °C until use.

2.7. *Quantification of the rSsEno-Antibody Response by Enzyme-Linked Immunosorbent Assay (ELISA)*

rSsEno IgG antibody titration was conducted as described previously [22]. Briefly, a 96-well ELISA plate (Merck KGaA Darmstadt, Germany) was coated with 5 µg rSsEno/mL in PBS and at 4 °C (overnight). The plate was washed with washing buffer (0.1% Tween 20) and then blocked 1 h at room temperature with 5% dried skim milk in washing buffer. Dilutions of the serum samples (1:500 in blocking buffer) were added to each well and incubated at room temperature for 2 h. After washing, peroxidase-conjugated anti-mouse IgG (1/500) (Merck KGaA Darmstadt, Germany) was added and incubated at 37 °C for 1 h. After exhaustive washing, tetramethylbenzidine was added to reveal the antigen-antibody reactions (30 min at room temperature). The reaction was stopped by the addition of 50 µL/well 1M H_2SO_4, and the absorbance was read with an ELISA reader (Multiskan Ascent, Labsystem, Vantaa, Finland) at 450 nm.

2.8. *Th1-Th17 Phenotipagem*

Spleens were aseptically removed and splenocytes were extracted. Viable splenocytes were adjusted to 1×10^7 cells/mL in complete RPMI-1640 culture medium (Merck KGaA Darmstadt, Germany), which was supplemented with 2 mm L-glutamine, 100 U/mL penicillin, 100 µg/mL penicillin/streptomycin, and 10% fetal calf serum (RPMI complete). For study of Th1 and Th17 lymphocytes subpopulations, the following anti-mouse mAb were used: anti-CD16/CD32, anti-CD3-FITC, anti-CD4-APC, anti-IL-17-PE, anti-IFN-γ-Percp, and respective isotype controls (all purchased from BD Biosciences, (Franklin Lakes, NJ, USA). Splenocytes were assessed for the frequency of Th1(IFN-γ+), Th17 (IL-17+). Briefly, viable splenocytes were stained for the extracellular markers, then fixed and permeabilized using eBiosciences' intracellular fixation (Thermo Scientific, Waltham, MA, USA) and permeabilization buffer set, and then the intracellular IFN-γ and IL-17A were stained with a fluorescent respective marker. Intracellular cytokines were detected after in vitro stimulation with 10 µg/mL of rSsEno and Brefeldin A for intracellular retention of the induced cytokine. Events were acquired using a BD Accuri C6 flow cytometer (BD Biosciences) and analyzed with the flow cytometer's proprietary software.

2.9. *IFN-γ, IL-4, and IL-17 Measurement in Supernatant of Splenocytes Culture*

Splenocytes from immunized and non-immunized mice were cultured as previously described and stimulated with 10 µg/mL of rSsEno for 24 h. The levels of IFN-γ, IL-4, and IL-17 after rSsEno stimulation were measured in the supernatant of splenocytes culture by Cytometric Bead Array (CBA) (BD Biosciences) according to the manufacturer's instructions using a BD Accuri C6 flow cytometer (BD Biosciences).

2.10. *Fungal Challenge and Infection Assessment*

Either vaccinated or non-vaccinated mice were intraperitoneally inoculated with 10^6 conidia of either wild type (WT) or toluene-adapted (Tadap) *S. schenckii* suspended in 100 µL of PBS or with an equal volume of PBS alone as control. To confirm the fungal cell count and viability of the inoculum, appropriately diluted samples of the conidia suspension were plated onto Mycosel agar plates and after seven days of incubation growing colonies were counted. At seventh day post-infection the mice were euthanized in CO_2 chamber. The liver and spleen of each animal were removed to measure the relative organ weight and assess the systemic fungal load. The relative weight of livers and spleens was calculated by the following formula:

$$\text{Related weight} = \text{organ weight (g)}/\text{body weight (kg)}.$$

To evaluate the fungal load, liver and spleen were macerated under sterile conditions and adequate dilutions of the macerate in PBS were cultured in duplicate, on Mycosel agar plates and the growing CFU were counted after three and six days. The final count was adjusted according to the dilution used.

2.11. Statistical Analysis

Statistical analysis was performed in GraphPad Prism ver. 6.01 (San Diego, CA, USA). A one-way analysis of variance (ANOVA) with Tukey comparisons test was used. The confidence interval was set at 95% for all tests. The significance level and *p*-values were shown as * ($p < 0.05$); ** ($p < 0.01$); *** ($p < 0.001$); **** ($p < 0.0001$).

3. Results

3.1. Production and Purification of rSsEno

Figure 1C,D show that the production and purification of rSsEno was effective. SDS-PAGE showed a unique band stained with Coomassie blue with the expected molecular mass of 47 kDa previously characterized as rSsEno [13]. In addition, a pooled anti-rSsEno serum obtained from mice immunized with Freund´s Adjuvants/rSsEno recognized specifically the rSsEno band in the immunoblotting while there were not detected non-specific binding in the control strip treated with a serum from non-immunized mice.

3.2. Post-Vaccination rSsEno-Antibody Response

The rSsEno-specific IgG antibody reaction after the second immunization with or without the PGA are displayed in Figure 2 as optical density (OD) measured at 450 nm. Immunization with PGA+rSsEno markedly enhanced the IgG antibody response to rSsEno compared to the response induced by the non-adjuvanted vaccine, seven days after the second immunization ($p < 0.0001$).

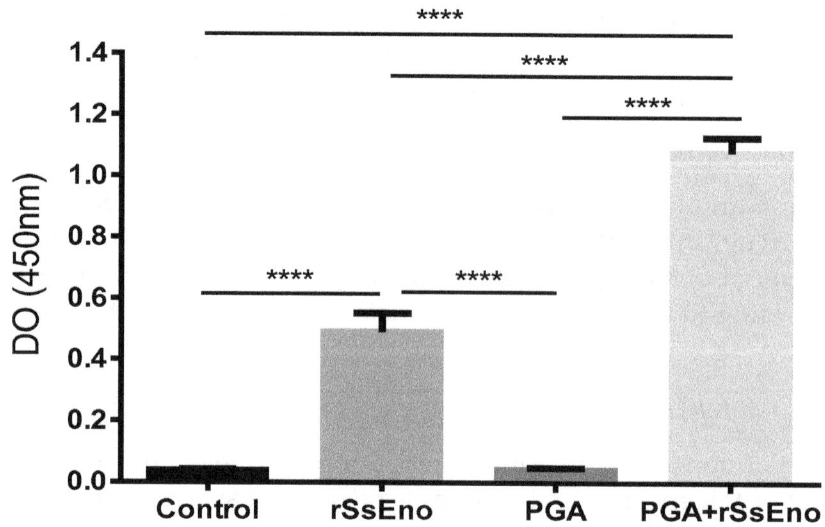

Figure 2. Immunization with PGA+rSsEno markedly enhanced the IgG antibody response to rSsEno. Balb/c mice were immunized (s.c.) twice with rSsEno, PGA, PGA+rSsEno, or PBS as negative control. Serum collected seven days after the second immunization was used to determine rSsEno-specific IgG antibody. **** ($p < 0.0001$).

3.3. *Th1 and Th17 Response*

The response Th1 and Th17 are determinant in the immune response against *S. schenckii*. Mice vaccinated with rSsEno+PGA induced a significant response of Th1 lymphocytes after in vitro stimulation with rSsEno compared with the other groups ($p < 0.0001$). However, the response of Th17 lymphocytes was not modified in any experimental group (Figure 3). A similar response was observed when the concentration of IFN-ɣ, IL-4, and IL-17A were measured by CBA. A high production of IFN-ɣ, belonging to the Th1 pattern was detected in the group vaccinated with rSsEno+PGA compared with non-adjuvanted *rSsEno* vaccination ($p < 0.001$) and with the control groups ($p < 0.0001$) (Figure 4).

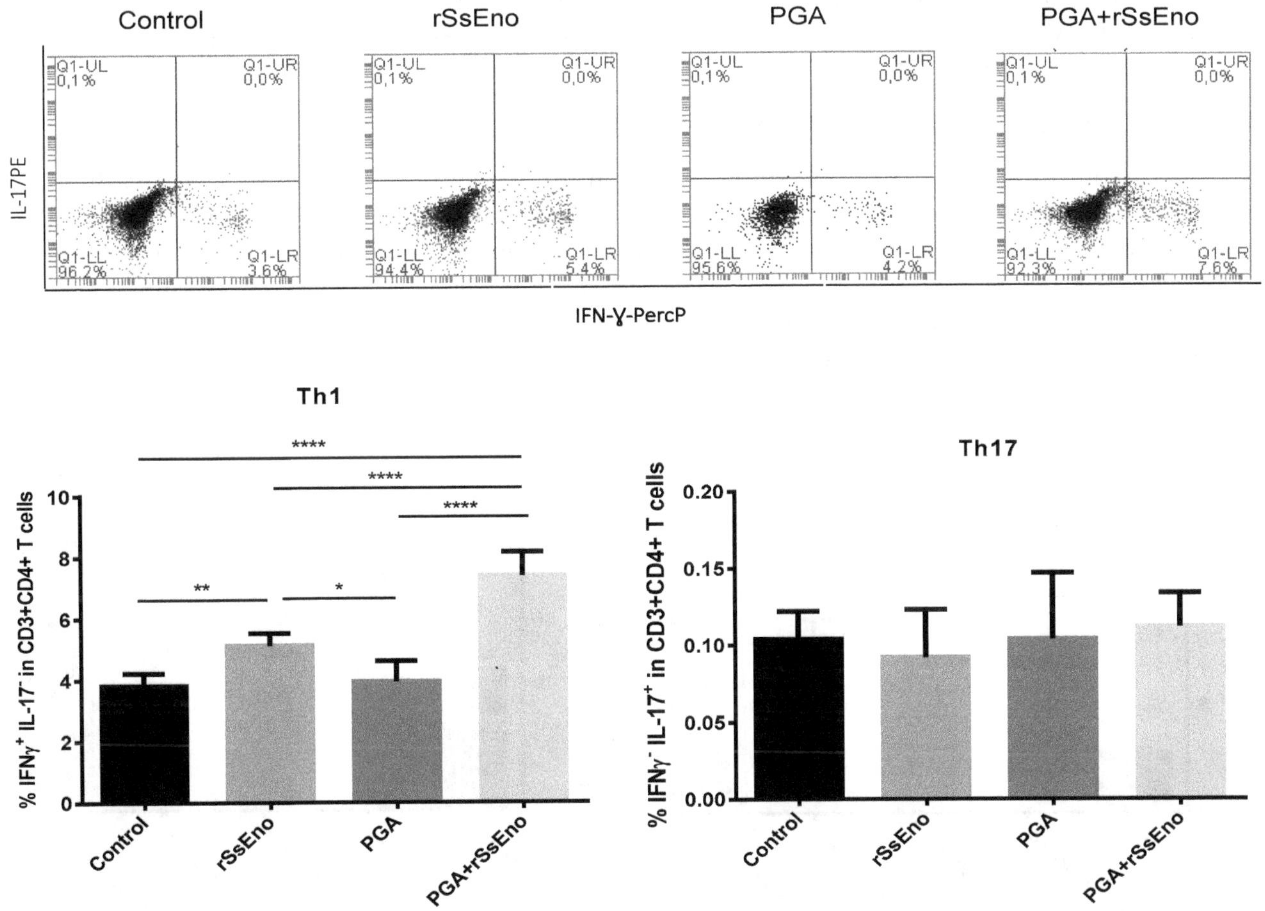

Figure 3. Response of Th1 (intracellular IFN-ɣ+) and Th17 (intracellular IL-17A+) cells induced by immunization with the PGA+rSsEno. Balb/c mice were immunized (s.c.) twice with rSsEno, PGA, PGA+rSsEno, or PBS as negative control. Splenocytes of each animal were collected seven days after the second immunization and purified cells were stimulated in vitro with rSsEno and Brefeldin A. The frequency of Th1 and Th17 cells was detected using a BD Accuri C6 flow cytometer. Upper figure shows representative dot plots of Th1 and Th17 frequency collected from each group. * ($p < 0.05$); ** ($p < 0.01$); *** ($p < 0.001$): **** ($p < 0.0001$).

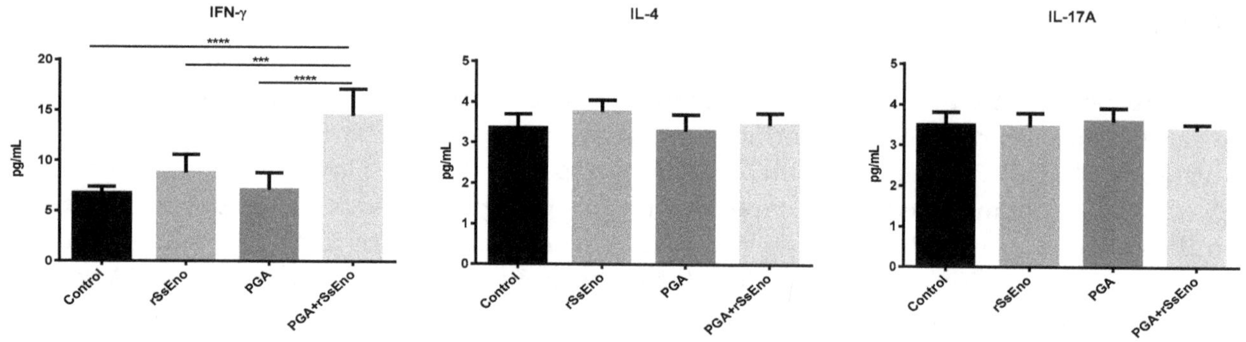

Figure 4. Cytokine profile in supernatant of splenocytes stimulated in vitro with rSsEno. Balb/c mice were immunized (s.c.) twice with rSsEno, PGA, PGA+rSsEno, or PBS as negative control. Splenocytes of each animal were collected seven days after the second immunization and purified cells were stimulated in vitro with rSsEno. Cytokine were quantified by cytometric bead array (CBA). * ($p < 0.05$); ** ($p < 0.01$); *** ($p < 0.001$): **** ($p < 0.0001$).

3.4. Fungal Challenge and Infection Assessment

The aim of this study was to investigate if the immune response induced by rSsEno adjuvanted with PGA was able to protect against a challenge with either WT or Tadap *S. schenckii.* We analyzed the spleen and the liver as representative organs to evaluate the fungal load. All the infected mice developed hepatomegaly that was observed by measuring the relative weight of the liver. However, splenomegaly was also observed in mice vaccinated and infected. Those animals vaccinated and infected with highly virulent toluene-adapted *S. schenckii* developed the greatest hepato- and splenomegaly compared with the control group ($p < 0.0001$) (Figure 5).

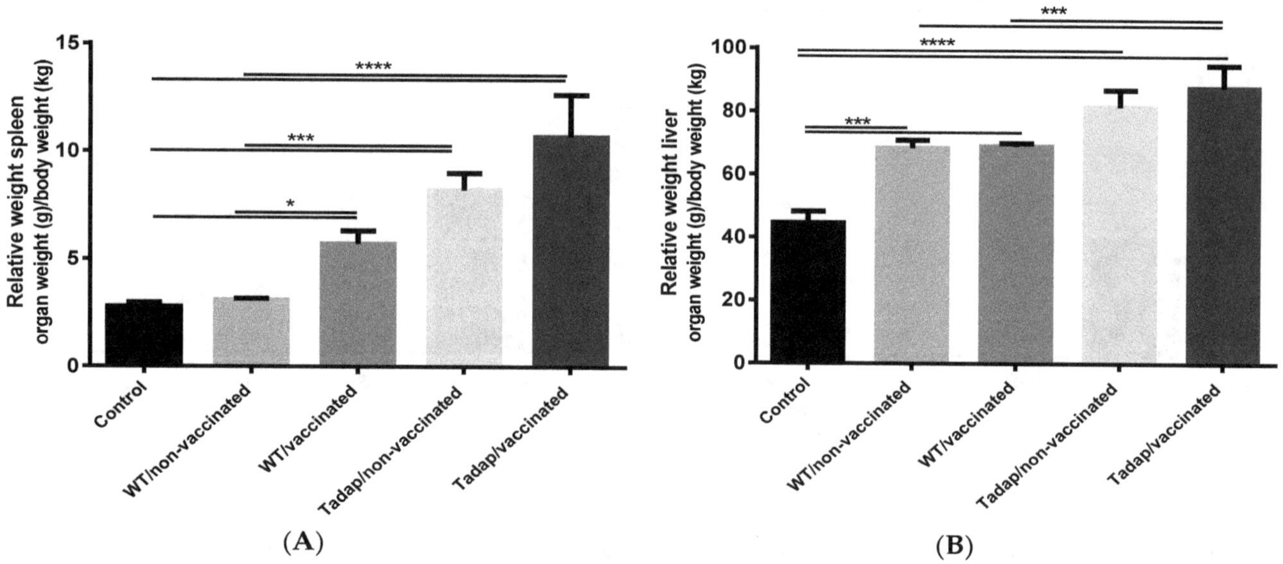

Figure 5. Relative (**A**) spleen and (**B**) liver weight. Balb/c mice were injected (s.c.) twice with PGA+rSsEno (vaccinated) or PBS (non-vaccinated). Seven days after the second dose of administration of PGA+rSsEno or PBS, mice were infected intraperitoneally with 1×10^6 conidia of either wild type (WT) or toluene adapted *S. schenckii* (Tadap). The spleen and the liver of each animal were collected seven days after the second immunization and the relative weight (organ weight/animal weight) was measured. * ($p < 0.05$); *** ($p < 0.001$); **** ($p < 0.0001$).

The protective effect induced by the adjuvanted vaccine after the fungal challenge is shown in Figure 6. The immune response induced by PGA+ rSsEno was able to reduce the fungal burden in spleen and liver of mice infected with either WT or Tadap *S. schenckii* in a similar way. However, owing to the higher virulence of Tadap *S. schenckii*, this finding suggests that PGA+rSsEno can be effective against fungus with different levels of virulence.

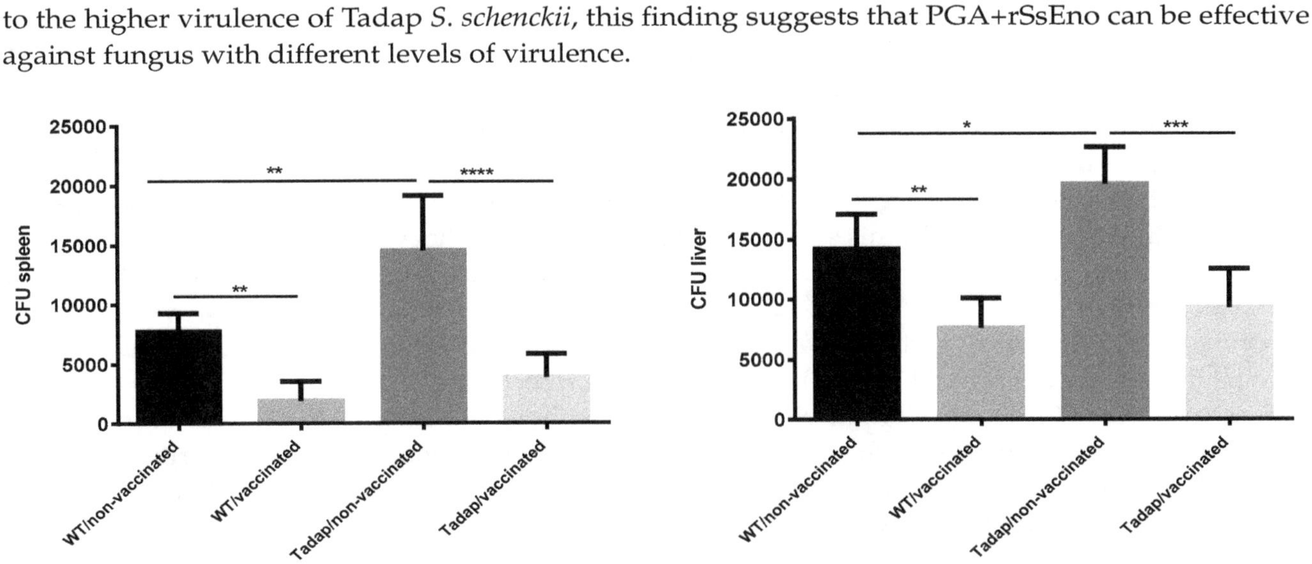

Figure 6. Vaccination with PGA+rSsEno was able to reduce the fungal burden in spleen and liver of mice infected with either wild type (WT) or toluene adapted *S. schenckii* (Tadap). Balb/c mice were injected (s.c.) twice with PGA+rSsEno (vaccinated) or PBS (non-vaccinated). One week after the boost, mice were i.p. challenged with *S. schenckii* and seven days after infection the protection was assessed by the number of CFUs recovered from the spleen and liver. * ($p < 0.05$); ** ($p < 0.01$); *** ($p < 0.001$); **** ($p < 0.0001$).

4. Discussion

Recent advances in the understanding of relevant immunological mechanisms against pathogenic fungi favor the development of prophylactic and therapeutic antifungal vaccines [23–25]. In contrast to classical antifungal medications, vaccines can be administered to large populations with low potential risks or side-effects [26]. Currently, there is a growing tendency to develop subunit vaccines, based in well-defined microbial components, in order to increase vaccine safety [27]. Unfortunately, pure antigens are poorly immunogenic, and they should be formulated with adjuvants to improve the vaccine efficacy [14,28].

Several non-toxic polymer adjuvants are being used for sustained delivery of protein subunit vaccines [29,30]. Polymeric adjuvants act through slow release of the antigen for the selective targeting to antigen presenting cells, promoting different signaling pathways including, activation of toll-like receptor(s) and inflammasome pathway or directly interacting with B cells. Polymer–antigen complex can be phagocytosed, and the antigen effectively presented to naive T cells via major histocompatibility complex (MHC) molecules [31].

Recently, we compared AH with the polymeric adjuvant PGA in a vaccine candidate against *S. schenckii* containing proteins extracted from the fungal cell wall. PGA induced a protective immune response against both *S. schenckii* and *S. brasiliensis* with lesser local toxicity than AH in vaccinated mice [21]. In other recent work, we developed recombinant enolase that was a key antigen in SsCWPs and it was evaluated in a vaccine formulated with PGA as an adjuvant. Again, protective immune response in vaccinated mice after a challenge with *S. brasiliensis* was observed with a survival rate above 90% after 45 days of intravenous fungal challenge [22].

Here, we evaluated the protective effect of PGA formulated with rSsEno against a highly virulent *S. schenckii*. The enhanced virulence was acquired after fungal exposure to 0.1% of toluene, which induced adaptive changes previously described, including enhanced melanosome formation and stronger antioxidant mechanism compared with the wild type strain [7].

Before the evaluation of the protective effect of vaccination, the immunogenicity of the vaccine after two subcutaneous doses of PGA+rSsEno was evaluated. In the aforementioned work [22], we evaluated the immunogenicity and efficacy of this vaccine candidate using three subcutaneous administrations and PGA 10%. However, here the immunogenicity of the vaccine was evaluated after two doses and PGA 5%, as we used in another vaccine candidate with SsCWPs [21]. As expected, the formulation of PGA+rSsEno induced elevated production of specific IgG antibodies and a strong Th1 response after in vitro stimulation of splenocytes with rSsEno. However, we did not observe a significant Th17 response analyzed by both intracellular and released IL-17A.

Several studies revealed that Th1 response plays a decisive role in the defense against *S. schenckii* infection [32–35]. In this sense, activation of Th1 lymphocytes is becoming an interesting immunomodulatory strategy against sporotrichosis. Flores-García et al. (2015) reported that treatment with recombinant murine IL-12 (rmIL-12) promotes Th1 immunity and clinical improvement in an experimental sporotrichosis gerbil model [36]. In other study, Batista-Duharte et al. (2016) evaluated the therapeutic effect of adjuvant Finlay cochleates 3 (AFCo3), a cochleate containing purified and non-toxic LPS derived from *Neisseria meningitidis B* as vehicle of Amphotericin B (AmB) to evaluate the combined effect of immunomodulation induced by AFCo3 and the antifungal effect in a murine model of *S. schenckii* infection. AFCo3 stimulated a strong Th1- and Th17 response associated with the antifungal effect of AmB, which significantly improved the fungal clearance [37]. Regarding vaccination, studies suggest that Th1 response is associated with anti-sporothrix vaccine protection [20–22,38,39] and the activation of dendritic cells by fungal wall proteins seems to be important in theTh1 bias [34]. However, the role of Th17 response to prevent sporotrichosis is controversial. Some studies reveal that anti-sporothrix vaccination can induce Th17- combined with Th1 response [20,38–40]. However, two studies using PGA as an adjuvant with either SsCWPs [21] or rSsEno [22], showed that Th1 response is sufficient to achieve protection against a challenge with *S. schenckii* or *S. brasiliensis*. In the previous comparative study, using SsCWPs as antigen with either AH or PGA as adjuvant revealed that the adjuvant is the main component that drives the quality of the immune response since AH induced a balanced Th1/Th2/Th17 response while PGA induced a Th1 response [21]. Interestingly, the reduction of fungal load in both groups was very similar despite having different overall Th cell pattern.

In this work, we observed that the anti- rSsEno Th1 response induced by PGA confers protection against Tadap *S. schenckii* after an intraperitoneal fungal challenge. Previously, we showed that infected mice with Tadap *S. schenckii* produced high levels of IFN-ɣ and, to a lesser extent, IL-17 [7]. This finding reinforces the criterion of the role of Th1-mediated response for protection against *S. schenckii* infection. Here, we observed significant production of IFN-ɣ after in vitro stimulation with rSsEno, compared to non-vaccinated mice, although the cytokine production was low in general. However, unlike infection where multiple lymphocyte clones are activated, vaccination stimulates specific clones, but they are sufficient in the booster phase to prevent infection. In this way, the role of vaccination is the expansion of specific lymphocytes to maintain a basal level of memory cell able to rapidly respond against microbial infection [41].

These results are important as part of the studies of the efficacy of the recombinant enolase-Montanide™ PetGel A vaccine, due to the environment can exert a direct influence on fungal virulence [4,5]. Ideally, a prophylactic vaccine should be able to prevent infections caused by microorganisms with different levels of virulence since imperfect vaccination can enhance the transmission of highly virulent pathogens [42]. In this sense, the choice of potent and safe adjuvants driving effective immunological mechanisms against the target microorganism is one of the most important factors for vaccine efficacy [28]. However, keeping in mind that besides the antigen and the adjuvant mode of action, vaccine efficacy and toxicity are strongly influenced by the genetic background of the host [43,44], additional studies in different mouse strains and non-rodent species will be performed.

5. Conclusions

In this work, we provide evidence that vaccination with a recombinant enolase-based vaccine formulated with PGA as an adjuvant promotes a protective immune response in mice, against a highly virulent *S. schenckii* by toluene exposure. To the best of our knowledge, this is the first experimental approach to assess the role of vaccination in providing protective immunity against pathogenic fungus with enhanced virulence by exposure to environmental contaminants. Further studies are necessary in order to evaluate the memory response, including other mouse strains and using a model of subcutaneous infection.

Author Contributions: Conceptualization, D.T.-M.; D.L.P.; A.B.-D.; I.Z.C. methodology, D.T.-M.; A.B.-D. D.L.P. M.L.L. formal analysis D.T.-M.; D.L.P.; A.B.-D.; investigation, D.T.-M.; A.B.-D. D.L.P., M.L.L.; resources, D.T.-M.; D.L.P.; A.B.-D.; data curation, A.B.-D.; writing—original draft preparation, D.T.M.; D.L.P.; A.B.-D.; writing—review and editing, D.T.-M.; D.L.P.; A.B.-D.; I.Z.; supervision, A.B.-D.; I.Z.C. project administration, I.Z.C.; A.B.-D.; funding acquisition, I.Z.C.

References

1. De Beer, Z.W.; Duong, T.A.; Wingfield, M.J. The divorce of *Sporothrix* and *Ophiostoma*: Solution to a problematic relationship. *Stud. Mycol.* **2016**, *83*, 165–191. [CrossRef]
2. Gremião, I.D.; Miranda, L.H.; Reis, E.G.; Rodrigues, A.M.; Pereira, S.A. Zoonotic Epidemic of Sporotrichosis: Cat to Human Transmission. *PLoS Pathog.* **2017**, *13*, e1006077. [CrossRef] [PubMed]
3. Barros, M.B.; de Almeida Paes, R.; Schubach, A.O. *Sporothrix schenckii* and Sporotrichosis. *Clin. Microbiol. Rev.* **2011**, *24*, 633–654. [CrossRef] [PubMed]
4. Téllez, M.D.; Batista-Duharte, A.; Portuondo, D.; Quinello, C.; Bonne-Hernández, R.; Carlos, I.Z. *Sporothrix schenckii* complex biology: Environment and fungal pathogenicity. *Microbiology* **2014**, *160 Pt 11*, 2352–2365. [CrossRef]
5. Ramírez-Soto, M.C.; Aguilar-Ancori, E.G.; Tirado-Sánchez, A.; Bonifaz, A. Ecological Determinants of Sporotrichosis Etiological Agents. *J. Fungi* **2018**, *4*, 95. [CrossRef] [PubMed]
6. Batista-Duharte, A.; Téllez-Martínez, D.; Aparecida Jellmayer, J.; Leandro Portuondo Fuentes, D.; Campos Polesi, M.; Martins Baviera, A.; Zeppone Carlos, I. Repeated Exposition to Mercury (II) Chloride Enhances Susceptibility to *S. schenckii sensu stricto* Infection in Mice. *J. Fungi* **2018**, *4*, 64. [CrossRef]
7. Tellez-Martinez, D.; Batista-Duharte, A.; Silva, V.P.; Portuondo, D.F.; Ferreira, L.S.; Marisa Polesi, C.; Costa, C.; Carlos, I.Z. Adaptive stress response induced by toluene increases *Sporothrix schenckii* virulence and host immune response. *bioRxiv* **2019**. [CrossRef]
8. Kauffman, C.A.; Bustamante, B.; Chapman, S.W.; Pappas, P.G. Clinical practice guidelines for the management of sporotrichosis: 2007 update by the Infectious Diseases Society of America. *Clin. Infect. Dis.* **2007**, *45*, 1255–1265. [CrossRef]
9. De Almeida, J.R.F.; Kaihami, G.H.; Jannuzzi, G.P.; de Almeida, S.R. Therapeutic vaccine using a monoclonal antibody against a 70-kDa glycoprotein in mice infected with highly virulent *Sporothrix schenckii* and *Sporothrix brasiliensis*. *Med. Mycol.* **2015**, *53*, 42–50. [CrossRef]
10. Batista-Duharte, A.; Pereira, S.A.; Freitas, D.F.S.; Gutierrez-Galhardo, M.C.; Fuentes, D.P.; Carlos, I.Z. Therapeutic and Prophylactic Tools for Sporotrichosis: Current Strategies and Future Tendencies. In *Sporotrichosis: New Developments and Future Prospects*; Carlos, I.Z., Ed.; Springer: Cham, Switzerland, 2015; pp. 147–177.
11. Edwards, J.E. Fungal cell wall vaccines: An update. *J. Med. Microbiol.* **2012**, *6*, 895–903. [CrossRef] [PubMed]
12. Portuondo, D.L.; Ferreira, L.S.; Urbaczek, A.C.; Batista-Duharte, A.; Carlos, I.Z. Adjuvants and delivery systems for antifungal vaccines: Current state and future developments. *Med. Mycol.* **2015**, *53*, 69–89. [CrossRef]
13. Di Pasquale, A.; Preiss, S.; Tavares Da Silva, F.; Garçon, N. Vaccine Adjuvants: From 1920 to 2015 and beyond. *Vaccines* **2015**, *3*, 320–343. [CrossRef] [PubMed]
14. Pérez, O.; Batista-Duharte, A.; González, E.; Zayas, C.; Balboa, J.; Cuello, M.; Cabrera, O.; Lastre, M.; Schijns, V.E. Human prophylactic vaccine adjuvants and their determinant role in new vaccine formulations. *Braz. J. Med. Biol. Res.* **2012**, *45*, 681–692. [CrossRef] [PubMed]

15. Hendrick, M.J.; Goldschmidt, M.H.; Shofer, F.S.; Wang, Y.Y.; Somlyo, A.P. Postvaccinal sarcomas in the cat: Epidemiology and electron probe microanalytical identification of aluminum. *Cancer Res.* **1992**, *52*, 5391–5394. [PubMed]
16. Coffman, R.L.; Sher, A.; Seder, R.A. Vaccine adjuvants: Putting innate immunity to work. *Immunity* **2010**, *33*, 492–503. [CrossRef] [PubMed]
17. Batista-Duharte, A.; Téllez-Martínez, D.; Fuentes, D.L.P.; Carlos, I.Z. Molecular adjuvants that modulate regulatory T cell function in vaccination: A critical appraisal. *Pharmacol. Res.* **2018**, *129*, 237–250. [CrossRef] [PubMed]
18. Han, J.; Zhao, D.; Li, D.; Wang, X.; Jin, Z.; Zhao, K. Polymer-based nanomaterials and applications for vaccines and drugs. *Polymers* **2018**, *10*, 31. [CrossRef]
19. Deville, S.; Carneaux, E.; Bertrand, F.; Cauchard, S.; Cauchard, J.; Dupuis, L. Adjuvant formulation for companion animals vaccines. *Procedia Vaccinol.* **2011**, *4*, 104–112. [CrossRef]
20. Portuondo, D.L.; Batista-Duharte, A.; Ferreira, L.S.; Martínez, D.T.; Polesi, M.C.; Duarte, R.A.; de Paula, E.; Silva, A.C.; Marcos, C.M.; Almeida, A.M.; et al. A cell wall protein-based vaccine candidate induce protective immune response against *Sporothrix schenckii* infection. *Immunobiology* **2016**, *221*, 300–309. [CrossRef] [PubMed]
21. Portuondo, D.L.; Batista-Duharte, A.; Ferreira, L.S.; de Andrade, C.R.; Quinello, C.; Téllez-Martínez, D.; de Aguiar Loesch, M.L.; Carlos, I.Z. Comparative efficacy and toxicity of two vaccine candidates against *Sporothrix schenckii* using either Montanide™ Pet Gel A or aluminum hydroxide adjuvants in mice. *Vaccine* **2017**, *35*, 4430–4436. [CrossRef] [PubMed]
22. Portuondo, D.L.; Dores-Silva, P.R.; Ferreira, L.S.; Téllez-Martínez, D.; Marcos, C.M.; de Aguiar Loesch, M.L.; Guzman, Q.F.; Borges, J.C.; Batista-Duharte, A.; Carlos, I.Z. Immunization with recombinant enolase of Sporothrix spp (rSsEno) confers effective protection against sporotrichosis in mice. *bioRxiv* **2019**. [CrossRef]
23. Taborda, C.P.; Nosanchuk, J.D. Vaccines, Immunotherapy and New Antifungal Therapy against Fungi: Updates in the New Frontier. *Front. Microbiol.* **2017**, *8*, 1743. [CrossRef]
24. Nami, S.; Mohammadi, R.; Vakili, M.; Khezripour, K.; Mirzaei, H.; Morovati, H. Fungal vaccines, mechanism of actions and immunology: A comprehensive review. *Biomed. Pharmacother.* **2019**, *109*, 333–344. [CrossRef]
25. Spellberg, B. Vaccines for invasive fungal infections. *F1000 Med. Rep.* **2011**, *3*, 13. [CrossRef] [PubMed]
26. Di Pasquale, A.; Bonanni, P.; Garçon, N.; Stanberry, L.R.; El-Hodhod, M.; Tavares Da Silva, F. Vaccine safety evaluation: Practical aspects in assessing benefits and risks. *Vaccine* **2016**, *34*, 6672–6680. [CrossRef] [PubMed]
27. Moyer, T.J.; Zmolek, A.C.; Irvine, D.J. Beyond antigens and adjuvants: Formulating future vaccines. *J. Clin. Investig.* **2016**, *126*, 799–808. [CrossRef] [PubMed]
28. Batista-Duharte, A.; Martínez, D.T.; Carlos, I.Z. Efficacy and safety of immunological adjuvants. Where is the cut-off? *Biomed. Pharmacother.* **2018**, *105*, 616–624. [CrossRef]
29. Adams, J.R.; Haughney, S.L.; Mallapragada, S.K. Effective polymer adjuvants for sustained delivery of protein subunit vaccines. *Acta Biomater.* **2015**, *14*, 104–114. [CrossRef] [PubMed]
30. Shakya, A.K.; Nandakumar, K.S. Polymers as immunological adjuvants: An update on recent developments. *J. BioSci. Biotechnol.* **2012**, *1*, 99–210.
31. Shakya, A.K.; Nandakumar, K.S. Applications of polymeric adjuvants in studying autoimmune responses and vaccination againstinfectious diseases. *J. R. Soc. Interface* **2013**, *10*, 20120536. [CrossRef]
32. Uenotsuchi, T.; Takeuchi, S.; Matsuda, T.; Urabe, K.; Koga, T.; Uchi, H.; Nakahara, T.; Fukagawa, S.; Kawasaki, M.; Kajiwara, H.; et al. Differential induction of Th1-prone immunity by human dendritic cells activated with Sporothrix schenckii of cutaneous and visceral origins to determine their different virulence. *Int. Immunol.* **2006**, *18*, 1637–1646. [CrossRef]
33. Maia, D.C.; Sassá, M.F.; Placeres, M.C.; Carlos, I.Z. Influence of Th1/Th2 cytokines and nitric oxide in murine systemic infection induced by Sporothrix schenckii. *Mycopathologia* **2006**, *161*, 11–19. [CrossRef]
34. Quinello, C.; Ferreira, L.S.; Picolli, I.; Loesch, M.L.; Portuondo, D.L.; Batista-Duharte, A.; Carlos, I.Z. Sporothrix schenckii Cell Wall Proteins-Stimulated BMDCs Are Able to Induce a Th1-Prone Cytokine Profile In Vitro. *J. Fungi* **2018**, *4*, 106. [CrossRef] [PubMed]
35. Batista-Duharte, A.; Téllez-Martínez, D.; Roberto de Andrade, C.; Portuondo, D.L.; Jellmayer, J.A.; Polesi, M.C.; Carlos, I.Z. Sporothrix brasiliensis induces a more severe disease associated with sustained

Th17 and regulatory T cells responses than Sporothrix schenckii sensu stricto in mice. *Fungal Biol.* **2018**, *122*, 1163–1170. [CrossRef]

36. Flores-García, A.; Velarde-Félix, J.S.; Garibaldi-Becerra, V.; Rangel-Villalobos, H.; Torres-Bugarín, O.; Zepeda-Carrillo, E.A.; Ruíz-Bernés, S.; Ochoa-Ramírez, L.A. Recombinant murine IL-12 promotes a protective Th1/cellular response in Mongolian gerbils infected with Sporothrix schenckii. *J. Chemother.* **2015**, *27*, 87–93. [CrossRef]
37. Batista-Duharte, A.; Lastre, M.; Romeu, B.; Portuondo, D.L.; Téllez-Martínez, D.; Manente, F.A.; Pérez, O.; Carlos, I.Z. Antifungal and immunomodulatory activity of a novel cochleate for amphotericin B delivery against Sporothrix schenckii. *Int. Immunopharmacol.* **2016**, *40*, 277–287. [CrossRef] [PubMed]
38. De Almeida, J.R.F.; Jannuzzi, G.P.; Kaihami, G.H.; Breda, L.C.D.; Ferreira, K.S.; de Almeida, S.R. An immunoproteomic approach revealing peptides from Sporothrix brasiliensis that induce a cellular immune response in subcutaneous sporotrichosis. *Sci. Rep.* **2018**, *8*, 4192. [CrossRef]
39. Chen, F.; Jiang, R.; Wang, Y.; Zhu, M.; Zhang, X.; Dong, S.; Shi, H.; Wang, L. Recombinant Phage Elicits Protective Immune Response against Systemic S. globosa Infection in Mouse Model. *Sci. Rep.* **2017**, *7*, 42024. [CrossRef] [PubMed]
40. García-Lozano, A.; Toriello, C.; Antonio-Herrera, L.; Bonifaz, L.C. Sporothrix schenckii Immunization, but Not Infection, Induces Protective Th17 Responses Mediated by Circulating Memory CD4+ T Cells. *Front. Microbiol.* **2018**, *9*, 1275. [CrossRef]
41. Li Causi, E.; Parikh, S.C.; Chudley, L.; Layfield, D.M.; Ottensmeier, C.H.; Stevenson, F.K.; Di Genova, G. Vaccination expands antigen-specific CD4+ memory T cells and mobilizes bystander central-memory T cells. *PLoS ONE* **2015**, *10*, e0136717. [CrossRef] [PubMed]
42. Read, A.F.; Baigent, S.J.; Powers, C.; Kgosana, L.B.; Blackwell, L.; Smith, L.P.; Kennedy, D.A.; Walkden-Brown, S.W.; Nair, V.K. Imperfect Vaccination Can Enhance the Transmission of Highly Virulent Pathogens. *PLoS Biol.* **2015**, *13*, e1002198. [CrossRef] [PubMed]
43. Alba-Fierro, C.A.; Pérez-Torres, A.; Toriello, C.; Pulido-Camarillo, E.; López-Romero, E.; Romo-Lozano, Y.; Gutiérrez-Sánchez, G.; Ruiz-Baca, E. Immune Response Induced by an Immunodominant 60 kDa Glycoprotein of the Cell Wall of Sporothrix schenckii in Two Mice Strains with Experimental Sporotrichosis. *J. Immunol. Res.* **2016**, *2016*, 6525831. [CrossRef] [PubMed]
44. Batista-Duharte, A.; Portuondo, D.; Pérez, O.; Carlos, I.Z. Systemic immunotoxicity reactions induced by adjuvanted vaccines. *Int. Immunopharmacol.* **2014**, *20*, 170–180. [CrossRef] [PubMed]

8

Antimicrobial Peptides from Plants

James P. Tam [1,*], Shujing Wang [1,2], Ka H. Wong [1] and Wei Liang Tan [1]

1 School of Biological Sciences, Nanyang Technological University, Singapore, Singapore; wangshujing@mail.tsinghua.edu.cn (S.W.); hwka@ntu.edu.sg (K.H.W.); TANW0209@e.ntu.edu.sg (W.L.T.)
2 Department of Pharmacology and Pharmaceutical Sciences, School of Medicine, Tsinghua University, Beijing 100084, China
* Author to whom correspondence should be addressed; jptam@ntu.edu.sg;

Academic Editor: Guangshun Wang

Abstract: Plant antimicrobial peptides (AMPs) have evolved differently from AMPs from other life forms. They are generally rich in cysteine residues which form multiple disulfides. In turn, the disulfides cross-braced plant AMPs as cystine-rich peptides to confer them with extraordinary high chemical, thermal and proteolytic stability. The cystine-rich or commonly known as cysteine-rich peptides (CRPs) of plant AMPs are classified into families based on their sequence similarity, cysteine motifs that determine their distinctive disulfide bond patterns and tertiary structure fold. Cystine-rich plant AMP families include thionins, defensins, hevein-like peptides, knottin-type peptides (linear and cyclic), lipid transfer proteins, α-hairpinin and snakins family. In addition, there are AMPs which are rich in other amino acids. The ability of plant AMPs to organize into specific families with conserved structural folds that enable sequence variation of non-Cys residues encased in the same scaffold within a particular family to play multiple functions. Furthermore, the ability of plant AMPs to tolerate hypervariable sequences using a conserved scaffold provides diversity to recognize different targets by varying the sequence of the non-cysteine residues. These properties bode well for developing plant AMPs as potential therapeutics and for protection of crops through transgenic methods. This review provides an overview of the major families of plant AMPs, including their structures, functions, and putative mechanisms.

Keywords: plant antimicrobial peptides; cysteine-rich peptides; cystine knot; thionin; defensin; hevein; knottin

---

1. Introduction

Higher plants have a broad range of defense mechanisms to counter physical, chemical and biological stress such as drought, cold, heavy metal, pollutants and pathogen attacks from fungi, bacteria and viruses. In response to infection by a variety of pathogens, plants display up-regulation of a set of genes associated with systemic acquired resistance [1]. General resistance is accomplished by the release of secondary metabolites like phytoalexins, tannins and polyphenolic compounds, and the generation of pathogenesis-related (PR) proteins. PR proteins were first discovered in the early 1970s in tobacco leaves in response totobacco mosaic virus infections and were later defined as the induced proteins that are released during pathogenic attacks [2,3]. According to a recent review, there are at least 17 families that have been detected and isolated that possess a wide range of defense-related properties, including antibacterial, antifungal, antiviral, anti-oxidative activity, chitinase and proteinase inhibitory activities [1–4]. This review will focus on peptides which possess antimicrobial activity, namely thionin (PR-13 family), defensin (PR-12 family), hevein-like peptide, knottin, α-hairpinin, lipid transfer protein (PR-14 family) and snakin.

Antimicrobial peptides (AMPs) are ubiquitous and found as host defenses against pathogens and pests in diverse organisms ranging from microbes to animals [5]. AMPs exist in different molecular forms, although the majority of them are linear peptides from insects, animals, and plants. Nevertheless, bacteria produce polycyclic peptides such as lantibiotics, and all major forms of life produce circular peptides which include bacteriocins from bacteria, cyclotides from plants and theta-defensins from animals [6–9]. In plants, the majority of AMPs are Cys-rich [10], a feature that enables the formation of multiple disulfide bonds (usually two to six) that contribute to a compact structure and resistance to chemical and proteolytic degradation.

In general, plant AMPs share several common characteristics with those from microbes, insects and animals. They include features such as their molecular forms, positive charge and amphipathic nature, all of which are primarily related to their defensive role(s) as membrane-active antifungals, antibacterials, and antivirals. These features, in addition to being Cys-rich, are well represented by two plant AMP families, thionins and plant defensins. Other families of plant AMPs act on pathogens differently from animal AMPs. For example, hevein-like peptides bind chitins, knottin-type peptides inhibit enzymes such as proteases, and lipid transfer proteins bind lipids to disrupt microbial penetration into cell membranes.

Classification of plant AMP families is largely based on their Cys motifs which exhibit a characteristic Cys pattern with a defined number of non-Cys residues between the two neighboring Cys. Currently, the number of AMPs isolated from a limited number of plants already exceeds a thousand and is likely to increase in the future. Sequence analysis and genomic data mining using these Cys motifs have revealed that Cys-rich peptides (CRPs) with AMP characteristics are under-predicted [11]. In model plants, such as rice and *Arabidopsis*, CRPs may account for about 3% of the expressed proteins.

Like animal AMPs, AMP expression in plants is constitutive or induced and often tissue-specific. Moreover, plant AMPs are evolvable with hypervariable sequences encased in a particular scaffold characteristic of a given family of AMPs, which is analogous, but to a much lesser extent, to the molecular diversity of vertebrate immunoglobulin-based immunity.

This review aims to provide a general overview of the major families of plant AMPs, including their structures, functions, and putative mechanisms of defense. Additional details on plant AMPs can be found in a number of excellent previous reviews [12–25]. Furthermore, information on AMPs from diverse organisms can be accessed through several databases, such as APD, APD2 [26,27], YADAMP [28], DAMPD [29], and PhytAMP (specific for plant AMPs) [10].

2. Classification and Characteristics

Plant AMPs are divided into families based on their sequence similarity, Cys motifs, and distinctive disulfide bond patterns which, in turn, determine their tertiary structure folding. Table 1 lists the major families of plant AMPs based on these criteria; families include thionins, defensins, hevein-like peptides, knottin-type peptides (linear and cyclic), lipid transfer proteins, α-hairpinin families, snakins, and unclassified CRP-AMPs. In addition, non-CRP AMPs, which may be rich in other amino acids, are also described in this review, including the Gly-rich peptide (GRP) Pg-AMP1, the Gly- and His-rich peptide shepherins, and peptides of less than 10 amino acids (aa), such as Cn-AMP1 and Cr-ACP1. The following defining features are found in plant AMPs:

1. Mostly characterized as moderate-size (MW of 2–6 kDa), basic, CRPs with two to six intra-molecular disulfide bonds.
2. Members within a family are classified based on Cys motif, sequence similarity and are conserved in secondary and tertiary structure.

3. One or two additional disulfide bonds are found in members of thionins, defensins, and hevein-like peptides. These additional bonds bolster structural stability without affecting the general scaffold. Because the varying number of Cys residues can create confusion, we refer to AMPs within a family based on the number of Cys when necessary throughout this review (e.g., 6C-thionins contain six Cys and 8C-thionins have eight Cys).
4. In addition to being antimicrobial, AMPs also display "peptide promiscuity", which refers to the multiple functions displayed by a single peptide.
5. All are ribosomally derived and bioprocessed from precursors, which often contain three domains: N- and C-terminal pro-domains and a mature AMP domain. Mature sequences are often hypervariable and display more variation than the conserved terminal domains in the preproprotein to give sequence diversity for adaptation.
6. Because of cross-bracing by multiple disulfide bonds, most CRP-AMPs with a molecular weight (MW) of 2–6 kDa are structurally compact with high thermal, chemical, and enzymatic stability.

Table 1. Major families of plant AMPs.

Peptide	S-S No.	Representative Member			Structural Motif
		Name	AA No.	Disulfide Motif	
6C-Thionin	3	Crambin	46	2-C-0-C-11-C-8-C-5-C-7-C-6	Gamma (Γ) fold
8C-Thionin	4	β-Purothionin	45	2-C-0-C-7-C-3-C-8-C-3-C-1-C-7-C-6	β1-α1-α2-β2-coil motif
8C-Defensin	4	NaD1	47	2-C-10-C-5-C-3-C-9-C-6-C-1-C-3-C	CSαβ motif
10C-Defensin	5	PhD1	47	2-C-3-C-6-C-5-C-2-C-0-C-9-C-6-C-1-C-3-C	β1-coil-α-β2-β3
6C-Hevein	3	Ac-AMP1	29	3-C-4-C-4-C-0-C-5-C-6-C-1	Gly & Cys rich Central β
8C-Hevein	4	Hevein	43	2-C-8-C-4-C-0-C-5-C-6-C-5-C-3-C-2	strands & (short helical)
10C-Hevein	5	EAFP1	41	2-C-3-C-3-C-4-C-0-C-5-C-6-C-5-C-1-C-1-C-2	side coils
Knottin	3	PAFP-S	38	2-C-6-C-8-C-0-C-3-C-10-C-3	Cystine knot Short β
Cyclic Knottin	3	Kalata B1	29	4-C-3-C-4-C-4-C-1-C-4-C-3	strand & coil
α-Hairpinin	2	Ec-AMP1	37	6-C-3-C-13-C-3-C-8	α1-turn-α2
LTP	4	Maize LTP1	93	3-C-9-C-14-C-0-C-19-C-1-C-22-C-13-C-4	Hydrophobic cavity
LTP	4	Wheat LTP2	67	1-C-7-C-13-C-0-C-8-C-1-C-23-C-6-C	α1-α2-α3-α4-coil
Snakin *	6	Snakin-1	63	4-C-3-C-3-C-8-C-3-C-2-CC-2-C-1-C-11-C-1-C-12-C-1	α -helices

* The disulfide and structural motif of Snakin-1 is predicted based on homology modelling.

2.1. *Thionins*

α-/β-Thionins are the prototypic plant AMP; they are cationic peptides of 45–48 aa with three or four disulfide bonds [12]. Initially, they were known as plant toxins because of their toxicity towards bacteria [30], fungi [31], plant and animal cells [32], as well as insect larvae [33]. The prototypic thionin with antimicrobial activity, α-purothionin, was isolated in the endosperm of wheat [30,34]. Following the discovery of α-purothionin, subsequent thionins isolated from other plants are labeled with descending letters of the Greek alphabet in the order of their discovery (e.g., α-thionins, β-thionins, and γ1/γ1-thionins).

Classification of thionins is largely based on α-purothionin and includes the α-/β-thinoins of crambin, viscotoxins, phoratoxin A, hordothionins, and purothinoins. However, γ-thionins are considered part of the plant defensin family based on structural considerations. Thus, α-/β-thionins share a similar structural fold different from that of γ-thionins. For convenience, α/β-thionins with eight Cys residues will be hereafter referred to as 8C-thionins and those with six Cys designated 6C-thionins (Figure 1A,B).

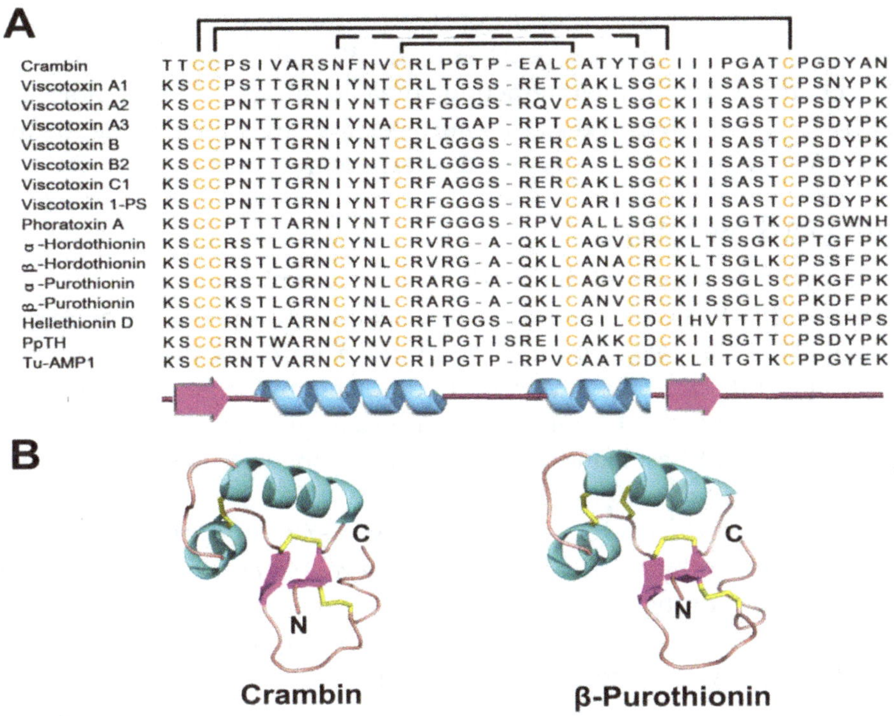

Figure 1. Sequences (**A**) and structures (**B**) of representative thionins. The secondary structure is represented by different colors: cyan-α helix; magenta-β strand; pink-random coil and yellow-disulfide bonds.

2.1.1. Occurrences, Distribution, and Biosynthesis

Thionins have been identified from monocots and dicots and are expressed in different tissues, such as seeds, leaves, and roots [35–37]. The expression of thionins can be induced by infection with various microbes [38,39] and has been shown to be related to the release of the hormone methyl jasmonate upon plant wounding or microorganism invasion [38,40,41]. Thionins are ribosomally derived and expressed as preproproteins, wherein the prothionin domain is flanked by two conserved sequences, the N-terminal signaling peptide and C-terminal acidic domain [35,38,42]. Mature thionin sequences display more variation than the conserved terminal domains in the preproprotein due to evolutionary pressure [43]. The three-domain precursor of plant AMPs in CRP families is typical and found in other CRP families, including defensins, hevein-like peptides, and knottin-type peptides.

2.1.2. Structure

From the limited number of members identified thus far, thionins have relatively conserved amino acid sequences compared to other plant defense peptides (Figure 1A). They also share a conserved β1-α1-α2-β2-coil secondary structural motif, which forms a gamma (Γ) fold, a special turn consists of three amino acid residues with the first and third residue connected by a hydrogen bond in the tertiary structure (Figure 1A,B).

Thionins can be loosely classified as pseudocyclics because of an end-to-end disulfide bond linking the N- and C-termini, conferring a circular structural topology. They are, however, not true pseudocyclics because there are additional non-cysteine amino acids located at both the N- and C-termini. 8C-Thionins contain four conserved stabilizing disulfide bonds between CysI-CysVIII (Cys numbering in Roman numerals from N-to-C-termini) linking β1 to the C-terminal coil, CysII-CysVII linking the end of β1 with the beginning of β2, CysIII-CysVI linking α1 and the loop after α2, and CysIV-CysV linking α1 and α2. The 6C-thionins have the same Cys pairing as 8C-thionins except for the absence of the CysII-CysVII disulfide bond. The structure of 8C-thionins, including α-/β-purothionins, α-/β-hordothionin, and hellethionin D, are similar to that of 6C-thionins with the Γ-shape but with minor differences in the C-terminal coil region [44–46]. The long arm of the Γ fold comprises the α1-α2 region, and the short arm consists of β1 and the β2-coil. The large groove between the two arms is proposed to be important for the interaction between thionins and membrane lipids [43]. Most hydrophobic side chains cluster around the outer surface of the long arm, while the hydrophilic chains are located on the surface within the groove or outer face of the short arm (Figure 2A).

2.1.3. Structure-Function Relationship

The 6C-thionins with three disulfide bonds include crambin, viscotoxins, and phoratoxin A. Most 6C-thionins are highly basic, amphipathic, and toxic, with the exception of crambin. Crambin is a neutral, hydrophobic, non-toxic peptide identified from *Crambe abyssinica* with two isomers, P22/L25 and S22/I25 [47,48]. High resolution structures of crambin have been determined by NMR and X-ray/neutron crystallography in both water and detergent [47,49–53]. Viscotoxins (including A1, A2, A3, B, B2, C1, and 1-PS) and phoratoxins from the mistletoes share a similar Γ-shape with β1-α1-α2-β2-coil motif [54–60].

8C-Thionins with four disulfide bonds include α-/β-purothionins, α-/β-hordothionins, hellethionin-D, *Pyrularia Pubera* thionin (PpTH), and *Tulipa gensneriana* bulb-purified AMPs (Tu-AMPs). The monomeric conformation of the 45-aa α-hordothionin isolated from barley [61,62] was previously determined by NMR [62], while X-ray crystallography revealed a dimeric structure [61]. A study by Vila-Perello showed that removal of one disulfide bond from PpTH is sufficient to significantly alter its folding [63]. A 45% size-reduced form of PpTH was synthesized, which only contains residues 7–32 with the two antiparallel α-helices stabilized by two disulfide bonds. Size-reduced PpTH appeared to display the same antimicrobial activity and mechanism of action as intact PpTH in selected test microorganisms [64].

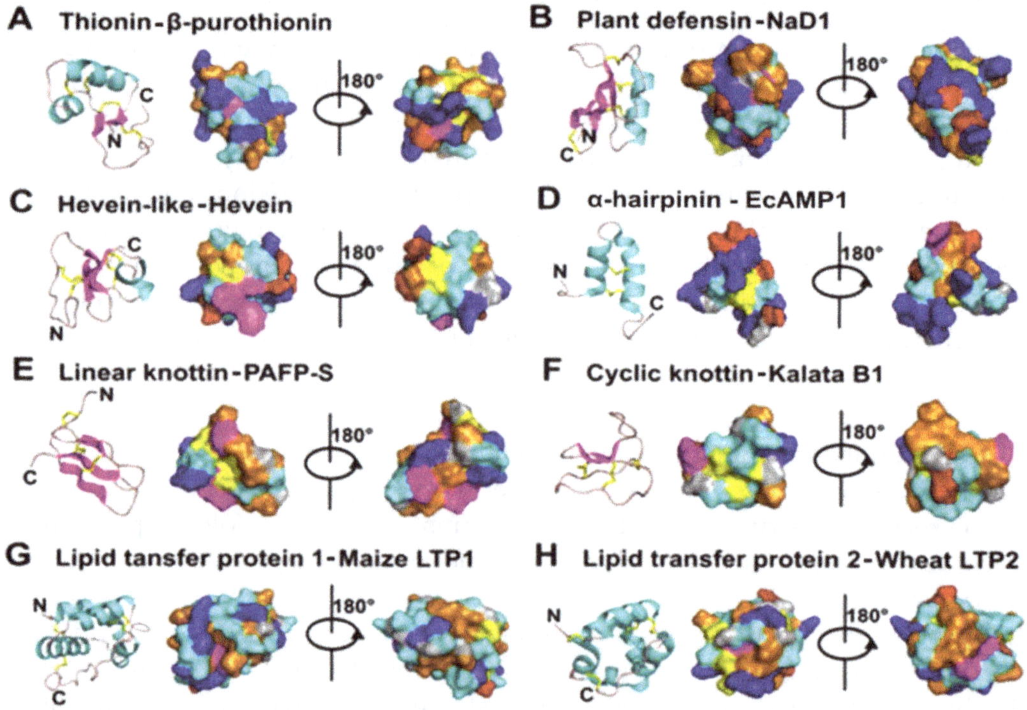

Figure 2. Cartoon illustration and surface plot of representative members of different antimicrobial peptides. The orientation of surface plot (left) of each representative member is the same as the cartoon illustration, while that of the right one is evolved from the left one by 180° turn around the y axis. Color representation rules for different amino acids are as follows: blue-positively charged (R, K & H), red-negatively charged (D & E), orange-hydrophobic (I, L, V, A, P & M), cyan-hydrophilic (S, T, E & Q), magenta-aromatic (F, Y & W), yellow-cysteine (C) and gray-glycine (G).

Tu-AMP1 and Tu-AMP2 are antibacterial, antifungal, and can reversibly bind chitin, a key constituent of the cell wall of fungi and exoskeletons of invertebrates, such as insects, anthropods, and nematodes. Initially, they were suggested to be thionin-like peptides, although Tu-AMP2 is a heterodimer of two chains joined by disulfide bonds [65]. However, it is worthwhile to point out that in our review of plant CRPs, the occurrence of heterodimer is exceedingly rare. In our view, it remains to be determined whether the heterodimeric formation occurs during the isolation process.

2.1.4. Mechanism of Action

Thionins are hydrophobic and likely elicit their toxicity to bacteria, fungi, and animal and plant cells via membrane interactions with their hydrophobic residues or/and positive surface charge [12,13,18,66–68]. The proposed mechanism of toxicity is attributed to lysis of cell membranes, but it is still under investigation [30,39,68–70]. Stec proposed a structural model of the thionin-phospholipid interaction to explain the solubilization and lysis of cell membranes [43].

Thionins are known to directly interact with membrane lipids apart from protein receptors [67,71,72]. *Pyrularia* thionin from the nuts of *Pyrularia pubera* mediates the influx of Ca^{2+} during certain cellular responses, while Tyr iodination reduces its hemolysis, phospholipase A2 activation, and cytotoxicity [32]. Structure-function studies have demonstrated that Lys1 and Tyr13 in thionins are highly conserved and proposed to be crucial to their toxicity, with the exception of non-toxic, non-lytic crambin. Instead, crambin contains Thr1 and Phe13 residues [32,43,73,74]. Furthermore, Arg10 is suggested to be important to the folding stability of all thionins, as it is an abundant source of hydrogen bonds between β1, α1, and the C-terminal coil [75].

2.2. *Plant Defensins*

Plant defensins are the best known, and likely most abundant, of all plant AMPs with membranolytic functions, according to data mining of selected plant genomes. They are cationic peptides of 45–54 aa with four to five disulfide bonds [76]. Plant defensins have diverse biological functions which include antifungal [77–81], antibacterial [82,83], and α-amylase and trypsin inhibitory activity [84,85]. In addition to being antimicrobial, plant defensins are also involved in the biotic stress response, as well as plant growth and development.

Plant defensins were first identified as γ-thionins, γ1-hordothionin, and γ1-/γ2-purothionins from wheat and barley grains [86,87]. Thus, they were initially classified as γ-thionins due to their limited sequence identity (25%) with α-/β-thionins. Later, they were found to be unrelated to thionins based on structural features [88]. In 1995, they were grouped as plant defensins based on their sequence, structure, and function similarities with mammalian and insect defensins [76,78,88,89].

2.2.1. Occurrences, Distribution, and Biosynthesis

Plant defensins include over 100 members from a wide range of plants, including wheat, barley, tobacco, radish, mustard, turnip, arabidopsis, potato, sorghum, soybean, cowpea, and spinach, among others [15,90]. They have been identified in multiple tissues, tubers [79,91], leaves [79], pods [92], and flowers [93–95], with the majority identified from seeds and roots [96]. Two types of precursors have been identified in plant defensins, wherein the dominant group is composed of the N-terminal signal peptide and a mature plant defensin domain [97], while the minor group is composed of an extra C-terminal acidic pro-domain of 33 aa reportedly associated with the vacuolar sorting mechanism since defensins with this domain were found in vacuoles and those without were found in the outer cell layers [16,79,95].

2.2.2. Structures

Plant defensins are generally characterized by four conserved disulfide bonds (except for PhDs, a 10C-plant defensin isolated from *Petunia hydrida*) with the outer disulfide pair as an end-to-end inner disulfide bridge and the inner three pairs of disulfide bonds forming a cystine knot (see knottins).

A secondary structure characteristic of plant defensins is a Cys-stabilized αβ (CSαβ) motif of the cysteine knot. The CSαβ motif was first characterized in charybdotoxin, a K^+ channel blocker isolated from scorpions [98] and named by Cornet *et al.* [99]. This motif forms a β1-coil-α-β2-β3 pattern in the secondary structure, where the α-helix is parallel to three antiparallel β-strands (Figure 3A,B). The CSαβ scaffold is stabilized and characterized by: (1) two disulfide bonds between the CXXXC motif from the α-helix and the CXC motif in the central β3 strand; (2) one disulfide bond between the β2 strand and the first loop before the α-helix; and (3) an end-to-end disulfide bond between the N- and C-termini, a disulfide connective similar to thionins. However, plant defensins (γ-thionins) differ greatly from α-/β-thinoins in their secondary and tertiary structures. In the secondary structure, α-/β-thionins show a typical β1-α1-α2-β2-coil motif, whereas γ-thionins display a β1-coil-α-β2-β3 motif. At the tertiary structural level, β1 and β2 orient antiparallel in α-/β-thinoins, whereas the corresponding β1and β3 in γ-thionins are oriented in parallel.

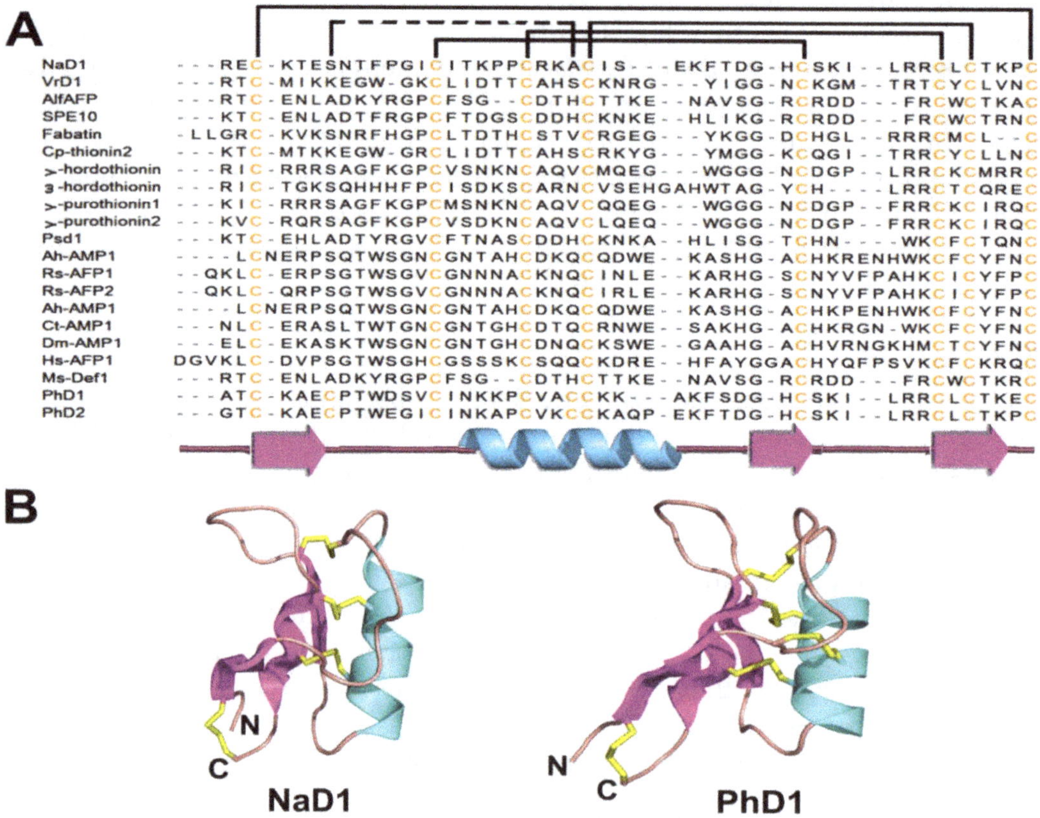

Figure 3. Sequences (**A**) and structures (**B**) of representative plant defensins. The secondary structure is represented by different colors: cyan-α helix; magenta-β strand; pink-random coil and yellow-disulfide bonds.

Similar to thionins, plant defensins are pseudocyclics (see thionins), with conservation of the disulfide bond between the first and last Cys, conferring a circular structural topology by connecting the side chains of the N- and C- termini.

Plant defensins have been reported to be stable in harsh conditions that mimic the digestive system and decoction process, including high temperature (~85 °C), low pH (~2.0), and oxidative and proteolytic environments [100–102]. Although defensins show conservation of the CSαβ motif, there are variations in the number of disulfide bonds, primary sequences, and tertiary structures [89,103,104]. It has been shown that Ala substitutions of non-Cys residues on VrD1 are tolerated in the CSαβ motif although the structural stability and inhibitory effects vary among the mutants [105].

2.2.3. Structure-Function Relationship

Based on the number of Cys, plant defensins are further divided into 8C-plant defensins with four disulfides and 10C-plant defensins with five disulfide bonds.

The 8C-plant defensins include NaD1, VrD1, AlfAFP, ω-hordothionin, Cp-thionin II, Rs-AFPs, Psd1, Fabatins, and Ms-Def1 (Figure 3A,B). NaD1 (47 aa) was identified from the outer cell layers of different flower parts of the ornamental tobacco *Nicotiana alata*. Its distribution is consistent with its protective roles in reproductive organs. *In vitro* results showed that NaD1 inhibits the growth of plant pathogens *Botrytis cinerea* and *Fusarium oxysporus* [95,106]. VrD1 (46 aa) from the mung bean *Vigna radiata* not only inhibits protein synthesis, but is also antimicrobial and insect (bruchids)-resistant [107, 108]. ω-Hordothionin (48 aa) purified from barley endosperm inhibits translational activity in both eukaryotic and prokaryotic cell-free systems [109]. The crystal structure of SPE10, identified from *Pachyrrhizus erosus* seeds [110], shows a dimer with each unit adopting the typical CSαβ motif [111]. Based on structural analysis and mutation studies, the dimeric conformation of SPE10 was suggested to be associated with its function, while the hydrophobic patch on the molecular head is necessary for its antifungal activity.

AlfAFP from *Medicago sativa* seeds is an antifungal peptide that provides robust resistance to the fungal pathogen *Verticillium dahliae* in transgenic potato plants [77,106]. Rs-AFPs (51 aa) purified from *Raphanus sativus* radish seeds are highly basic oligomeric proteins with an N-terminal pyroglutamic acid. They have a broad antifungal spectrum with an IC_{50} = 0.3–100 μg/mL [78,79,81]. Rs-AFPs are abundant in near-mature and mature seeds and released to create a fungal-suppressing microenvironment after disruption of the seed coat [79]. Ms-Def1 from *Medicago sativa* seeds strongly inhibits the fungal growth of *Fusarium graminearum in vitro* [112]; the inhibitory effect is reduced in the presence of Ca^{2+} ions. Homologous antifungal peptides were also reported from seeds of *Aesculus hippocastanum*, *Clitoria ternatea* (Ct-AMP1), *Dahlia merckii* (Dm-AMP1), *Lens culinaris* (Lc-def) and *Heuchera sanguine* (Hs-AFP1) [80,97,113].

Cp-thionin II (47 aa) was identified from *Vigna unguiculata* cowpea seeds and is antibacterial against both Gram-positive and Gram-negative bacteria such as *Staphylococcus aureus*, *Escherichia coli*, and *Pseudomonas syringae* with minimal inhibitory concentrations of 128, 64, and 42 μg/mL, respectively [90]. Psd1, a 46 aa peptide identified from seeds of the pea *Pisum sativum*, is antibacterial and acts as a K^+ channel inhibitor based on a surface charge distribution analysis [114]. Fabatins isolated from the broad bean *Vicia faba* are active against both Gram-positive and Gram-negative bacteria, but inactive against the yeasts *Saccharomyces cerevisiae* and *Candida albicans* [115].

PhDs are 10C-plant defensins. From flowers of *Petunia* hybrids, Lay *et al.* reported two AMPs with antifungal activity, PhD1 (47 aa) and PhD2 (49 aa) [95]. A fifth disulfide bond exists between the α-helix and the loop after β1 within these defensins that do not alter the typical CSαβ topology [108]. The fifth disulfide bond appears only to change the corresponding hydrophobic interaction and hydrogen bond, as in 8C-plant defensins, to a covalent disulfide bond in PhD1 without altering the side-chain orientation of substituted residues.

The γ-thionins which have been reclassified as defensins, γ-hordothionin and ω-hordothionin from *Hordeum vulgare*, were shown to inhibit protein translation in rabbit reticulocytes and mouse liver extracts [87]. However, this inhibitory effect was not observed on plants, such as *Triticum aestivum*, *Cucumis sativus*, *Vicea sativa* and *H. vulgare*, and which may indicate a certain specificity in its mechanism of action. Similarly, no direct interaction was observed between the plant defensins and nucleic acids, which is the proposed mechanism of the inhibitory activity of protein synthesis by the plant thionin family [116]. Instead of protein translation, Mendez *et al.* suggested that ω-hordothionin may act on protein synthesis at the initiation and elongation step [109].

Defensins isolated from the seeds of *Sorghum bicolor*, S1α_1, S1α_2 and S1α_3, were demonstrated to display inhibitory activity against α-amylase activity [84]. They are able to inhibit α-amylase obtained from the gut of the insects *Periplaneta americana* and *Locusta migratoria migratorioides*, and weakly inhibit the α-amylase from human saliva. Defensins from *Vigna unguiculata* and ω-hordothionin, from *H.*

vulgare, also exhibit similar inhibitory activity against insect α-amylase [109,117,118], however, no significant inhibitory effect was observed on porcine α-amylase by plant defensins [119]. Several plant defensins exhibit the ability to inhibit ion channels. Kushmerick *et al.* showed that γ1-zeathionin and γ2-zeathionin from maize kernels block voltage-gated Na^+ channels reversibly in intact mammalian GH3 cells using the patch-clamp technique [120]. These authors postulated that the ion channel inhibitory effect of defensins may be related to the similar 3D structure with scorpion neurotoxin, a well-known Na^+ channel blocker. Plant defensins were also shown to inhibit Ca^{2+} channels [112]. However, no significant inhibitory effect was observed on K^+ channels by plant defensins [119].

Two homologous peptides that display high sequence similarity to plant defensins were isolated from the plant *Cassia fistula*, denoted 5459 and 5144 according to their molecular weight [85]. The 5459 defensin was demonstrated to exhibit trypsin inhibitory activity, whereas no inhibitory effect was observed by the 5144 defensin. Another defensin peptide, Cp-thionin from *V. uguiculata* seeds, was reported to display inhibitory activity against pancreatic bovine trypsin [121].

An enzymatic activity was attributed to a plant defensin. Huang *et al.* cloned the defensin SPD1 from the roots of Ipomoea batatas and showed that it has the ability to regenerate dehydroascorbate (DHA) to ascorbic acid (AsA) in the presence of glutathione [122]. The peptide is also able to convert monodehydroascrobate (MDA) to AsA in the presence of NADH, functioning as a glutathione-dependent dehydroascorbate reductase. SPD1 is likely to function as a regulator of the redox state of AsA, which has been implicated in the response of the plant cell to reactive oxidative stress [123].

2.2.4. Mechanism of Action

The structure-function relationship of plant defensins has been suggested to correlate with their positive charge and amphipathic nature, as illustrated by the structure-surface plot of NaD1 in Figure 2B. Thus, plant defensins could initially bind to microbial membranes through interactions with specific binding sites ("receptors"), as reported for Rs-AFP2, Hs-AFP1, and Dm-AMP1 [16,124,125]. Binding of plant defensins, such as Rs-AFP2 and Dm-AMP1, to the cell membrane results in the influx and efflux of positive ions like Ca^{2+} and K^+ [126,127]. Lastly, Ms-Def1 is able to block the Ca^{2+} channel in a manner similar to the Ca^{2+} channel blocker KP4 [112]. Van der Weerden *et al.* demonstrated that NaD1 does not cause membranes permeabilization via a canonical mechanism which involves nonspecific insertion into membranes [128] but rather a cell wall dependent process, likely requiring a specific receptor. The mechanism of the fungicidal action of NaD1 is likely through permeabilization of the hyphae of *Fusarium oxysporum*, entering into the cytoplasm of the cell and inducing ROS oxidative stress [129]. Hayes *et al.* reported that the high-osmolarity glycerol (HOG) pathway is involved in the protection of the cell against NaD1 [130], indicating that the inhibition of the HOG pathway increases the activity of antimicrobial peptides against *Candida albicans*. Several reviews have discussed in detail the plant defensin mechanism of action [16,101,131,132].

2.3. Hevein-Like Peptides

Hevein-like peptides are basic peptides of 29–45 aa with three to five disulfide bonds. They are rich in Gly and contain conserved aromatic residues found in the hevein domain of lectins. Hevein domains bind to chitin [133–135], which is their primary target.

Hevein was first identified as the most abundant protein component from the latex of the rubber tree *Hevea brasiliensis* and displays strong antifungal activity *in vitro* [136,137]. It was also reported to be a major allergen from latex involved in human latex-fruit syndrome [138,139]. Similar to hevein, hevein-like peptides inhibit the growth of chitin-containing fungi and defend plants against attack from a wide range of fungal pathogens [133,140].

2.3.1. Occurrences, Distribution and Biosynthesis

As a chitin-binding domain, the hevein domain is found in several plant lectins, natural variants of heveins (pseudo-hevein, wheat germ agglutinin, *Urtica dioica* agglutinin), and AMPs [134,141,142].

Similar to other families of CRP-AMPs, the hevein-like peptide is processed from a three-domain precursor. For example, the cDNA of the Ar-AMP precursor comprises a 25 aa N-terminal signal sequence, 30 aa mature peptide, and 34 aa C-terminal region which is cleaved during post-translational processing [143]. In 10C-hevein (hevein-like peptide containing 10 cysteine residues), there are two different precursor peptide structures in the C-terminal prodomain. The WAMP 10C-hevein from *Triticum kiharae* have precursor similar to other families CRP-AMPs, with a 45aa C-terminal region [144], while Ee-CBP 10C-hevein from *Euonymus europaeus* is produced as a chimeric precursor consisting of the mature peptide domain linked to a long C-terminal chitinase-like domain [145]. Andreev *et al.* [144] also showed that the WAMP-1 and WAMP-2 gene may have originated from ancestral chitinase genes and that a frame-shift deletion of the coding region for the catalytic domain led to the WAMP gene formation.

2.3.2. Structure

Hevein-like peptides share conserved Cys, Gly, and several aromatic amino acid residues. They vary substantially in their primary sequences and number of disulfide bonds (from three to five; Figure 4A,B). Thus, hevein-like peptides can be divided into 6C-, 8C-, and 10C-hevein-like peptide subgroups based on the number of Cys they contain. All hevein-like peptides has a cysteine knot motif (see knottins). The solid-state and solution structures of the hevein domain, as determined by X-ray crystallography and NMR, respectively [142,146,147], provide the basis for analyzing the carbohydrate binding ability of this domain. Generally, hevein-like peptides contain a coil-β1-β2-coil-β3 secondary structural motif with variations based on the presence of short turns in the two long coils and β3 strand. Antiparallel β-strands form the central β-sheet of the hevein motif with the two long coils located on each side stabilized by disulfide bonds.

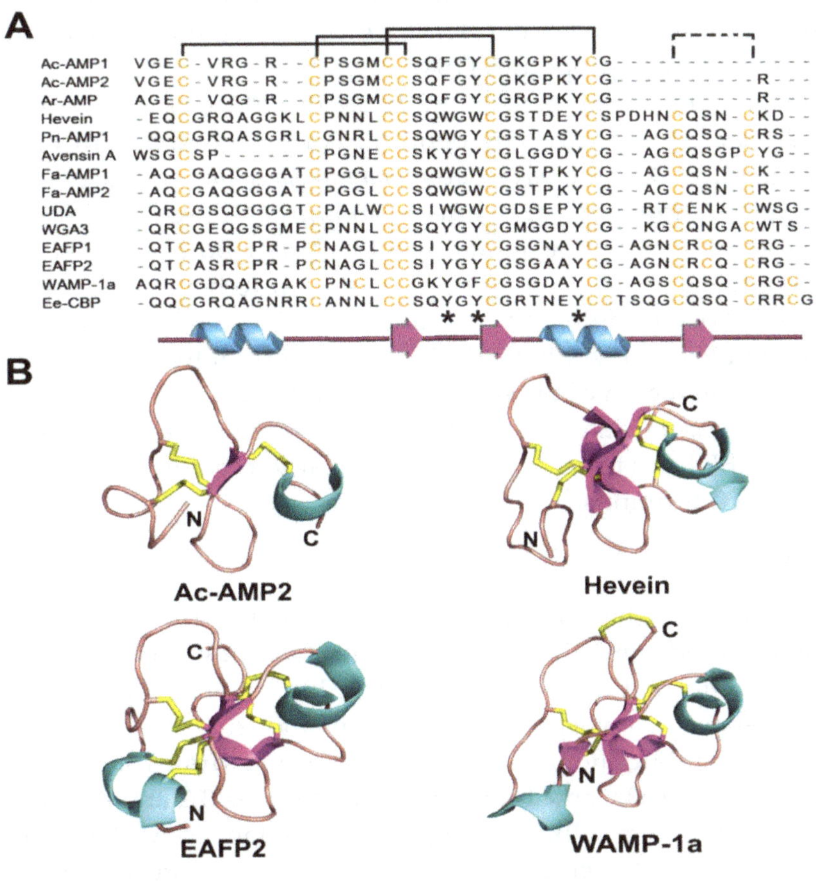

Figure 4. Sequences (**A**) and structures (**B**) of representative hevein-like peptides. The secondary structure is represented by different colors: cyan-α helix; magenta-β strand; pink-random coil and yellow-disulfide bonds.

2.3.3. Structure-Function Study

6C-Hevein-like peptides Ac-AMP1 and Ac-AMP2 isolated from *Amaranthus caudatus* seeds exhibit antimicrobial activity against both Gram-positive bacteria and plant pathogenic fungi with an IC_{50} 2–10 μg/mL [148]. Interestingly, their antimicrobial activity is antagonized by cations. Both Ac-AMP1 and Ac-AMP2 are similar to chitin-binding proteins and known to reversibly bind chitin in the C-terminal truncated fold of hevein [149]. This structure consists of a β-sheet with two antiparallel β-strands as the main central element, an N-terminal coil region, and C-terminal helical turn. The N-terminal coil region is linked to the two central β-strands by two disulfide bonds, while the C-terminal helical coil is connected to the first β-strand through a third disulfide bond. Ar-AMP (30 aa) purified from the seeds of amaranth (*Amaranthus retroflexus*) is another 6C-hevein-like peptide with antifungal activity [143].

Compared to Ac-AMPs, most hevein-like AMPs, including hevein, are 8C-hevein-like peptides with an additional C-terminal sequence containing the fourth disulfide bond. Thus, 8C-hevein contains a central β-sheet of three antiparallel β-stands, wherein the last β-strand is formed from the additional C-terminal sequences and oriented parallel to the fourth disulfide bond. The 6C-hevein32, a truncated form of hevein with the N-terminal 32 aa of hevein similar to Ac-AMP2, is defined as the minimum hevein domain since it presents comparable binding affinity for chito-oligosaccharides as native hevein [150]. Pn-AMP1 and Pn-AMP2 from seeds of the morning glory *Pharbitis nil* are highly basic (pI 12.02) and thermally stable. They exhibit potent antifungal activity against both chitin-containing and non-chitin-containing fungi with an IC_{50} 0.6–75 μg/mL, but lose their antifungal activity in acidic (pH 2.0) or reducing conditions [151]. As the first hevein-like peptides reported antifungal activity similar to thionins, Pn-AMPs have been successfully cloned into tomato and tobacco plants, endowing these transgenic plants with potent antifungal activities [152,153]. Fa-AMP1 and Fa-AMP2 from seeds of the buckwheat *Fagopyrum esculentum,* have antifungal and antibacterial activities with an IC_{50} of 11–36 μg/mL [82]. Avesin A from seeds of the oat *Avena sativa* represents another chitin-binding peptide with weak to moderate antifungal properties [154].

Several hevein-like AMPs contain five disulfide bonds (10C-hevein-like peptides), although the location of the fifth disulfide bond varies by peptide. For example, EAFP1 and EAFP2, each 41 aa long, were purified from the bark of the olive *Eucommia ulmoides Oliv* with an N-terminal pyroglutamic acid [155]. These peptides show inhibitory effects on both chitin-containing and chitin-free fungi with an IC_{50} 18–155 μg/mL and can be antagonized by Ca^{2+}. Both solution and crystal structures indicate that EAFPs contain a chitin-binding domain similar to hevein-like peptides with a distinct Cys7-Cys37 fifth disulfide bond bridging the N-terminal coiled region with the third β-strand [156,157]. In contrast, the fifth disulfide bond within WAMP-1a isolated from the wheat *Triticum kiharae* connects the C-terminus to the central region of the structure [158,159]. Similarly, Ee-CBP from the bark of the spindle tree *Euonymus europaeus* is a potent antifungal peptide with an IC_{50} 1 μg/mL for the fungus *Botrytis cinerea* [160]. Ee-CBP has a primary sequence similar to other hevein-like peptides but with the fifth disulfide bond at the C-terminus.

2.3.4. Mechanism of Action

As a chitin-binding domain, hevein is an excellent model for studying the carbohydrate-peptide interaction, which is reportedly mediated by hydrogen bonding and van der Waals forces. The carbohydrate-induced conformational change to the hevein domain is small based on NMR investigations of pseudo-hevein, a wheat germ agglutinin and truncated hevein mutant [142,161,162]. The interaction between the hydrophobic C-H groups of carbohydrates and the π-electron systems of aromatic amino acids (Trp21, Trp23, and Tyr30 in hevein; Figures 3A and 8C) of hevein-like peptides appear to play an important role in chitin binding, as observed in Ac-AMP synthetic mutants, hevein, and a truncated form of hevein (hevein32) at key interacting positions [150,161,163,164]. Studies on Pn-AMPs showed that they rapidly penetrate fungal hyphae, leading to hyphal tip bursting, which disrupts the fungal membrane causing leakage of cytoplasmic materials [151].

In addition to the chitin binding function of hevein, Slavokhotova *et al.* showed an alternative function in which hevein plays a role in the plant defense against fungal infection [165]. WAMPs which contains an additional Ser at position 36 is able to inhibit the proteolytic activity of the secreted fungal protease fungalysin (Fv-cmp), a Zn-metalloproteinase, isolated from *Fusarium verticillioides*. This protease is able to truncate corn and Arabidopsis class IV chitinases by cleaving within the Gly-Cys site located in the chitin-binding domain of the plant chitinase. The presence of Ser36 prevents WAMP from being digested by Fv-cmp, allowing it to bind to fungalysin, and displace the plant chitinase, thus enabling the chitinase to remain intact and active [165].

2.4. *Knottin-Type Peptides*

Plant knottins belong to a superfamily, with members containing approximately 30 aa. They include inhibitors of α-amylase, trypsin and carboxypeptidase families as well as cyclotides. In general, they are among the smallest in size, but most diverse in functions of plant CRP-AMPs. Knottins typically comprise six Cys residues with conserved disulfide bonds between CysI-CysIV, CysII-CysV, and CysIII-CysVI, forming a cystine knot, but their Cys motifs differ among different subfamilies. Both plant defensins and hevein-like peptides also contain a cysteine-knot motif but they differ in their cysteine spacing.

One characteristic of this family is that they display a very broad range of bioactive functions which include hormone-like functions as well as enzyme-inhibitory, cytotoxic, antimicrobial, insecticidal, and anti-HIV activities [166]. Certain cystine-knot (CK) peptides with identical scaffold structures involved in multiple biological functions has been viewed as "peptide promiscuity" [167].

Historically, the knottin-type peptides were discovered as protease inhibitors sharing in common only in a cystine knot motif, and they are named collectively as cystine-knot inhibitor peptides, knottins. The prototypic knottin scaffold was first discovered in the subfamily of potato carboxypeptidase inhibitor (PCI) in 1982 [168]. The use of knottins also distinguishes the CK-CRPs from those initially described in the structures of the protein growth factors found in animals [169]. As a superfamily, they are believed to be the largest group of plant peptides associated with AMPs, surpassing defensins in the number of molecular forms and sequence diversity.

Knottins in the cyclotide and trypsin inhibitor families are found in two molecular forms, cyclic and linear, based on the presence or absence of backbone (head-to-tail) cyclization. In literature, cyclic knottins of the squash trypsin subfamily are often included in the cyclotide subfamily. Apart from their Cys residues, cyclic knottins and cyclotides share little sequence identity. Currently, both linear (acyclotides) and cyclic (cyclotides) forms of the cyclotide subfamily are found in plants.

2.4.1. Occurrences, Distribution, and Biosynthesis

Linear knottins are found not only in plants, but also in other biological sources, including fungi, insects, and spiders. Thus, CK peptides with identical or related scaffold structures found in diverse life forms provide an example of parallel evolution of protein structures. Cyclotides and their acyclic variants are found only in plants, from the dicot plants of the *Rubiaceae*, *Violaceae*, *Cucurbitaceae*, *Fabaceae*, and *Solanaceae* families to a monocot plant of the *Poaceae* family, with predicted wide and abundant distribution [170–177].

Cyclotides and certain members of cyclic knottins of the squash family are produced from precursor proteins encoding one or more cyclotide domains. The precursor is composed of an endoplasmic reticulum signal region, pro-domain, one (or more) mature cyclotide domain(s), and a short C-terminal tail [172]. However, there are variations in their biosynthesis. A recent report on cyclotides such as cliotides (cT1-cT12) identified from *Clitoria ternatea* showed that they originate from chimeric precursors consisting of Albumin-1 chain A and cyclotide domains [173]. Studies have shown that an asparaginyl endoproteinase could be involved in the backbone cyclization of cyclotides [178–181]. Our laboratory has isolated one of the bioprocessing enzymes responsible for the backbone cyclization process from *C. ternatea*, butelase 1 [181]. Butelase 1 acts as a transamidase, cyclase and ligase and is C-terminal specific to produce Asx-Xaa bonds, with Xaa being a diverse group of residues. Butelase 1 cyclizes various peptides of plant and animal origin efficiently and is the fastest peptide ligase known. Linear variants of cyclotides share high sequence identity and contain a similar knottin scaffold but are biosynthetically unable to cyclize from their precursors [173,182]. Violacin A, a naturally occurring linear cyclotide from *Viola odorata*, lacks the essential bioprocessing signal, the C-terminal Asn residue required for cyclization due to the presence of a stop codon earlier in the C-terminal sequence [177].

Cystine knot α-amylase inhibitors (CKAIs) are plant-derived α-amylase inhibitors originally isolated from *Amaranthus hypocondriacus* [183]. They are the smallest family of proteinacous α-amylase inhibitors among the seven known families [184]. Unlike other knottins, these peptides are rich in proline residues, with at least one of them existing in a *cis-* configuration [185]. In recent studies, Nguyen *et al.* have isolated an additional three members of CKAIs from the leaves and flowers of *Wrightia religiosa* [186] and another five members from the leaves of *Allamanda cathartica* [187]. These CKAIs contain 30 residues, two residues shorter than AAI, and share high sequence homology to each other.

2.4.2. Structure

A common knottin structural motif was initially defined in 1994 as a CK and triple-stranded β-sheet with a long loop connecting the first and second β-strand [166]. The first two disulfide bonds (between CysI-CysIV and CysII-CysV), together with their connecting backbone, form an embedded ring that is penetrated by the third disulfide bond (between CysIII-CysVI). Studies on the subfamily of squash trypsin inhibitors and PCIs showed that only two disulfide bonds (between CysII-CysV and CysIII-CysVI) in the knottin scaffold are highly conserved and sufficient to maintain the Cys-stabilized β-sheet motif [188,189]. It is worthwhile to point out that cystine-knot motifs appear to be common occurrence in plant CRP-AMPs. They are found, at the primary structure level, in plant defensins and heveins. However, they differ in the secondary and tertiary structure levels.

Despite the common knottin motif, knottin-type peptides have hypervariable sequences, differing by their amino acid sequences, the length between CysIII-CysIV and CysIV-CysV, and the linear and cyclic nature of the peptide backbone (Figures 4 and 5). Owing to the high sequence tolerance of the knottin scaffold and its diverse biological functions, the knottin scaffold has been used as a template for drug design. Knottins engineered by substitution of individual or several consecutive amino acids and/or insertion of additional amino acids without changing the structural integrity have been shown to provide novel bioactivity or increase stability [190].

Plant knottin-type peptides, particularly the subfamily of cyclotides, have been reported to possess high thermal, chemical, and enzymatic stability [186,191,192]. Cyclotides are also resistant to gastrointestinal proteases like trypsin, chymotrypsin, pepsin, or elastase [191,193], and certain members of cyclotide family can even penetrate the intestinal mucosa excised from rats [194,195]. Disulfide bonds in the knottin scaffold are crucial to its chemical and enzymatic stability based on studies of various members of cyclotides such as violacin A, kalata B1, and kalata B2 [177,191], whereas the cyclized backbone is important for exopeptidase resistance. For example, stability tests show that acyclic vilacin A is resistant to endopeptidase, trypsin, and thermolysin, comparable to cyclotides. The exoprotease aminopeptidase M cleaves the first two N-terminal residues of violacin A but leaves the third and fourth residues intact due to their proximity to the disulfide bond. Although no large differences are observed in the structure and flexibility between cyclotides and their corresponding linear analogs under standard conditions, simulation studies of linear and circular squash inhibitors revealed that cyclization increases resistance to high temperatures by limiting structure unfolding [192].

CKAIs exhibit another method in which these peptides are able to maintain stability against exopeptidases without a cyclic backbone structure, a pseudocyclic structure [186]. In wrightides, CKAIs isolated from the plant *W. religiosa*, the N-terminus and C-terminus are protected by the formation of disulfide bonds at the ultimate or penultimate residues. Structural analysis showed that this arrangement allows the termini to loop back to the peptide chain via the disulfide bonds especially at the N-terminal, forming a pseudocyclic structure. Allotides, CKAIs from *A. cathartica*, and AAI also exhibit similar structural features [183,187].

2.4.3. Structure-Function Relationship

With the exception of the cyclotide subfamily, the majority of knottins, are linear. They include the subfamilies of PAFP-S, Mj-AMPs, insect α-amylase inhibitor, squash trypsin inhibitor CMTI-1 and carboxypeptidase A inhibitor, as well as several linear homology analogs of cyclotides (violacin A and panitide L2; Figure 5A,B). Several knottin-type peptides were identified as plant AMPs, such as PAFP-S, Mj-AMPs, and Psacotheasin (Ps). PAFP-S was identified from seeds of *Phytolacca americana* and models the typical knottin structure of antifungal peptides [196]. Mj-AMP1 and Mj-AMP2 extracted from *Mirabilis jalapa* seeds have a broad spectrum of antimicrobial activity, being active against all 13 tested fungal pathogens and two tested Gram-positive bacteria but inactive against Gram-negative bacteria and cultured human cells. Reduced and non-reduced SDS-PAGE results suggest that Mj-AMP1 and Mj-AMP2 exist as dimers in their native form [197]. Ps from *Psacothea hilaris* is a 34 aa antibacterial peptide with a minimal inhibitory concentration of 12.5–25 μM [198].

Knottin-type peptides act as α-amylase or protease (carboxypeptidase A or trypsin) inhibitors (Figure 5A,B) and propagate plant defense mechanisms by conferring resistance to insects, pests, and pathogens [199]. The α-amylase inhibitor identified from *A. cathartica* and *W. religiosa* are the smallest peptide inhibitor of α-amylase activity (30 aa) [186,187]. Wr-AI1 and Wr-AI2, CKAIs from the plant *W. religiosa*, have been demonstrated to inhibit the α-amylase activity isolated from *Tenebrio molitor* (yellow mealworm), but no inhibitory was observed in fungal or mammalian α-amylase. Similar α-amylase inhibitory activity was observed from allotide Ac4. However, it was found that allotides interact with TMA differently from AAI and wrightides due to variation in the N-terminal sequences and high content of *cis*-proline. AAI confers pest resistance to plants by targeting insect α-amylase, but does not interfere with α-amylase from mammalian digestive systems, suggesting that amaranth seed AAI could be an attractive candidate to endow pest resistance to transgenic plants.

Squash trypsin inhibitors are 27–32 aa knottin-type peptides (e.g., CMTI-II of both pumpkin *Cucurbita maxima* and fig leaf gourd *Cucurbita ficifolia* seeds) [200]. The first squash inhibitor containing the knottin scaffold was reported from the seeds from squash of the *Cucurbitaceae* family [201]. Most squash trypsin inhibitors have linear backbones, except for MCoTI-I and MCoTI-II. However, not all the protease inhibitor peptides are knottin-type, such as sun flower trypsin inhibitor, a 14 aa cyclic peptide braced by a central disulfide bond [202]. Another type of knottin with protease inhibitory function includes carboxypeptidase inhibitors from potatoes [145] and tomatoes [203]. Potato carboxypeptidase inhibitor (PCI) (39 aa) has long loops instead of the typical β-strands observed in other knottin-type peptides. It binds the active site of carboxypeptidase A with the C-terminal tail as an active fragment binding to protease in a stopper-like manner and uses some aromatic residues as secondary binding sites [204,205].

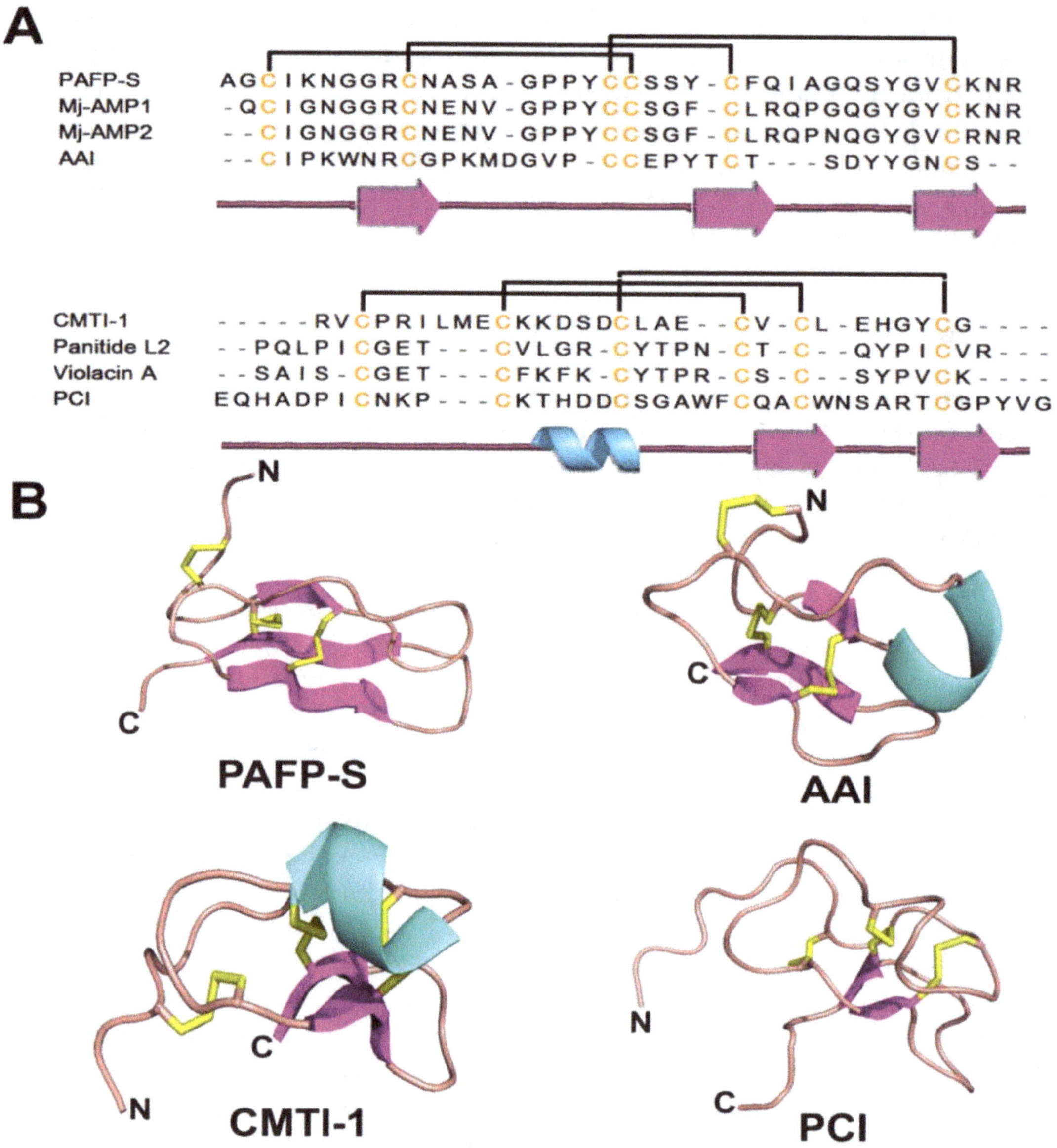

Figure 5. Sequences (**A**) and structures (**B**) of representative linear knottin-type peptides. The secondary structure is represented by different colors: cyan-α helix; magenta-β strand; pink-random coil and yellow-disulfide bonds.

A few linear variants of cyclotides have also been identified from the monocot rice plant *Panicum laxum* of the *Poaceae* family as Panitide L1-12 [175]. Several Panitides are active against *Escherichia coli* and cytotoxic to HeLa cells. The other subgroup of knottin-type peptides is cyclotides, including typical cyclotides and cyclic knotttins such as MCoTIs (Figure 6A,B). Cyclotides are 29–37 aa in length with a CK arrangement of three disulfide bonds which are widely involved in plant defense, as deduced from their activity against insects, nematodes, and mollusks [206–208]. The first cyclotide was identified in 1973 as an uterotonic agent from the African plant *Oldenlandia affinis*, a main component of medicinal tea used to accelerate childbirth [209]. Cyclotides have potential pharmacological functions, considering their antimicrobial, anti-HIV, anti-tumor, and neurotensin activities [22]. Cyclotides are found mainly in *Rubiaceae* (coffee), Violaceae (violet) and families. They are highly variable in sequence, but conserved in structure, and are divided into two types: Möbius and bracelet. Möbius types contain one *cis*-Pro in loop 5 and a twist in the cyclic backbone, while the bracelet type does not [210]. Yet, both types do not significantly differ from one another in the general scaffold structure.

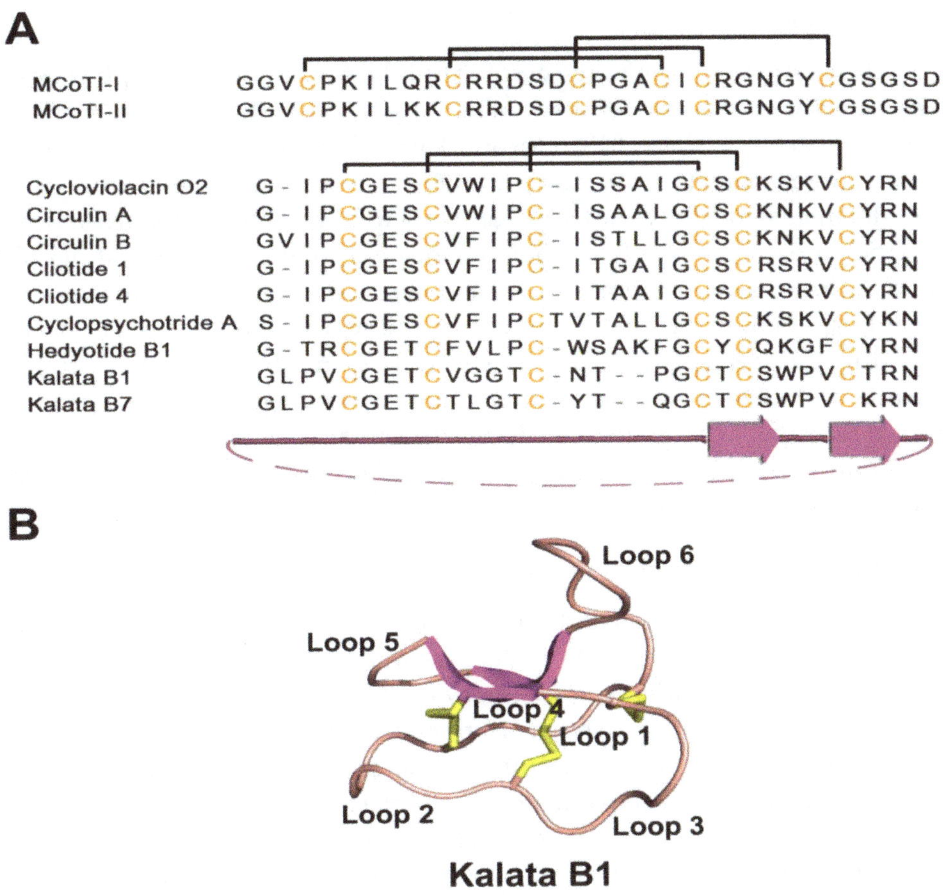

Figure 6. Sequences (**A**) and structures (**B**) of representative cyclic knottin-type peptides. The secondary structure is represented by different colors: magenta-β strand; pink-random coil and yellow-disulfide bonds.

Antimicrobial activity of cyclotides was first reported for four synthetically produced cyclotides isolated from coffee plants, kalata B1, circulin A, circulin B, and cyclopsychotride [211]. Subsequently, more cyclotides were reported to have antimicrobial activity. Cyclotides kalata B1 and B7 (29 aa each) from the tropical plant *Oldenlandia affinis* display antibiotic effects both in salt and salt-free medium [212]. While the 30 aa cycloviolacin O2 from *Viola odorata* is resistant to Gram-negative bacteria [213], cliotides cT1 and cT4 from *Clitoria ternatea* show antimicrobial activity against Gram-negative bacteria and cytotoxicity to HeLa cells [173]. Hedyotide B1, on the other hand, is a positively charged bracelet cyclotide from *Hedyotis biflora*, rich in aromatic residues and active against both Gram-positive and Gram-negative bacteria [214].

MCoTI-I and MCoTI-II are two squash trypsin inhibitors from *Momordica cochinchinensis* that contain a cyclized backbone [215] and have large sequences differences from typical cyclotides, as discussed above (Figure 6A). The C- to N-cyclization in MCoTI-II has no significant impact on the protein structure, though cyclized squash inhibitors are postulated to be less sensitive to exopeptidases [216]. Based on structural studies of MCoTI-II in free and complex forms, Heitz revealed that the cyclization and active site loops of MCoTI-II are flexible in solution, but converge into a single, well-defined conformation upon binding trypsin [217]. Compared to previously defined cyclotides, such as kalata B1 or circulin A, MCoTI-I and MCoTI-II share similar motifs wherein two disulfide bonds stabilize the β-sheet but differ greatly in their amino acid sequences and in loops 3 and 6 [217]. Furthermore, MCoTIs have an entirely charged surface *versus* the amphipathic nature of circulin A. These differences may explain functional disparities such as squash inhibitor MCoTIs having no antibacterial activity, unlike circulins and kalata B1.

2.4.4. Mechanism of Action

Generally, knottin-type peptides with membranolytic functions are amphipathic in nature like other AMPs, a characteristic necessary for membrane interactions which implement their antimicrobial effects. For example, the surface plots of PAFP-S and kalata B1 show hydrophobic patches surrounded by several hydrophilic residues (Figure 2E,F). However, in contrast the strongly cationic-charged thionins and plant defensins, most cyclotides are unlikely to have a strong electrostatic interaction with membranes since they are normally weakly positive or neutral at physiological pH (Figure 2F) [218]. The interaction of cyclotides with membranes has been previously investigated *in vitro* using the detergent dodecylphosphocholine [219]. In this study, the structure of kalata B1 was not significantly altered upon binding the detergent; binding was largely mediated by the strong hydrophobic interactions between cyclotide loops and lipid tails of the detergent, as well as favored by the weak interactions between positively charged kalata B1 and the polar head of the detergent However, similar studies on kalata B2 and cycloviolacin O2 suggest that different cyclotides have different membrane binding modalities because of the varied location of hydrophobic patches in cyclotides [220].

2.4.5. Knottin Scaffold in Pharmaceutical Engineering

The knottin scaffold is an excellent candidate for peptide-based pharmaceutical engineering [221] as a result of several features: (1) remarkable proteolytic, thermal, and chemical stability due to the CK and backbone cyclization of cyclotides; (2) feasibility of chemical synthesis due to small size; and (3) excellent sequence tolerance due to sequence variation in loop regions.

Synthesis of cyclotides and cyclic knottins. To exploit cyclotides and cyclic knottins for agricultural and medical use, it is necessary to develop efficient methods for their production. Methods employed to date include solid phase peptide synthesis [9,211,222–227], as well as chemo-enzymatic and biological methods using modified inteins [210–213] and Asn-endoprotease such as butelase-1 [228–231].

Irrespective of the means of its preparation, a linear precursor containing a macrocycle sequence is first generated, followed by a macrocyclizaion step to give a head-to-tail backbone-cyclized compound. The head-to-tail cyclization poses a substantial hurdle and challenge because it is highly entropy-disfavored due to the great distance between the N- and C-termini, but has been solved elegantly by the discovery of the thia zip cyclization reaction in 1997 [232]. Thia zip cyclization is an entropic reaction, characterized by a series of entropic ring expansion by making use of the multiple Cys residues in a CRP-linear precursor functionalized with an N-terminal Cys and a C-terminal thioester. This construct enables a thiol-thioester to form a thiolactone and then thiol-thiolactone exchange reactions in tandem, ending with a head-to-tail thiolactone which spontaneously forms a peptide bond through an S, N-acyl shift. In 1997, the first report on both Möbius and bracelet cyclotides have been synthesized by the thia zip reaction and regio-selective disulfide bond formation to guarantee the correct knottin scaffold [225]. Since then, many successful syntheses of cyclic CRPs based on thia zip cyclization have been reported. We have recently reviewed the progress of macrocyclization relevant to cyclotides and cyclic knottins [9]. Since 2012, new advances based on amide-to-amide transpeptidation reaction have made preparation of cyclotides, cyclic knottins and other macrocycles possible through chemical or biological means [181].

2.5. α-Hairpinin Family

The α-hairpinin family is composed of Lys/Arg-rich plant defense peptides. α-Hairpinin AMPs share a characteristic C1XXXC2-(X)n-C3XXXC4 motif in their primary sequence and, more importantly, a helix-loop-helix secondary structure (Figure 7A,B). The helix-loop-helix or α1-turn-α2 motif has both α-helices oriented antiparallel and is stabilized by two disulfide bonds in the tertiary structure. This structure is a surprise finding in plant CRPs, and the α-hairpinin family is structurally distinguished from the β-strand decorated CRP-AMPs, such as thionins, defensins, and knottin-type peptides.

Thus far, only a limited number of α-hairpinin AMPs have been reported, including MBP-1, MiAMP2s, Ec-AMP1, Luffin P1, VhT1, BWI-2c, Tk-AMP-Xs, and Sm-AMP-X. MBP-1, a 33 aa peptide isolated from the maize kernel, inhibits spore germination and hyphal enlongation of several plant pathogenic fungi and bacteria *in vitro* [233]. MiAMP2 peptides (50 aa) isolated from the nut kernel of *Macadamia integrifolia* inhibit various plant pathogenic fungi *in vitro* [234]. They are produced from a 666 aa precursor protein homologous to vicilin 7S globulin. Ec-AMP1 from the seeds of the baryard grass *Echinochloa crus-gali* was reported to have antifungal activity against several phytopathogenic fungi with an IC_{50} = 1–10 μM. A confocal microscopy study showed that Ec-AMP1 binds the fungal conidia surface and then internalizes and accumulates in the cytoplasm without disturbing membrane integrity [235].

Tk-AMP-X1 and Tk-AMP-X2 extracted from the wheat *Triticum kiharae* and Sm-AMP-X from seeds of the chickweed *Stellaria media* are another two α-hairpinin members with antifungal activity [236,237]. Both are produced from multimodular precursor proteins. The Tk-AMP-X-related sequences have been shown to be widespread in crops such as barley, rice, and maize, which suggest the importance of this type of plant defense peptide. VhT1 from the seeds of *Veronica hederifolia* and BWI-2c from seeds of the buckwheat *Fagopyrum esculentum* represent a new family of trypsin inhibitors with an α-hairpinin structure and act as defensive peptides in plants [238,239]. Luffin P1, extracted from the seeds of the sponge gourd *Luffa cylindrical*, has been shown to have anti-HIV-1 activity in HIV-1-infected C8166 T-cell lines *in vitro* [240]. This study proposed that Luffin P1 displays a novel inhibitory mechanism owing to its charge complementation with viral and cellular proteins.

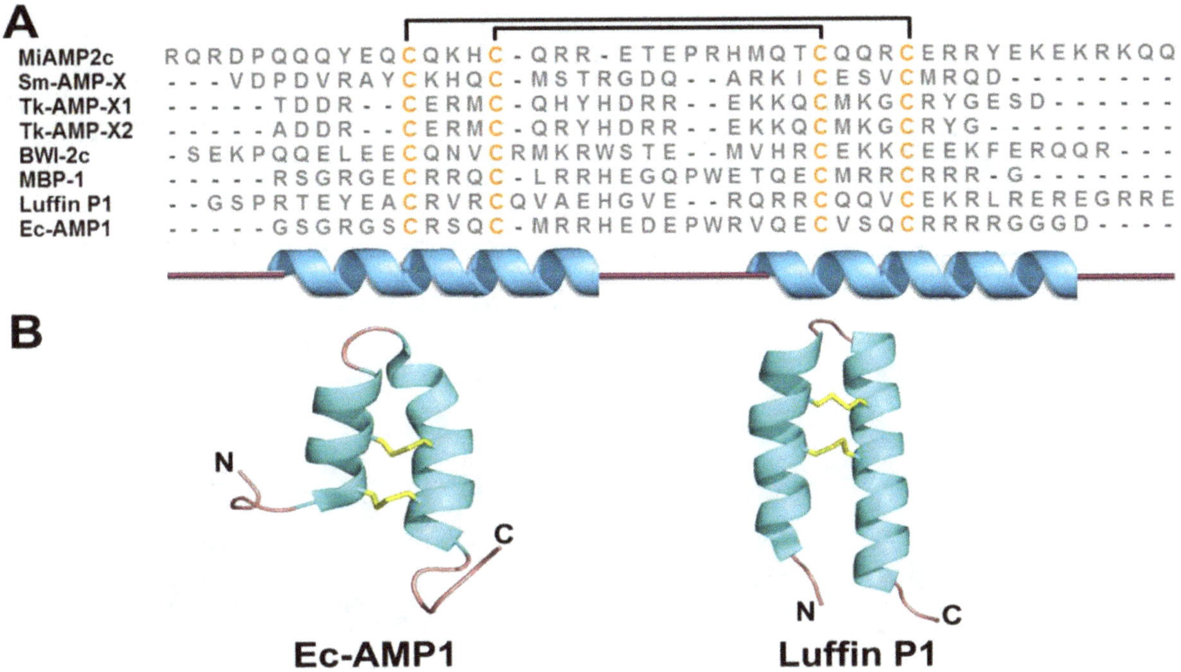

Figure 7. Sequences (**A**) and structures (**B**) of representative α-hairpinins. The secondary structure is represented by different colors: cyan-α helix; pink-random coil and yellow-disulfide bonds.

2.6. Lipid Transfer Proteins

Plant lipid transfer proteins (LTPs) and snakins (described in the following section) are two families of CRP-AMPs with MW >7 kDa, and are considered proteins. LTPs are cationic proteins of approximately 70 and 90 aa with eight Cys residues. They are distinguished from other CRP-AMPs by their lipid transfer activity, in which they bind a wide range of lipids including fatty acids (C10–C14), phospholipids, prostaglandin B2, lyso-derivatives, and acyl-coenzyme A. Consequently, they are also called non-specific LTPs [4,241,242]. LTPs can inhibit growth of fungus and some bacterial pathogens and are involved in the plant defense system. LTPs are subdivided into LTP1s (MW = 9 kDa) and LTP2s (MW = 7 kDa) based on their molecular mass.

2.6.1. Occurrences, Distribution, and Biosynthesis

Plant LTPs have been identified in various species, such as seeds of the radish, barley, maize, *Arabidopsis*, spinach, grapevine, wheat, and onion [4,241–246]. They are synthesized as precursors containing a signal peptide of 20–25 aa and a mature protein with eight Cys [247].

2.6.2. Structure

Although LTPs vary in their primary sequence, they share a defining structural feature, a conserved inner hydrophobic cavity surrounded by α-helices (Figure 8A,B). Surface plots of LTP1 and LTP2 representatives are illustrated in Figure 2G, H. LTP1s and LTP2s share the same Cys signature and similar tertiary fold, but vary in amino acid sequence and disulfide bonding at the CXC motif [248,249]. LTP1 contains four α-helices stabilized by four disulfide bonds (between CysI-CysVI, CysII-CysIII, CysIV-CysVII, and CysV-CysVIII) and a flexible C-terminal coil. In contrast to LTP1, LTP2 contains three extended helices, two single-turn helices, and four disulfide bonds between CysI-CysV, CysII-CysIII, CysIV-CysVII, and CysVI-CysVIII (Figure 8A) [249,250]. The helices in LTP1 and LTP2 form a hydrophobic cavity which accommodates a variety of lipids [251–254].

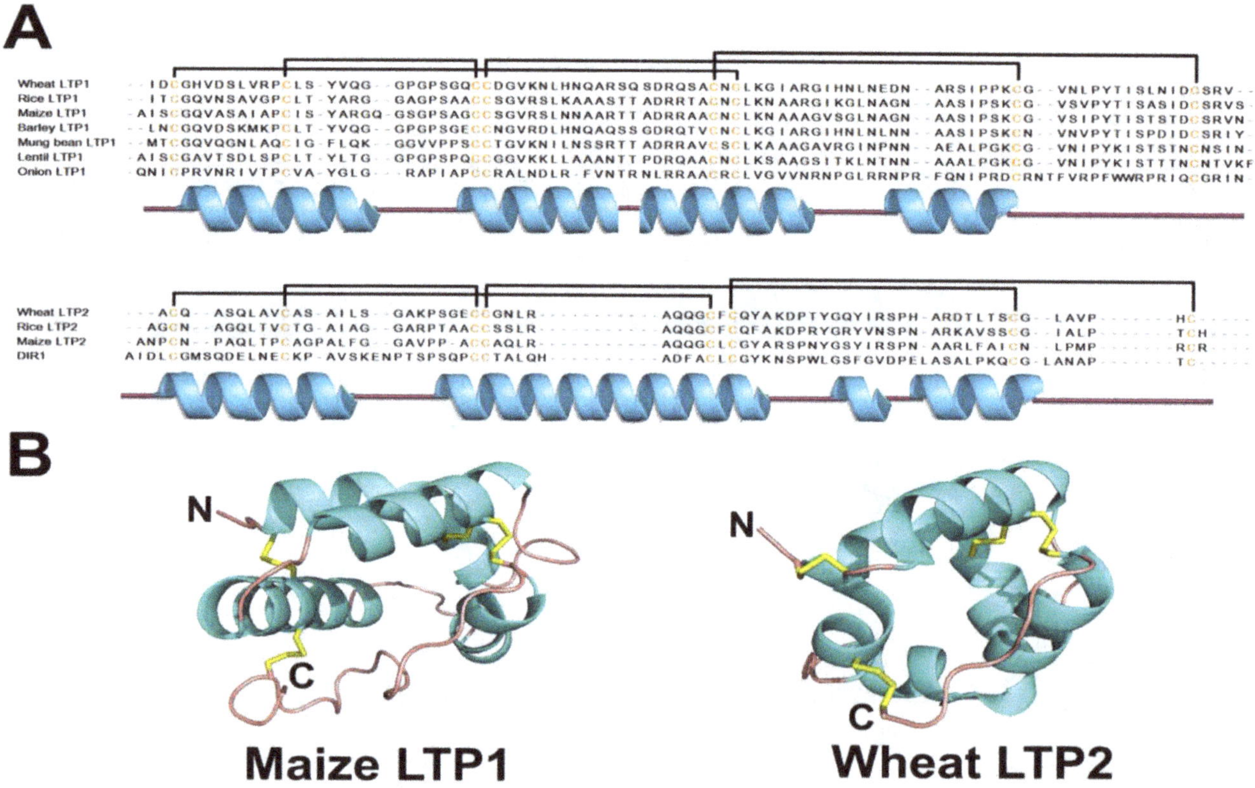

Figure 8. Sequences (**A**) and structures (**B**) of representative lipid transfer proteins. The secondary structure is represented by different colors: cyan-α helix; pink-random coil and yellow-disulfide bonds.

LTP1s and LTP2s have a conserved structure reported in rice [253,255,256], wheat [257,258], barley [259,260], maize [261,262], lentils [263], and mung beans [264]. Their lipid-binding properties can be modulated by subtle changes in their conserved global structure, as evidenced by structural and functional differences of LTP1s in tobacco, wheat, and maize [265]. Mutagenesis studies have revealed that different residues forming the hydrophobic cavity of LTP2 play various roles in maintaining structure and conferring function [266]. Although LTP2 is found to have a similar but smaller hydrophobic cavity compared to LTP1 [249,250,253,254,259], it is quite flexible and can accommodate voluminous sterol molecules [267].

2.6.3. Structure-Function Relationship

Plant LTPs inhibit the growth of bacterial and fungal pathogens to different degrees [243,246,268]. Transgenic expression of barley LTP2 in tobacco and *Arabidopsis thaliana* leaves endows higher tolerance to bacterial pathogens [269]. The antifungal activity of LTPs from *Brassica* and mung beans is found to be thermally, pH-, and pepsin/trypsin treatment-stable [268].

Ace-AMP1 (onion LTP1; Figure 8A) isolated from onion seeds, exhibits a higher antimicrobial activity than the LTP extracted from radish seeds [89,243]. Ace-AMP1 shares a similar global fold as LTP1s, but does not possess a continuous cavity for lipid binding nor does it bind fluorescently labeled phospholipids in solution [252]. In addition, Ace-AMP1 does not exhibit characteristic LTP behavior, such as transferring lipids between membranes *in vitro*. While DIR1 from *Arabidopsis thaliana* shares similar structural and lipid binding properties with plant LTP2, it is distinguished by its acidic pI and ability to bind two long-chain fatty acid derivatives in its cavity, suggesting DIR1 could be a new type of plant LTP [270]. The functions of plant LTPs, such as defensive signaling, cuticle deposition and plant defense, have been previously reviewed by Yeats and Rose [271].

2.6.4. Mechanism of Action

Initially, LTPs were reported to facilitate lipid transfer between membranes of vesicles or organelles *in vitro* [272,273]. However, later discoveries have shown that LTP1s are extracellular cell wall proteins, making *in vivo* intracellular lipid transfer activity unlikely [274,275]. Thus, LTPs promote membrane permeabilization in pathogens rather than host cells [246,276]. Although structural studies have shown that LTPs can "cage" lipid molecules in their hydrophobic cavity, a detailed mechanism of antimicrobial activity mediated by lipid transport remains unclear [271].

2.7. Snakins

Snakin-1 (63 aa) and snakin-2 (66 aa) are AMPs with 12 Cys isolated from potato tubers (*Solanum tuberosum*) [277,278] found to be active against fungal and bacterial pathogens at 1–20 μM. Snakins induce the aggregation of both Gram-positive and Gram-negative bacteria and therefore, are recognized as components of constitutive and inducible plant defense barriers. The structure of snakin is predicted to have two long α-helices with disulfide bonds between CysI-CysIX, CysII-CysVII, CysIII-CysIV, CysV-CysXI, CysVI-CysXII, and CysVIII-CysX, which demonstrates a small degree of structural similarity to thionins and α-hairpinins [279].

A 64 aa homolog of snakin-2, also containing 12 Cys, was identified from the French bean to be a domain of a 42 kDa Pro-rich protein with chitin-binding ability that is involved in plant-pathogen interactions [280]. Snakin-Z (31 aa), identified from the fruit of *Zizyphus jujuba*, contains a sequence similar to the C-terminal region of Snakin-2. It has antimicrobial activity against different bacterial and fungal strains at minimal concentrations (7.65–28.8 μg/mL) [281].

2.8. Other Plant CRP-AMPs

In addition to the different classes of CRP-AMPs mentioned above, there are several unclassified Cys-containing AMPs, such as Ps-AFP1, Ib-AMPs, Pp-AMPs, ToAMPs, and MiAMP1 that contain two to eight Cys. Ps-AFP1 (38 aa) from the pea *Pisum sativum* root contains two disulfide bonds between CysI-CysII and CysIII-CysIV, has been proposed to adopt a novel αβ-trumpet fold, and is capable of binding the cell wall of fungi [282]. Ib-AMPs1-4, purified from the seed of *Impatiens balsamina*, are four basic 20 aa peptides encoded by a single transcript. Ib-AMPs represent a novel class of AMPs that lack homology to other peptides [283,284]. They contain four Cys which share a common CC and CXXXC sequence motif and form two disulfide bonds between CysI-CysIII and CysII-CysIV. The structure of Ib-AMP1 is well-defined, with loops and turns stabilized by two disulfide bonds [285]. Ib-AMPs can inhibit the growth of a range of fungi and Gram-positive bacteria but is not cytotoxic to most Gram-negative bacteria or cultured human cells. Studies of Ib-AMP1 analogs without disulfide bonds have shown these bonds are not essential for its antimicrobial activity, and that Ib-AMP1 targets intracellular components instead of bacterial cell membranes [286].

Pp-AMP1 and Pp-AMP2 are two chitin-binding AMPs from the shoots of the Japanese bamboo *Phyllostachys pubescens* that have antimicrobial activity against pathogenic bacteria and fungi [287]. Pp-AMP1 contains four Cys in its 44 aa sequence, while Pp-AMP2 (45 aa) is composed of six Cys. Although they share relatively high sequence homology with thionins, especially the N-terminal continuous CC motif, their differences in the C-terminal sequence and Cys distribution pattern do not suggest Pp-AMPs are thionins. ToAMPs1-4 are four basic 38–44 aa AMPs identified from *Taraxacum officinale* flowers that have antifungal and antibacterial activity [288,289]. Sequence analysis has shown that ToAMP1, ToAMP2, and ToAMP4 possess a novel peptide motif of six Cys with a –CC– motif between CysII and CysIII, while ToAMP3 has eight Cys with a –CC– motif between CysVI and CysVII.

MiAMP1 is a 76 aa basic AMP identified from the nut kernel of *Macadamia integrifolia*. MiAMP1 inhibits several plant microbial pathogens *in vitro* [290], yet presents no sequence homology with other plant AMPs and has a β-barrelin structure. The β-barrelins contain eight β-strands forming two Greek key motifs that are stabilized by three disulfide bonds. MiAMP1 has a structure similar to that of a yeast killer toxin from *Williopsis mrakii*, which inhibits β-glucan synthesis and thereby disturbs the cell wall of yeast. The structural similarity between these two peptides suggests a similar antimicrobial mode of action.

2.9. Non-CRP Plant AMPs

Although the majority of known plant AMPs are stabilized by multiple disulfide bonds, exceptions include Cn-AMPs, Cr-ACP1, as well as GRPs Pg-AMP1 and shepherins. All of these plant AMPs either do not contain Cys or contain only one and thus, possess high structural flexibility. Cn-AMP1 is a 9 aa Cys-free AMP identified from green coconut (*Cocos nucifera*) water with "promiscuous" activity, as it is antibacterial, antifungal, and immune stimulatory [291]. Cr-ACP1 is a 9 aa AMP from the seeds of *Cycas revoluta* with pro-apoptotic and antimicrobial activities [292]. A previous bioinformatics study suggests that these Cr-AMP1 activities are likely mediated by hydrogen bond-mediated DNA binding within cells.

Pg-AMP1 is a 55 aa GRP extracted from seeds of the guava *Psidium guajava*. It contains 14 Gly and only one Cys [293] and inhibits the growth of both Gram-positive and Gram-negative bacteria, pathogens involved in urinary and gastro-intestinal infections [294]. Shepherins I and II are Gly- and His-rich AMPs identified from the roots of Shepherd's Purse, *Capsella bursa-pastoris* [295]. Shepherin I (28 aa) and shepherin II (38 aa) are produced from a single 120 aa propeptide precursor composed of an N-terminal signal peptide, shepherin I, a linker dipeptide, shepherin II, and a C-terminal peptide. Both exhibit antimicrobial activity against Gram-negative bacteria and fungi with an IC_{50} of 2.5–8 μg/mL.

2.10. Mechanism of AMP Action

AMPs are generally moderate-to-large size, positively charged, amphipathic CRPs. Structurally, AMPs fall into diverse and distinct groups (Table 1; Figure 2), including α-helical peptides (α-hairpinin family and lipid transfer proteins), β-sheet peptides (hevein and knottin-type peptides) as well as mixed α-helical and β-sheet peptides (thionins and plant defensins). Generally, the mechanism of AMP interaction with microbes is believed to be associated with cell lysis due to membrane disruption and/or peptide penetration of lipid membranes followed by attack of intracellular targets [14]. Various mechanistic models have been proposed, such as the barrel-stave model, toroidal pore model, and carpet model, in previous reviews by Barbosa, Rahnamaeian, and Nawrot [14,296,297]. Besides perturbing the lipid membrane, AMPs can also form ion channels, which can induce ion leakage (e.g., K^+) in addition to other intracellular contents [298,299]. All of these actions lead to inhibition of microbial cell growth and cell death.

3. Conclusions and Perspective

A striking feature of plant AMPs is that the majority are families of CRPs, with each family sharing a characteristic motif. In turn, these cysteinyl motifs enable plant AMPs to organize into specific families with conserved structural folds that enable sequence variation of non-Cys residues encased in the same scaffold within a particular family to play multiple functions. This evolvable phenomenon is particularly evident in the family of knottins, and to a lesser extent, in the defensins. Knottins are known to play diverse roles, being antimicrobial, insecticidal, enzyme inhibitory, and agonistic/antagonistic to hormones. The ability of plant AMPs to tolerate hypervariable sequences using a conserved scaffold mimic is, in certain respects, similar to that of immunoglobulins, which recognize diverse targets by varying the sequence of complementary binding regions.

The presence of multiple disulfide bonds in a particular CRP family gives plant AMPs a compact structure and a specific scaffold. In turn, they confer stability against thermal and chemical denaturation and enzymatic degradation. These properties bode well for developing plant AMPs as potential therapeutics and for protection of crops through transgenic methods [300,301]. A cystine-stabilized structure opens the possibility to use it as a stable scaffold for grafting biological active peptides sequences to intracellular targets. Specifically, the backbone portions between cysteine residues can be modified to incorporate bioactive peptides which are normally unstable against digestive enzymes and other physiological conditions [302,303]. This technique has successfully been applied to graft bradykinin B1 antagonists onto kalata B1 as an orally active analgesic [221], human kallikrein-related peptidase 4 inhibitor onto sunflower trypsin inhibitor-1 [228], angiogenic peptides, laminin and osteopontin, onto *Momordica cochinca cochinchinensis* trypsin inhibitor-II [304] and melanocortin onto kalata B1 [305]. More importantly, these grafted peptides have been shown to possess the same biological property with similar potency as compared with the original bioactive peptides, as well as resistance to digestive enzymes due to the robust scaffold. In addition, plants AMPs, in particular defensin, have been shown to protect transgenic plants against microorganism infection. Expression of alfalfa antifungal peptide defensin, from the seeds of *Medicago sativa*, in transgenic potato plants has been found to provide resistance against phyto-pathogen *Verticillium dahilae* [77,306].

AMPs offer several advantages as compared to current antibiotic drugs as they represent a naturally occurring defense mechanism that has been used by plants for thousands of years in combating external pathogenic challenges. Most of the recent studies included in this review were focused on the anti-fungal and anti-bacterial effect of AMPs, while the anti-viral property of AMPs was still under-explored. Further investigation in tackling this issue is urgently warranted. Since plant AMPs have been identified in only a small fraction of plants, it is anticipated that many more plant AMPs, both in molecular form and sequence, will be forthcoming.

Acknowledgments: This work was supported in part by the Singapore National Research Foundation grant NRF-CRP8-2011-05.

Author Contributions: All the authors contributed to manuscript preparation.

References

1. Stintzi, A.; Heitz, T.; Prasad, V.; Wiedemann-Merdinoglu, S.; Kauffmann, S.; Geoffroy, P.; Legrand, M.; Fritig, B. Plant "pathogenesis-related" proteins and their role in defense against pathogens. *Biochimie* **1993**, *75*, 687–706. [CrossRef]
2. Sinha, M.; Singh, R.P.; Kushwaha, G.S.; Iqbal, N.; Singh, A.; Kaushik, S.; Kaur, P.; Sharma, S.; Singh, T.P. Current overview of allergens of plant pathogenesis related protein families. *Sci. World J.* **2014**, *2014*, 543195.

3. Ebrahim, S.; Usha, K.; Singh, B. Pathogenesis related (pr) proteins in plant defense mechanism. *Sci. Against Microb. Pathog.* **2011**, *2*, 1043–1054.
4. Sels, J.; Mathys, J.; De Coninck, B.M.; Cammue, B.P.; De Bolle, M.F. Plant pathogenesis-related (pr) proteins: A focus on pr peptides. *Plant Physiol. Biochem.* **2008**, *46*, 941–950. [CrossRef] [PubMed]
5. Egorov, T.A.; Odintsova, T.I.; Pukhalsky, V.A.; Grishin, E.V. Diversity of wheat anti-microbial peptides. *Peptides* **2005**, *26*, 2064–2073. [CrossRef] [PubMed]
6. Rao, A.G. Antimicrobial peptides. *Mol. Plant Microbe Interact.* **1995**, *8*, 6–13. [CrossRef] [PubMed]
7. Reddy, K.V.; Yedery, R.D.; Aranha, C. Antimicrobial peptides: Premises and promises. *Int. J. Antimicrob. Agents* **2004**, *24*, 536–547. [CrossRef] [PubMed]
8. Montalban-Lopez, M.; Sanchez-Hidalgo, M.; Cebrian, R.; Maqueda, M. Discovering the bacterial circular proteins: Bacteriocins, cyanobactins, and pilins. *J. Biol. Chem.* **2012**, *287*, 27007–27013. [CrossRef] [PubMed]
9. Tam, J.P.; Wong, C.T. Chemical synthesis of circular proteins. *J. Biol. Chem.* **2012**, *287*, 27020–27025. [CrossRef] [PubMed]
10. Hammami, R.; Ben Hamida, J.; Vergoten, G.; Fliss, I. Phytamp: A database dedicated to antimicrobial plant peptides. *Nucleic Acids Res.* **2009**, *37*, D963–D968. [CrossRef] [PubMed]
11. Silverstein, K.A.; Moskal, W.A., Jr.; Wu, H.C.; Underwood, B.A.; Graham, M.A.; Town, C.D.; VandenBosch, K.A. Small cysteine-rich peptides resembling antimicrobial peptides have been under-predicted in plants. *Plant. J.* **2007**, *51*, 262–280. [CrossRef] [PubMed]
12. Stec, B. Plant thionins–the structural perspective. *Cell. Mol. Life Sci.* **2006**, *63*, 1370–1385. [CrossRef] [PubMed]
13. Garcia-Olmedo, F.; Molina, A.; Alamillo, J.M.; Rodriguez-Palenzuela, P. Plant defense peptides. *Biopolymers* **1998**, *47*, 479–491. [CrossRef]
14. Nawrot, R.; Barylski, J.; Nowicki, G.; Broniarczyk, J.; Buchwald, W.; Gozdzicka-Jozefiak, A. Plant antimicrobial peptides. *Folia Microbiol. (Praha)* **2013**, *59*, 181–196. [CrossRef] [PubMed]
15. Padovan, L.; Scocchi, M.; Tossi, A. Structural aspects of plant antimicrobial peptides. *Curr. Protein Pept. Sci.* **2010**, *11*, 210–219. [CrossRef] [PubMed]
16. Lay, F.T.; Anderson, M.A. Defensins–components of the innate immune system in plants. *Curr. Protein Pept. Sci.* **2005**, *6*, 85–101. [CrossRef] [PubMed]
17. Das, S.N.; Madhuprakash, J.; Sarma, P.V.; Purushotham, P.; Suma, K.; Manjeet, K.; Rambabu, S.; Gueddari, N.E.; Moerschbacher, B.M.; Podile, A.R. Biotechnological approaches for field applications of chitooligosaccharides (cos) to induce innate immunity in plants. *Crit. Rev. Biotechnol.* **2013**, *35*, 29–43. [CrossRef] [PubMed]
18. Mander, L.N.; Liu, H.-W. *Comprehensive Natural Products ii Chemistry and Biology*; Elsevier Science: Oxford, England, 2010; p. 1.
19. Tavares, L.S.; Santos Mde, O.; Viccini, L.F.; Moreira, J.S.; Miller, R.N.; Franco, O.L. Biotechnological potential of antimicrobial peptides from flowers. *Peptides* **2008**, *29*, 1842–1851. [CrossRef] [PubMed]
20. De Lucca, A.J.; Cleveland, T.E.; Wedge, D.E. Plant-derived antifungal proteins and peptides. *Can. J. Microbiol.* **2005**, *51*, 1001–1014. [CrossRef] [PubMed]
21. Gruber, C.W.; Cemazar, M.; Anderson, M.A.; Craik, D.J. Insecticidal plant cyclotides and related cystine knot toxins. *Toxicon* **2007**, *49*, 561–575. [CrossRef] [PubMed]
22. Craik, D.J. Host-defense activities of cyclotides. *Toxins (Basel)* **2012**, *4*, 139–156. [CrossRef] [PubMed]
23. van der Weerden, N.L.; Bleackley, M.R.; Anderson, M.A. Properties and mechanisms of action of naturally occurring antifungal peptides. *Cell. Mol. Life Sci.* **2013**, *70*, 3545–3570. [CrossRef] [PubMed]
24. Ng, T.B. Antifungal proteins and peptides of leguminous and non-leguminous origins. *Peptides* **2004**, *25*, 1215–1222. [CrossRef] [PubMed]
25. Harris, F.; Dennison, S.R.; Phoenix, D.A. Anionic antimicrobial peptides from eukaryotic organisms. *Curr. Protein Pept. Sci.* **2009**, *10*, 585–606. [CrossRef] [PubMed]
26. Wang, G.S.; Li, X.; Wang, Z. Apd2: The updated antimicrobial peptide database and its application in peptide design. *Nucleic Acids Res.* **2009**, *37*, D933–D937. [CrossRef] [PubMed]
27. Wang, Z.; Wang, G.S. Apd: The antimicrobial peptide database. *Nucleic Acids Res.* **2004**, *32*, D590–D592. [CrossRef] [PubMed]
28. Piotto, S.P.; Sessa, L.; Concilio, S.; Iannelli, P. Yadamp: Yet another database of antimicrobial peptides. *Int. J. Antimicrob. Agents* **2012**, *39*, 346–351. [CrossRef] [PubMed]

29. Sundararajan, V.S.; Gabere, M.N.; Pretorius, A.; Adam, S.; Christoffels, A.; Lehvaslaiho, M.; Archer, J.A.C.; Bajic, V.B. Dampd: A manually curated antimicrobial peptide database. *Nucleic Acids Res.* **2012**, *40*, D1108–D1112. [CrossRef] [PubMed]
30. Fernandez de Caleya, R.; Gonzalez-Pascual, B.; Garcia-Olmedo, F.; Carbonero, P. Susceptibility of phytopathogenic bacteria to wheat purothionins *in vitro*. *Appl. Microbiol.* **1972**, *23*, 998–1000. [PubMed]
31. Ebrahimnesbat, F.; Behnke, S.; Kleinhofs, A.; Apel, K. Cultivar-related differences in the distribution of cell-wall-bound thionins in compatible and incompatible interactions between barley and powdery mildew. *Planta* **1989**, *179*, 203–210. [CrossRef] [PubMed]
32. Evans, J.; Wang, Y.D.; Shaw, K.P.; Vernon, L.P. Cellular responses to pyrularia thionin are mediated by Ca^{2+} influx and phospholipase a2 activation and are inhibited by thionin tyrosine iodination. *Proc. Natl. Acad. Sci. USA* **1989**, *86*, 5849–5853. [CrossRef] [PubMed]
33. Kramer, K.J.; Klassen, L.W.; Jones, B.L.; Speirs, R.D.; Kammer, A.E. Toxicity of purothionin and its homologues to the tobacco hornworm, manduca sexta (l.) (lepidoptera:Sphingidae). *Toxicol. Appl. Pharmacol.* **1979**, *48*, 179–183. [CrossRef]
34. Balls, A.K.; Hale, W.S.; Harris, T.H. A crystalline protein obtained from a lipoprotein of wheat flour. *Cereal Chem.* **1942**, *19*, 951–961.
35. Ponz, F.; Paz-Ares, J.; Hernandez-Lucas, C.; Carbonero, P.; Garcia-Olmedo, F. Synthesis and processing of thionin precursors in developing endosperm from barley (hordeum vulgare l.). *EMBO J.* **1983**, *2*, 1035–1040. [PubMed]
36. Steinmuller, K.; Batschauer, A.; Apel, K. Tissue-specific and light-dependent changes of chromatin organization in barley (hordeum vulgare). *Eur. J. Biochem.* **1986**, *158*, 519–525. [CrossRef] [PubMed]
37. Gausing, K. Thionin genes specifically expressed in barley leaves. *Planta* **1987**, *171*, 241–246. [CrossRef] [PubMed]
38. Epple, P.; Apel, K.; Bohlmann, H. An arabidopsis-thaliana thionin gene is inducible via a signal-transduction pathway different from that for pathogenesis-related proteins. *Plant. Physiol.* **1995**, *109*, 813–820. [CrossRef] [PubMed]
39. Bohlmann, H.; Clausen, S.; Behnke, S.; Giese, H.; Hiller, C.; Reimann-Philipp, U.; Schrader, G.; Barkholt, V.; Apel, K. Leaf-specific thionins of barley-a novel class of cell wall proteins toxic to plant-pathogenic fungi and possibly involved in the defence mechanism of plants. *EMBO J.* **1988**, *7*, 1559–1565. [PubMed]
40. Andresen, I.; Becker, W.; Schluter, K.; Burges, J.; Parthier, B.; Apel, K. The identification of leaf thionin as one of the main jasmonate-induced proteins of barley (hordeum vulgare). *Plant. Mol. Biol.* **1992**, *19*, 193–204. [CrossRef] [PubMed]
41. Penninckx, I.A.; Eggermont, K.; Terras, F.R.; Thomma, B.P.; De Samblanx, G.W.; Buchala, A.; Metraux, J.P.; Manners, J.M.; Broekaert, W.F. Pathogen-induced systemic activation of a plant defensin gene in arabidopsis follows a salicylic acid-independent pathway. *Plant Cell.* **1996**, *8*, 2309–2323. [CrossRef] [PubMed]
42. Castagnaro, A.; Marana, C.; Carbonero, P.; Garciaolmedo, F. Extreme divergence of a novel wheat thionin generated by a mutational burst specifically affecting the mature protein domain of the precursor. *J. Mol. Biol.* **1992**, *224*, 1003–1009. [CrossRef]
43. Stec, B.; Markman, O.; Rao, U.; Heffron, G.; Henderson, S.; Vernon, L.P.; Brumfeld, V.; Teeter, M.M. Proposal for molecular mechanism of thionins deduced from physico-chemical studies of plant toxins. *J. Pept. Res.* **2004**, *64*, 210–224. [CrossRef] [PubMed]
44. Rao, U.; Stec, B.; Teeter, M.M. Refinement of purothionins reveals solute particles important for lattice formation and toxicity. Part 1: Alpha1-purothionin revisited. *Acta Crystallogr. D Biol. Crystallogr.* **1995**, *51*, 904–913. [CrossRef] [PubMed]
45. Stec, B.; Rao, U.; Teeter, M.M. Refinement of purothionins reveals solute particles important for lattice formation and toxicity. Part 2: Structure of beta-purothionin at 1.7 a resolution. *Acta Crystallogr. D Biol. Crystallogr.* **1995**, *51*, 914–924. [CrossRef] [PubMed]
46. Milbradt, A.G.; Kerek, F.; Moroder, L.; Renner, C. Structural characterization of hellethionins from helleborus purpurascens. *Biochemistry* **2003**, *42*, 2404–2411. [CrossRef] [PubMed]
47. Yamano, A.; Heo, N.H.; Teeter, M.M. Crystal structure of ser-22/ile-25 form crambin confirms solvent, side chain substate correlations. *J. Biol. Chem.* **1997**, *272*, 9597–9600. [PubMed]
48. Yamano, A.; Teeter, M.M. Correlated disorder of the pure pro22/leu25 form of crambin at 150 k refined to 1.05-a resolution. *J. Biol. Chem.* **1994**, *269*, 13956–13965. [PubMed]

49. Hendrickson, W.A.; Teeter, M.M. Structure of the hydrophobic protein crambin determined directly from the anomalous scattering of sulfur. *Nature* **1981**, *290*, 107–113. [CrossRef]
50. Ahn, H.C.; Juranic, N.; Macura, S.; Markley, J.L. Three-dimensional structure of the water-insoluble protein crambin in dodecylphosphocholine micelles and its minimal solvent-exposed surface. *J. Am. Chem. Soc.* **2006**, *128*, 4398–4404. [CrossRef] [PubMed]
51. Schmidt, A.; Teeter, M.; Weckert, E.; Lamzin, V.S. Crystal structure of small protein crambin at 0.48 a resolution. *Acta Crystallogr. Sect. F Struct. Biol. Cryst. Commun.* **2010**, *67*, 424–428. [CrossRef] [PubMed]
52. Chen, J.C.; Hanson, B.L.; Fisher, S.Z.; Langan, P.; Kovalevsky, A.Y. Direct observation of hydrogen atom dynamics and interactions by ultrahigh resolution neutron protein crystallography. *Proc. Natl. Acad. Sci. USA* **2012**, *109*, 15301–15306. [CrossRef] [PubMed]
53. Jelsch, C.; Teeter, M.M.; Lamzin, V.; Pichon-Pesme, V.; Blessing, R.H.; Lecomte, C. Accurate protein crystallography at ultra-high resolution: Valence electron distribution in crambin. *Proc. Natl. Acad. Sci. USA* **2000**, *97*, 3171–3176. [CrossRef] [PubMed]
54. Pal, A.; Debreczeni, J.E.; Sevvana, M.; Gruene, T.; Kahle, B.; Zeeck, A.; Sheldrick, G.M. Structures of viscotoxins a1 and b2 from european mistletoe solved using native data alone. *Acta Crystallogr. D Biol. Crystallogr.* **2008**, *64*, 985–992. [CrossRef] [PubMed]
55. Romagnoli, S.; Fogolari, F.; Catalano, M.; Zetta, L.; Schaller, G.; Urech, K.; Giannattasio, M.; Ragona, L.; Molinari, H. Nmr solution structure of viscotoxin c1 from viscum album species coloratum ohwi: Toward a structure-function analysis of viscotoxins. *Biochemistry* **2003**, *42*, 12503–12510. [CrossRef] [PubMed]
56. Coulon, A.; Mosbah, A.; Lopez, A.; Sautereau, A.M.; Schaller, G.; Urech, K.; Rouge, P.; Darbon, H. Comparative membrane interaction study of viscotoxins a3, a2 and b from mistletoe (viscum album) and connections with their structures. *Biochem. J.* **2003**, *374*, 71–78. [CrossRef] [PubMed]
57. Romagnoli, S.; Ugolini, R.; Fogolari, F.; Schaller, G.; Urech, K.; Giannattasio, M.; Ragona, L.; Molinari, H. Nmr structural determination of viscotoxin a3 from viscum album l. *Biochem. J.* **2000**, *350 (Pt. 2)*, 569–577. [CrossRef] [PubMed]
58. Debreczeni, J.E.; Girmann, B.; Zeeck, A.; Kratzner, R.; Sheldrick, G.M. Structure of viscotoxin a3: Disulfide location from weak sad data. *Acta Crystallogr. D Biol. Crystallogr.* **2003**, *59*, 2125–2132. [CrossRef] [PubMed]
59. Clore, G.M.; Sukumaran, D.K.; Nilges, M.; Gronenborn, A.M. 3-dimensional structure of phoratoxin in solution - combined use of nuclear-magnetic-resonance, distance geometry, and restrained molecular-dynamics. *Biochemistry* **1987**, *26*, 1732–1745. [CrossRef]
60. Mellstra, S.T.; Samuelss, G. Phoratoxin, a toxic protein from mistletoe phoradendron-tomentosum subsp. Macrophyllum (loranthaceae) - improvements in isolation procedure and further studies on properties. *Eur. J. Biochem.* **1973**, *32*, 143–147. [CrossRef]
61. Johnson, K.A.; Kim, E.; Teeter, M.M.; Suh, S.W.; Stec, B. Crystal structure of alpha-hordothionin at 1.9 angstrom resolution. *FEBS Lett.* **2005**, *579*, 2301–2306. [CrossRef] [PubMed]
62. Han, K.H.; Park, K.H.; Yoo, H.J.; Cha, H.; Suh, S.W.; Thomas, F.; Moon, T.S.; Kim, S.M. Determination of the three-dimensional structure of hordothionin-alpha by nuclear magnetic resonance. *Biochem. J.* **1996**, *313 (Pt. 3)*, 885–892. [CrossRef] [PubMed]
63. Vila-Perello, M.; Andreu, D. Characterization and structural role of disulfide bonds in a highly knotted thionin from pyrularia pubera. *Biopolymers* **2005**, *80*, 697–707. [CrossRef] [PubMed]
64. Vila-Perello, M.; Sanchez-Vallet, A.; Garcia-Olmedo, F.; Molina, A.; Andreu, D. Structural dissection of a highly knotted peptide reveals minimal motif with antimicrobial activity. *J. Biol. Chem.* **2005**, *280*, 1661–1668. [CrossRef] [PubMed]
65. Fujimura, M.; Ideguchi, M.; Minami, Y.; Watanabe, K.; Tadera, K. Purification, characterization, and sequencing of novel antimicrobial peptides, tu-amp 1 and tu-amp 2, from bulbs of tulip (tulipa gesneriana l.). *Biosci. Biotechnol. Biochem.* **2004**, *68*, 571–577. [CrossRef] [PubMed]
66. Florack, D.E.; Stiekema, W.J. Thionins: Properties, possible biological roles and mechanisms of action. *Plant Mol. Biol.* **1994**, *26*, 25–37. [CrossRef] [PubMed]
67. Osorio e Castro, V.R.; Vernon, L.P. Hemolytic activity of thionin from pyrularia pubera nuts and snake venom toxins of naja naja species: Pyrularia thionin and snake venom cardiotoxin compete for the same membrane site. *Toxicon* **1989**, *27*, 511–517. [CrossRef]
68. Hughes, P.; Dennis, E.; Whitecross, M.; Llewellyn, D.; Gage, P. The cytotoxic plant protein, beta-purothionin, forms ion channels in lipid membranes. *J. Biol. Chem.* **2000**, *275*, 823–827. [CrossRef] [PubMed]

69. Carrasco, L.; Vazquez, D.; Hernandez-Lucas, C.; Carbonero, P.; Garcia-Olmedo, F. Thionins: Plant peptides that modify membrane permeability in cultured mammalian cells. *Eur. J. Biochem.* **1981**, *116*, 185–189. [CrossRef] [PubMed]
70. Oka, T.; Murata, Y.; Nakanishi, T.; Yoshizumi, H.; Hayashida, H.; Ohtsuki, Y.; Toyoshima, K.; Hakura, A. Similarity, in molecular-structure and function, between the plant toxin purothionin and the mammalian pore-forming proteins. *Mol. Biol. Evol.* **1992**, *9*, 707–715. [PubMed]
71. Richard, J.A.; Kelly, I.; Marion, D.; Pezolet, M.; Auger, M. Interaction between beta-purothionin and dimyristoylphosphatidylglycerol: A p-31-nmr and infrared spectroscopic study. *Biophysic. J.* **2002**, *83*, 2074–2083. [CrossRef]
72. Richard, J.A.; Kelly, I.; Marion, D.; Auger, M.; Pezolet, M. Structure of beta-purothionin in membranes: A two-dimensional infrared correlation spectroscopy study. *Biochemistry* **2005**, *44*, 52–61. [CrossRef] [PubMed]
73. Wada, K.; Ozaki, Y.; Matsubara, H.; Yoshizumi, H. Studies on purothionin by chemical modifications. *J. Biochem.* **1982**, *91*, 257–263. [PubMed]
74. Fracki, W.S.; Li, D.; Owen, N.; Perry, C.; Naisbitt, G.H.; Vernon, L.P. Role of tyr and trp in membrane responses of pyrularia thionin determined by optical and nmr spectra following tyr iodination and trp modification. *Toxicon* **1992**, *30*, 1427–1440. [CrossRef]
75. Rao, A.G.; Hassan, M.; Hempel, J. Validation of the structure-function properties of alpha-hordothionin and derivatives through protein modeling. *Protein Eng.* **1993**, *6*, 117–117.
76. Pelegrini, P.B.; Franco, O.L. Plant gamma-thionins: Novel insights on the mechanism of action of a multi-functional class of defense proteins. *Int. J. Biochem. Cell. Biol.* **2005**, *37*, 2239–2253. [CrossRef] [PubMed]
77. Gao, A.G.; Hakimi, S.M.; Mittanck, C.A.; Wu, Y.; Woerner, B.M.; Stark, D.M.; Shah, D.M.; Liang, J.; Rommens, C.M. Fungal pathogen protection in potato by expression of a plant defensin peptide. *Nat. Biotechnol.* **2000**, *18*, 1307–1310. [PubMed]
78. Terras, F.R.; Schoofs, H.M.; De Bolle, M.F.; Van Leuven, F.; Rees, S.B.; Vanderleyden, J.; Cammue, B.P.; Broekaert, W.F. Analysis of two novel classes of plant antifungal proteins from radish (raphanus sativus l.) seeds. *J. Biol. Chem.* **1992**, *267*, 15301–15309. [PubMed]
79. Terras, F.R.; Eggermont, K.; Kovaleva, V.; Raikhel, N.V.; Osborn, R.W.; Kester, A.; Rees, S.B.; Torrekens, S.; Van Leuven, F.; Vanderleyden, J.; *et al.* Small cysteine-rich antifungal proteins from radish: Their role in host defense. *Plant Cell.* **1995**, *7*, 573–588. [CrossRef] [PubMed]
80. Fant, F.; Vranken, W.F.; Borremans, F.A. The three-dimensional solution structure of aesculus hippocastanum antimicrobial protein 1 determined by 1h nuclear magnetic resonance. *Proteins* **1999**, *37*, 388–403. [CrossRef]
81. Fant, F.; Vranken, W.; Broekaert, W.; Borremans, F. Determination of the three-dimensional solution structure of raphanus sativus antifungal protein 1 by 1h nmr. *J. Mol. Biol.* **1998**, *279*, 257–270. [CrossRef] [PubMed]
82. Fujimura, M.; Minami, Y.; Watanabe, K.; Tadera, K. Purification, characterization, and sequencing of a novel type of antimicrobial peptides, fa-amp1 and fa-amp2, from seeds of buckwheat (*Fagopyrum esculentum* Moench.). *Biosci. Biotechnol. Biochem.* **2003**, *67*, 1636–1642. [CrossRef] [PubMed]
83. Sitaram, N. Antimicrobial peptides with unusual amino acid compositions and unusual structures. *Curr. Med. Chem.* **2006**, *13*, 679–696. [CrossRef] [PubMed]
84. Bloch, C., Jr.; Richardson, M. A new family of small (5 kda) protein inhibitors of insect alpha-amylases from seeds or sorghum (*Sorghum bicolar* (L.) Moench.) have sequence homologies with wheat gamma-purothionins. *FEBS Lett.* **1991**, *279*, 101–104. [CrossRef]
85. Wijaya, R.; Neumann, G.M.; Condron, R.; Hughes, A.B.; Polya, G.M. Defense proteins from seed of cassia fistula include a lipid transfer protein homologue and a protease inhibitory plant defensin. *Plant Sci.* **2000**, *159*, 243–255. [CrossRef]
86. Colilla, F.J.; Rocher, A.; Mendez, E. Gamma-purothionins: Amino acid sequence of two polypeptides of a new family of thionins from wheat endosperm. *FEBS Lett.* **1990**, *270*, 191–194. [CrossRef]
87. Mendez, E.; Moreno, A.; Colilla, F.; Pelaez, F.; Limas, G.G.; Mendez, R.; Soriano, F.; Salinas, M.; de Haro, C. Primary structure and inhibition of protein synthesis in eukaryotic cell-free system of a novel thionin, gamma-hordothionin, from barley endosperm. *Eur. J. Biochem.* **1990**, *194*, 533–539. [CrossRef] [PubMed]
88. Bruix, M.; Jimenez, M.A.; Santoro, J.; Gonzalez, C.; Colilla, F.J.; Mendez, E.; Rico, M. Solution structure of gamma 1-h and gamma 1-p thionins from barley and wheat endosperm determined by 1h-nmr: A structural motif common to toxic arthropod proteins. *Biochemistry* **1993**, *32*, 715–724. [CrossRef] [PubMed]

89. Broekaert, W.F.; Terras, F.R.G.; Cammue, B.P.A.; Osborn, R.W. Plant defensins - novel antimicrobial peptides as components of the host-defense system. *Plant Physiol.* **1995**, *108*, 1353–1358. [CrossRef] [PubMed]
90. Franco, O.L.; Murad, A.M.; Leite, J.R.; Mendes, P.A.; Prates, M.V.; Bloch, C., Jr. Identification of a cowpea gamma-thionin with bactericidal activity. *FEBS J.* **2006**, *273*, 3489–3497. [CrossRef] [PubMed]
91. Moreno, M.; Segura, A.; Garcia-Olmedo, F. Pseudothionin-st1, a potato peptide active against potato pathogens. *Eur. J. Biochem.* **1994**, *223*, 135–139. [CrossRef] [PubMed]
92. Chiang, C.C.; Hadwiger, L.A. The fusarium solani-induced expression of a pea gene family encoding high cysteine content proteins. *Mol. Plant Microbe Interact.* **1991**, *4*, 324–331. [CrossRef] [PubMed]
93. Park, H.C.; Kang, Y.H.; Chun, H.J.; Koo, J.C.; Cheong, Y.H.; Kim, C.Y.; Kim, M.C.; Chung, W.S.; Kim, J.C.; Yoo, J.H.; *et al.* Characterization of a stamen-specific cdna encoding a novel plant defensin in chinese cabbage. *Plant Mol. Biol.* **2002**, *50*, 59–69. [CrossRef] [PubMed]
94. Milligan, S.B.; Gasser, C.S. Nature and regulation of pistil-expressed genes in tomato. *Plant Mol. Biol.* **1995**, *28*, 691–711. [CrossRef] [PubMed]
95. Lay, F.T.; Brugliera, F.; Anderson, M.A. Isolation and properties of floral defensins from ornamental tobacco and petunia. *Plant Physiol.* **2003**, *131*, 1283–1293. [CrossRef] [PubMed]
96. Sharma, P.; Lonneborg, A. Isolation and characterization of a cdna encoding a plant defensin-like protein from roots of norway spruce. *Plant Mol. Biol.* **1996**, *31*, 707–712. [CrossRef] [PubMed]
97. Finkina, E.I.; Shramova, E.I.; Tagaev, A.A.; Ovchinnikova, T.V. A novel defensin from the lentil lens culinaris seeds. *Biochem. Biophys. Res. Commun.* **2008**, *371*, 860–865. [CrossRef] [PubMed]
98. Bontems, F.; Roumestand, C.; Boyot, P.; Gilquin, B.; Doljansky, Y.; Menez, A.; Toma, F. Three-dimensional structure of natural charybdotoxin in aqueous solution by 1h-nmr. Charybdotoxin possesses a structural motif found in other scorpion toxins. *Eur. J. Biochem.* **1991**, *196*, 19–28. [CrossRef] [PubMed]
99. Cornet, B.; Bonmatin, J.M.; Hetru, C.; Hoffmann, J.A.; Ptak, M.; Vovelle, F. Refined three-dimensional solution structure of insect defensin A. *Structure* **1995**, *3*, 435–448. [CrossRef]
100. Broekaert, W.F.; Cammue, B.P.A.; DeBolle, M.F.C.; Thevissen, K.; DeSamblanx, G.W.; Osborn, R.W. Antimicrobial peptides from plants. *Crit. Rev. Plant. Sci.* **1997**, *16*, 297–323. [CrossRef]
101. Thomma, B.P.; Cammue, B.P.; Thevissen, K. Plant defensins. *Planta* **2002**, *216*, 193–202. [CrossRef] [PubMed]
102. Raj, P.A.; Dentino, A.R. Current status of defensins and their role in innate and adaptive immunity. *FEMS Microbiol. Lett.* **2002**, *206*, 9–18. [CrossRef] [PubMed]
103. Bulet, P.; Hetru, C.; Dimarcq, J.L.; Hoffmann, D. Antimicrobial peptides in insects; structure and function. *Dev. Comp. Immunol.* **1999**, *23*, 329–344. [CrossRef]
104. Carvalho Ade, O.; Gomes, V.M. Plant defensins and defensin-like peptides - biological activities and biotechnological applications. *Curr. Pharm. Des.* **2011**, *17*, 4270–4293. [CrossRef] [PubMed]
105. Yang, Y.F.; Cheng, K.C.; Tsai, P.H.; Liu, C.C.; Lee, T.R.; Lyu, P.C. Alanine substitutions of noncysteine residues in the cysteine-stabilized alphabeta motif. *Protein Sci.* **2009**, *18*, 1498–1506. [CrossRef] [PubMed]
106. Lay, F.T.; Schirra, H.J.; Scanlon, M.J.; Anderson, M.A.; Craik, D.J. The three-dimensional solution structure of nad1, a new floral defensin from nicotiana alata and its application to a homology model of the crop defense protein alfafp. *J. Mol. Biol.* **2003**, *325*, 175–188. [CrossRef]
107. Chen, K.C.; Lin, C.Y.; Kuan, C.C.; Sung, H.Y.; Chen, C.S. A novel defensin encoded by a mungbean cdna exhibits insecticidal activity against bruchid. *J. Agric. Food Chem.* **2002**, *50*, 7258–7263. [CrossRef] [PubMed]
108. Janssen, B.J.; Schirra, H.J.; Lay, F.T.; Anderson, M.A.; Craik, D.J. Structure of petunia hybrida defensin 1, a novel plant defensin with five disulfide bonds. *Biochemistry* **2003**, *42*, 8214–8222. [CrossRef] [PubMed]
109. Mendez, E.; Rocher, A.; Calero, M.; Girbes, T.; Citores, L.; Soriano, F. Primary structure of omega-hordothionin, a member of a novel family of thionins from barley endosperm, and its inhibition of protein synthesis in eukaryotic and prokaryotic cell-free systems. *Eur. J. Biochem.* **1996**, *239*, 67–73. [CrossRef] [PubMed]
110. Song, X.; Zhou, Z.; Wang, J.; Wu, F.; Gong, W. Purification, characterization and preliminary crystallographic studies of a novel plant defensin from pachyrrhizus erosus seeds. *Acta Crystallogr. D Biol. Crystallogr.* **2004**, *60*, 1121–1124. [CrossRef] [PubMed]
111. Song, X.; Zhang, M.; Zhou, Z.; Gong, W. Ultra-high resolution crystal structure of a dimeric defensin spe10. *FEBS Lett.* **2011**, *585*, 300–306. [CrossRef] [PubMed]

112. Spelbrink, R.G.; Dilmac, N.; Allen, A.; Smith, T.J.; Shah, D.M.; Hockerman, G.H. Differential antifungal and calcium channel-blocking activity among structurally related plant defensins. *Plant Physiol.* **2004**, *135*, 2055–2067. [CrossRef] [PubMed]
113. Osborn, R.W.; De Samblanx, G.W.; Thevissen, K.; Goderis, I.; Torrekens, S.; Van Leuven, F.; Attenborough, S.; Rees, S.B.; Broekaert, W.F. Isolation and characterisation of plant defensins from seeds of asteraceae, fabaceae, hippocastanaceae and saxifragaceae. *FEBS Lett.* **1995**, *368*, 257–262. [CrossRef]
114. Almeida, M.S.; Cabral, K.M.; Kurtenbach, E.; Almeida, F.C.; Valente, A.P. Solution structure of pisum sativum defensin 1 by high resolution nmr: Plant defensins, identical backbone with different mechanisms of action. *J. Mol. Biol.* **2002**, *315*, 749–757. [CrossRef] [PubMed]
115. Zhang, Y.; Lewis, K. Fabatins: New antimicrobial plant peptides. *FEMS Microbiol. Lett.* **1997**, *149*, 59–64. [CrossRef] [PubMed]
116. Garciaolmedo, F.; Carbonero, P.; Hernandezlucas, C.; Pazares, J.; Ponz, F.; Vicente, O.; Sierra, J.M. Inhibition of eukaryotic cell-free protein-synthesis by thionins from wheat endosperm. *Biochim. Biophys. Acta* **1983**, *740*, 52–56. [CrossRef]
117. Pelegrini, P.B.; Lay, F.T.; Murad, A.M.; Anderson, M.A.; Franco, O.L. Novel insights on the mechanism of action of alpha-amylase inhibitors from the plant defensin family. *Proteins* **2008**, *73*, 719–729. [CrossRef] [PubMed]
118. Dos Santos, I.S.; Carvalho Ade, O.; de Souza-Filho, G.A.; do Nascimento, V.V.; Machado, O.L.; Gomes, V.M. Purification of a defensin isolated from vigna unguiculata seeds, its functional expression in escherichia coli, and assessment of its insect alpha-amylase inhibitory activity. *Protein Expr. Purif.* **2010**, *71*, 8–15. [CrossRef] [PubMed]
119. Carvalho Ade, O.; Gomes, V.M. Plant defensins–prospects for the biological functions and biotechnological properties. *Peptides* **2009**, *30*, 1007–1020. [CrossRef] [PubMed]
120. Kushmerick, C.; de Souza Castro, M.; Santos Cruz, J.; Bloch, C., Jr.; Beirao, P.S. Functional and structural features of gamma-zeathionins, a new class of sodium channel blockers. *FEBS Lett.* **1998**, *440*, 302–306. [CrossRef]
121. Melo, F.R.; Rigden, D.J.; Franco, O.L.; Mello, L.V.; Ary, M.B.; Grossi de Sa, M.F.; Bloch, C., Jr. Inhibition of trypsin by cowpea thionin: Characterization, molecular modeling, and docking. *Proteins* **2002**, *48*, 311–319. [CrossRef] [PubMed]
122. Huang, G.J.; Lai, H.C.; Chang, Y.S.; Sheu, M.J.; Lu, T.L.; Huang, S.S.; Lin, Y.H. Antimicrobial, dehydroascorbate reductase, and monodehydroascorbate reductase activities of defensin from sweet potato [ipomoea batatas (l.) lam. 'Tainong 57'] storage roots. *J. Agric. Food Chem.* **2008**, *56*, 2989–2995. [CrossRef] [PubMed]
123. Chen, Z.; Gallie, D.R. Dehydroascorbate reductase affects leaf growth, development, and function. *Plant Physiol.* **2006**, *142*, 775–787. [CrossRef] [PubMed]
124. Thevissen, K.; Osborn, R.W.; Acland, D.P.; Broekaert, W.F. Specific binding sites for an antifungal plant defensin from dahlia (dahlia merckii) on fungal cells are required for antifungal activity. *Mol. Plant Microbe Interact.* **2000**, *13*, 54–61. [CrossRef] [PubMed]
125. Thevissen, K.; Warnecke, D.C.; Francois, I.E.; Leipelt, M.; Heinz, E.; Ott, C.; Zahringer, U.; Thomma, B.P.; Ferket, K.K.; Cammue, B.P. Defensins from insects and plants interact with fungal glucosylceramides. *J. Biol. Chem.* **2004**, *279*, 3900–3905. [CrossRef] [PubMed]
126. Thevissen, K.; Ghazi, A.; De Samblanx, G.W.; Brownlee, C.; Osborn, R.W.; Broekaert, W.F. Fungal membrane responses induced by plant defensins and thionins. *J. Biol. Chem.* **1996**, *271*, 15018–15025. [PubMed]
127. Thevissen, K.; Terras, F.R.; Broekaert, W.F. Permeabilization of fungal membranes by plant defensins inhibits fungal growth. *Appl. Environ. Microbiol.* **1999**, *65*, 5451–5458. [PubMed]
128. Van der Weerden, N.L.; Hancock, R.E.; Anderson, M.A. Permeabilization of fungal hyphae by the plant defensin nad1 occurs through a cell wall-dependent process. *J. Biol. Chem.* **2010**, *285*, 37513–37520. [CrossRef] [PubMed]
129. Van der Weerden, N.L.; Lay, F.T.; Anderson, M.A. The plant defensin, nad1, enters the cytoplasm of fusarium oxysporum hyphae. *J. Biol. Chem.* **2008**, *283*, 14445–14452. [CrossRef] [PubMed]
130. Hayes, B.M.; Bleackley, M.R.; Wiltshire, J.L.; Anderson, M.A.; Traven, A.; van der Weerden, N.L. Identification and mechanism of action of the plant defensin nad1 as a new member of the antifungal drug arsenal against candida albicans. *Antimicrob. Agents Chemother.* **2013**, *57*, 3667–3675. [CrossRef] [PubMed]

131. De Coninck, B.; Cammue, B.P.A.; Thevissen, K. Modes of antifungal action and in planta functions of plant defensins and defensin-like peptides. *Fungal Biol. Rev.* **2013**, *26*, 109–120. [CrossRef]
132. Gachomo, E.W.; Jimenez-Lopez, J.C.; Kayode, A.P.; Baba-Moussa, L.; Kotchoni, S.O. Structural characterization of plant defensin protein superfamily. *Mol. Biol. Rep.* **2012**, *39*, 4461–4469. [CrossRef] [PubMed]
133. Beintema, J.J. Structural features of plant chitinases and chitin-binding proteins. *FEBS Lett.* **1994**, *350*, 159–163. [CrossRef]
134. Jimenez-Barbero, J.; Javier Canada, F.; Asensio, J.L.; Aboitiz, N.; Vidal, P.; Canales, A.; Groves, P.; Gabius, H.J.; Siebert, H.C. Hevein domains: An attractive model to study carbohydrate-protein interactions at atomic resolution. *Adv. Carbohydr. Chem. Biochem.* **2006**, *60*, 303–354. [PubMed]
135. Kini, S.G.; Nguyen, P.Q.; Weissbach, S.; Mallagaray, A.; Shin, J.; Yoon, H.S.; Tam, J.P. Studies on the chitin binding property of novel cysteine-rich peptides from alternanthera sessilis. *Biochemistry* **2015**, *54*, 6639–6649. [CrossRef] [PubMed]
136. Archer, B.L. The proteins of hevea brasiliensis latex. 4. Isolation and characterization of crystalline hevein. *Biochem. J.* **1960**, *75*, 236–240. [CrossRef] [PubMed]
137. Van Parijs, J.; Broekaert, W.F.; Goldstein, I.J.; Peumans, W.J. Hevein: An antifungal protein from rubber-tree (*Hevea brasiliensis*) latex. *Planta* **1991**, *183*, 258–264. [CrossRef] [PubMed]
138. Diaz-Perales, A.; Collada, C.; Blanco, C.; Sanchez-Monge, R.; Carrillo, T.; Aragoncillo, C.; Salcedo, G. Cross-reactions in the latex-fruit syndrome: A relevant role of chitinases but not of complex asparagine-linked glycans. *J. Allergy Clin. Immunol.* **1999**, *104*, 681–687. [CrossRef]
139. Blanco, C.; Diaz-Perales, A.; Collada, C.; Sanchez-Monge, R.; Aragoncillo, C.; Castillo, R.; Ortega, N.; Alvarez, M.; Carrillo, T.; Salcedo, G. Class i chitinases as potential panallergens involved in the latex-fruit syndrome. *J. Allergy Clin. Immunol.* **1999**, *103*, 507–513. [CrossRef]
140. Gidrol, X.; Chrestin, H.; Tan, H.L.; Kush, A. Hevein, a lectin-like protein from hevea brasiliensis (rubber tree) is involved in the coagulation of latex. *J. Biol. Chem.* **1994**, *269*, 9278–9283. [PubMed]
141. Peumans, W.J.; Van Damme, E.J. Plant lectins: Specific tools for the identification, isolation, and characterization of o-linked glycans. *Crit. Rev. Biochem. Mol. Biol.* **1998**, *33*, 209–258. [PubMed]
142. Asensio, J.L.; Siebert, H.C.; von Der Lieth, C.W.; Laynez, J.; Bruix, M.; Soedjanaamadja, U.M.; Beintema, J.J.; Canada, F.J.; Gabius, H.J.; Jimenez-Barbero, J. Nmr investigations of protein-carbohydrate interactions: Studies on the relevance of trp/tyr variations in lectin binding sites as deduced from titration microcalorimetry and nmr studies on hevein domains. Determination of the nmr structure of the complex between pseudohevein and n,n',n''-triacetylchitotriose. *Proteins* **2000**, *40*, 218–236. [PubMed]
143. Lipkin, A.; Anisimova, V.; Nikonorova, A.; Babakov, A.; Krause, E.; Bienert, M.; Grishin, E.; Egorov, T. An antimicrobial peptide ar-amp from amaranth (*Amaranthus retroflexus* L.) seeds. *Phytochemistry* **2005**, *66*, 2426–2431. [CrossRef] [PubMed]
144. Andreev, Y.A.; Korostyleva, T.V.; Slavokhotova, A.A.; Rogozhin, E.A.; Utkina, L.L.; Vassilevski, A.A.; Grishin, E.V.; Egorov, T.A.; Odintsova, T.I. Genes encoding hevein-like defense peptides in wheat: Distribution, evolution, and role in stress response. *Biochimie* **2012**, *94*, 1009–1016. [CrossRef] [PubMed]
145. Van den Bergh, K.P.; Rouge, P.; Proost, P.; Coosemans, J.; Krouglova, T.; Engelborghs, Y.; Peumans, W.J.; Van Damme, E.J. Synergistic antifungal activity of two chitin-binding proteins from spindle tree (*Euonymus europaeus* L.). *Planta* **2004**, *219*, 221–232. [CrossRef] [PubMed]
146. Asensio, J.L.; Canada, F.J.; Bruix, M.; Gonzalez, C.; Khiar, N.; Rodriguez-Romero, A.; Jimenez-Barbero, J. Nmr investigations of protein-carbohydrate interactions: Refined three-dimensional structure of the complex between hevein and methyl beta-chitobioside. *Glycobiology* **1998**, *8*, 569–577. [CrossRef] [PubMed]
147. Harata, K.; Muraki, M. Crystal structures of urtica dioica agglutinin and its complex with tri-n-acetylchitotriose. *J. Mol. Biol.* **2000**, *297*, 673–681. [CrossRef] [PubMed]
148. Broekaert, W.F.; Marien, W.; Terras, F.R.; De Bolle, M.F.; Proost, P.; Van Damme, J.; Dillen, L.; Claeys, M.; Rees, S.B.; Vanderleyden, J.; *et al.* Antimicrobial peptides from amaranthus caudatus seeds with sequence homology to the cysteine/glycine-rich domain of chitin-binding proteins. *Biochemistry* **1992**, *31*, 4308–4314. [CrossRef] [PubMed]
149. Martins, J.C.; Maes, D.; Loris, R.; Pepermans, H.A.; Wyns, L.; Willem, R.; Verheyden, P. H nmr study of the solution structure of ac-amp2, a sugar binding antimicrobial protein isolated from amaranthus caudatus. *J. Mol. Biol.* **1996**, *258*, 322–333. [CrossRef] [PubMed]

150. Aboitiz, N.; Vila-Perello, M.; Groves, P.; Asensio, J.L.; Andreu, D.; Canada, F.J.; Jimenez-Barbero, J. Nmr and modeling studies of protein-carbohydrate interactions: Synthesis, three-dimensional structure, and recognition properties of a minimum hevein domain with binding affinity for chitooligosaccharides. *ChemBioChem* **2004**, *5*, 1245–1255. [CrossRef] [PubMed]
151. Koo, J.C.; Lee, S.Y.; Chun, H.J.; Cheong, Y.H.; Choi, J.S.; Kawabata, S.; Miyagi, M.; Tsunasawa, S.; Ha, K.S.; Bae, D.W.; *et al.* Two hevein homologs isolated from the seed of pharbitis nil l. Exhibit potent antifungal activity. *Biochim. Biophys. Acta* **1998**, *1382*, 80–90. [CrossRef]
152. Lee, O.S.; Lee, B.; Park, N.; Koo, J.C.; Kim, Y.H.; Prasad, D.T.; Karigar, C.; Chun, H.J.; Jeong, B.R.; Kim, D.H.; *et al.* Pn-amps, the hevein-like proteins from pharbitis nil confers disease resistance against phytopathogenic fungi in tomato, lycopersicum esculentum. *Phytochemistry* **2003**, *62*, 1073–1079. [CrossRef]
153. Koo, J.C.; Chun, H.J.; Park, H.C.; Kim, M.C.; Koo, Y.D.; Koo, S.C.; Ok, H.M.; Park, S.J.; Lee, S.H.; Yun, D.J.; *et al.* Over-expression of a seed specific hevein-like antimicrobial peptide from pharbitis nil enhances resistance to a fungal pathogen in transgenic tobacco plants. *Plant Mol. Biol.* **2002**, *50*, 441–452. [PubMed]
154. Li, S.S.; Claeson, P. Cys/gly-rich proteins with a putative single chitin-binding domain from oat (*Avena sativa*) seeds. *Phytochemistry* **2003**, *63*, 249–255. [CrossRef]
155. Huang, R.H.; Xiang, Y.; Liu, X.Z.; Zhang, Y.; Hu, Z.; Wang, D.C. Two novel antifungal peptides distinct with a five-disulfide motif from the bark of eucommia ulmoides oliv. *FEBS Lett.* **2002**, *521*, 87–90. [CrossRef]
156. Huang, R.H.; Xiang, Y.; Tu, G.Z.; Zhang, Y.; Wang, D.C. Solution structure of eucommia antifungal peptide: A novel structural model distinct with a five-disulfide motif. *Biochemistry* **2004**, *43*, 6005–6012. [CrossRef] [PubMed]
157. Xiang, Y.; Huang, R.H.; Liu, X.Z.; Zhang, Y.; Wang, D.C. Crystal structure of a novel antifungal protein distinct with five disulfide bridges from eucommia ulmoides oliver at an atomic resolution. *J. Struct. Biol* **2004**, *148*, 86–97. [CrossRef] [PubMed]
158. Odintsova, T.I.; Vassilevski, A.A.; Slavokhotova, A.A.; Musolyamov, A.K.; Finkina, E.I.; Khadeeva, N.V.; Rogozhin, E.A.; Korostyleva, T.V.; Pukhalsky, V.A.; Grishin, E.V.; *et al.* A novel antifungal hevein-type peptide from triticum kiharae seeds with a unique 10-cysteine motif. *FEBS J.* **2009**, *276*, 4266–4275. [CrossRef] [PubMed]
159. Dubovskii, P.V.; Vassilevski, A.A.; Slavokhotova, A.A.; Odintsova, T.I.; Grishin, E.V.; Egorov, T.A.; Arseniev, A.S. Solution structure of a defense peptide from wheat with a 10-cysteine motif. *Biochem. Biophys. Res. Commun.* **2011**, *411*, 14–18. [CrossRef] [PubMed]
160. Van den Bergh, K.P.; Proost, P.; Van Damme, J.; Coosemans, J.; Van Damme, E.J.; Peumans, W.J. Five disulfide bridges stabilize a hevein-type antimicrobial peptide from the bark of spindle tree (*Euonymus europaeus* L.). *FEBS Lett.* **2002**, *530*, 181–185. [CrossRef]
161. Chavez, M.I.; Vila-Perello, M.; Canada, F.J.; Andreu, D.; Jimenez-Barbero, J. Effect of a serine-to-aspartate replacement on the recognition of chitin oligosaccharides by truncated hevein. A 3d view by using nmr. *Carbohydr. Res.* **2010**, *345*, 1461–1468. [CrossRef] [PubMed]
162. Espinosa, J.F.; Asensio, J.L.; Garcia, J.L.; Laynez, J.; Bruix, M.; Wright, C.; Siebert, H.C.; Gabius, H.J.; Canada, F.J.; Jimenez-Barbero, J. Nmr investigations of protein-carbohydrate interactions binding studies and refined three-dimensional solution structure of the complex between the b domain of wheat germ agglutinin and n,n',n''-triacetylchitotriose. *Eur. J. Biochem.* **2000**, *267*, 3965–3978. [CrossRef] [PubMed]
163. Muraki, M. The importance of ch/pi interactions to the function of carbohydrate binding proteins. *Protein Pept. Lett.* **2002**, *9*, 195–209. [CrossRef] [PubMed]
164. Chavez, M.I.; Andreu, C.; Vidal, P.; Aboitiz, N.; Freire, F.; Groves, P.; Asensio, J.L.; Asensio, G.; Muraki, M.; Canada, F.J.; *et al.* On the importance of carbohydrate-aromatic interactions for the molecular recognition of oligosaccharides by proteins: Nmr studies of the structure and binding affinity of acamp2-like peptides with non-natural naphthyl and fluoroaromatic residues. *Chemistry* **2005**, *11*, 7060–7074. [CrossRef] [PubMed]
165. Slavokhotova, A.A.; Naumann, T.A.; Price, N.P.; Rogozhin, E.A.; Andreev, Y.A.; Vassilevski, A.A.; Odintsova, T.I. Novel mode of action of plant defense peptides - hevein-like antimicrobial peptides from wheat inhibit fungal metalloproteases. *FEBS J.* **2014**, *281*, 4754–4764. [CrossRef] [PubMed]
166. Pallaghy, P.K.; Nielsen, K.J.; Craik, D.J.; Norton, R.S. A common structural motif incorporating a cystine knot and a triple-stranded beta-sheet in toxic and inhibitory polypeptides. *Protein Sci.* **1994**, *3*, 1833–1839. [CrossRef] [PubMed]

167. Franco, O.L. Peptide promiscuity: An evolutionary concept for plant defense. *FEBS Lett.* **2011**, *585*, 995–1000. [CrossRef] [PubMed]
168. Rees, D.C.; Lipscomb, W.N. Refined crystal structure of the potato inhibitor complex of carboxypeptidase a at 2.5 a resolution. *J. Mol. Biol.* **1982**, *160*, 475–498. [CrossRef]
169. McDonald, N.Q.; Hendrickson, W.A. A structural superfamily of growth factors containing a cystine knot motif. *Cell* **1993**, *73*, 421–424. [CrossRef]
170. Craik, D.J.; Daly, N.L.; Bond, T.; Waine, C. Plant cyclotides: A unique family of cyclic and knotted proteins that defines the cyclic cystine knot structural motif. *J. Mol. Biol.* **1999**, *294*, 1327–1336. [CrossRef] [PubMed]
171. Gruber, C.W.; Elliott, A.G.; Ireland, D.C.; Delprete, P.G.; Dessein, S.; Goransson, U.; Trabi, M.; Wang, C.K.; Kinghorn, A.B.; Robbrecht, E.; *et al.* Distribution and evolution of circular miniproteins in flowering plants. *Plant Cell.* **2008**, *20*, 2471–2483. [CrossRef] [PubMed]
172. Poth, A.G.; Mylne, J.S.; Grassl, J.; Lyons, R.E.; Millar, A.H.; Colgrave, M.L.; Craik, D.J. Cyclotides associate with leaf vasculature and are the products of a novel precursor in petunia (solanaceae). *J. Biol. Chem.* **2012**, *287*, 27033–27046. [CrossRef] [PubMed]
173. Nguyen, G.K.; Zhang, S.; Nguyen, N.T.; Nguyen, P.Q.; Chiu, M.S.; Hardjojo, A.; Tam, J.P. Discovery and characterization of novel cyclotides originated from chimeric precursors consisting of albumin-1 chain a and cyclotide domains in the fabaceae family. *J. Biol. Chem.* **2011**, *286*, 24275–24287. [CrossRef] [PubMed]
174. Poth, A.G.; Colgrave, M.L.; Lyons, R.E.; Daly, N.L.; Craik, D.J. Discovery of an unusual biosynthetic origin for circular proteins in legumes. *Proc. Natl. Acad. Sci. USA* **2011**, *108*, 10127–10132. [CrossRef] [PubMed]
175. Mylne, J.S.; Chan, L.Y.; Chanson, A.H.; Daly, N.L.; Schaefer, H.; Bailey, T.L.; Nguyencong, P.; Cascales, L.; Craik, D.J. Cyclic peptides arising by evolutionary parallelism via asparaginyl-endopeptidase-mediated biosynthesis. *Plant Cell.* **2012**, *24*, 2765–2778. [CrossRef] [PubMed]
176. Nguyen, G.K.; Lian, Y.; Pang, E.W.; Nguyen, P.Q.; Tran, T.D.; Tam, J.P. Discovery of linear cyclotides in monocot plant panicum laxum of poaceae family provides new insights into evolution and distribution of cyclotides in plants. *J. Biol. Chem.* **2012**, *288*, 3370–3380. [CrossRef] [PubMed]
177. Ireland, D.C.; Colgrave, M.L.; Nguyencong, P.; Daly, N.L.; Craik, D.J. Discovery and characterization of a linear cyclotide from viola odorata: Implications for the processing of circular proteins. *J. Mol. Biol.* **2006**, *357*, 1522–1535. [CrossRef] [PubMed]
178. Gruber, C.W.; Cemazar, M.; Clark, R.J.; Horibe, T.; Renda, R.F.; Anderson, M.A.; Craik, D.J. A novel plant protein-disulfide isomerase involved in the oxidative folding of cystine knot defense proteins. *J. Biol. Chem.* **2007**, *282*, 20435–20446. [CrossRef] [PubMed]
179. Saska, I.; Gillon, A.D.; Hatsugai, N.; Dietzgen, R.G.; Hara-Nishimura, I.; Anderson, M.A.; Craik, D.J. An asparaginyl endopeptidase mediates *in vivo* protein backbone cyclization. *J. Biol. Chem.* **2007**, *282*, 29721–29728. [CrossRef] [PubMed]
180. Conlan, B.F.; Gillon, A.D.; Craik, D.J.; Anderson, M.A. Circular proteins and mechanisms of cyclization. *Biopolymers* **2010**, *94*, 573–583. [CrossRef] [PubMed]
181. Nguyen, G.K.T.; Wang, S.J.; Qiu, Y.B.; Hemu, X.; Lian, Y.L.; Tam, J.P. Butelase 1 is an asx-specific ligase enabling peptide macrocyclization and synthesis. *Nat. Chem. Biol.* **2014**, *10*, 732–738. [CrossRef] [PubMed]
182. Cao, Y.; Nguyen, G.K.; Tam, J.P.; Liu, C.F. Butelase-mediated synthesis of protein thioesters and its application for tandem chemoenzymatic ligation. *Chem. Commun. (Camb)* **2015**. [CrossRef] [PubMed]
183. Chagolla-Lopez, A.; Blanco-Labra, A.; Patthy, A.; Sanchez, R.; Pongor, S. A novel alpha-amylase inhibitor from amaranth (*Amaranthus hypocondriacus*) seeds. *J. Biol. Chem.* **1994**, *269*, 23675–23680. [PubMed]
184. Svensson, B.; Fukuda, K.; Nielsen, P.K.; Bonsager, B.C. Proteinaceous alpha-amylase inhibitors. *Biochim. Biophys. Acta* **2004**, *1696*, 145–156. [CrossRef] [PubMed]
185. Martins, J.C.; Enassar, M.; Willem, R.; Wieruzeski, J.M.; Lippens, G.; Wodak, S.J. Solution structure of the main alpha-amylase inhibitor from amaranth seeds. *Eur. J. Biochem.* **2001**, *268*, 2379–2389. [CrossRef] [PubMed]
186. Nguyen, P.Q.T.; Wang, S.J.; Kumar, A.; Yap, L.J.; Luu, T.T.; Lescar, J.; Tam, J.P. Discovery and characterization of pseudocyclic cystine-knot alpha-amylase inhibitors with high resistance to heat and proteolytic degradation. *FEBS J.* **2014**, *281*, 4351–4366. [CrossRef] [PubMed]
187. Nguyen, P.Q.; Luu, T.T.; Bai, Y.; Nguyen, G.K.; Pervushin, K.; Tam, J.P. Allotides: Proline-rich cystine knot alpha-amylase inhibitors from allamanda cathartica. *J. Nat. Prod.* **2015**, *78*, 695–704. [CrossRef] [PubMed]

188. Le-Nguyen, D.; Heitz, A.; Chiche, L.; el Hajji, M.; Castro, B. Characterization and 2d nmr study of the stable [9–21, 15–27] 2 disulfide intermediate in the folding of the 3 disulfide trypsin inhibitor eeti ii. *Protein Sci.* **1993**, *2*, 165–174. [CrossRef] [PubMed]
189. Heitz, A.; Le-Nguyen, D.; Chiche, L. Min-21 and min-23, the smallest peptides that fold like a cystine-stabilized beta-sheet motif: Design, solution structure, and thermal stability. *Biochemistry* **1999**, *38*, 10615–10625. [CrossRef] [PubMed]
190. Kolmar, H. Biological diversity and therapeutic potential of natural and engineered cystine knot miniproteins. *Curr. Opin. Pharmacol.* **2009**, *9*, 608–614. [CrossRef] [PubMed]
191. Colgrave, M.L.; Craik, D.J. Thermal, chemical, and enzymatic stability of the cyclotide kalata b1: The importance of the cyclic cystine knot. *Biochemistry* **2004**, *43*, 5965–5975. [CrossRef] [PubMed]
192. Heitz, A.; Avrutina, O.; Le-Nguyen, D.; Diederichsen, U.; Hernandez, J.F.; Gracy, J.; Kolmar, H.; Chiche, L. Knottin cyclization: Impact on structure and dynamics. *BMC Struct. Biol.* **2008**, *8*, 54. [CrossRef] [PubMed]
193. Ireland, D.C.; Colgrave, M.L.; Craik, D.J. A novel suite of cyclotides from viola odorata: Sequence variation and the implications for structure, function and stability. *Biochem. J.* **2006**, *400*, 1–12. [CrossRef] [PubMed]
194. Werle, M.; Kafedjiiski, K.; Kolmar, H.; Bernkop-Schnurch, A. Evaluation and improvement of the properties of the novel cystine-knot microprotein mcoeeti for oral administration. *Int. J. Pharm.* **2007**, *332*, 72–79. [CrossRef] [PubMed]
195. Werle, M.; Schmitz, T.; Huang, H.L.; Wentzel, A.; Kolmar, H.; Bernkop-Schnurch, A. The potential of cystine-knot microproteins as novel pharmacophoric scaffolds in oral peptide drug delivery. *J. Drug Target.* **2006**, *14*, 137–146. [CrossRef] [PubMed]
196. Gao, G.H.; Liu, W.; Dai, J.X.; Wang, J.F.; Hu, Z.; Zhang, Y.; Wang, D.C. Solution structure of pafp-s: A new knottin-type antifungal peptide from the seeds of phytolacca americana. *Biochemistry* **2001**, *40*, 10973–10978. [CrossRef] [PubMed]
197. Cammue, B.P.A.; Debolle, M.F.C.; Terras, F.R.G.; Proost, P.; Vandamme, J.; Rees, S.B.; Vanderleyden, J.; Broekaert, W.F. Isolation and characterization of a novel class of plant antimicrobial peptides from mirabilis-jalapa l seeds. *J. Biol. Chem.* **1992**, *267*, 2228–2233. [PubMed]
198. Hwang, J.S.; Lee, J.; Hwang, B.; Nam, S.H.; Yun, E.Y.; Kim, S.R.; Lee, D.G. Isolation and characterization of psacotheasin, a novel knottin-type antimicrobial peptide, from psacothea hilaris. *J. Microbiol. Biotechnol.* **2010**, *20*, 708–711. [CrossRef] [PubMed]
199. Konarev, A.V.; Anisimova, I.N.; Gavrilova, V.A.; Vachrusheva, T.E.; Konechnaya, G.Y.; Lewis, M.; Shewry, P.R. Serine proteinase inhibitors in the compositae: Distribution, polymorphism and properties. *Phytochemistry* **2002**, *59*, 279–291. [CrossRef]
200. Bode, W.; Greyling, H.J.; Huber, R.; Otlewski, J.; Wilusz, T. The refined 2.0 a x-ray crystal structure of the complex formed between bovine beta-trypsin and cmti-i, a trypsin inhibitor from squash seeds (*Cucurbita maxima*). Topological similarity of the squash seed inhibitors with the carboxypeptidase a inhibitor from potatoes. *FEBS Lett.* **1989**, *242*, 285–292. [PubMed]
201. Polanowski, A.; Wilusz, T.; Nienartowicz, B.; Cieslar, E.; Slominska, A.; Nowak, K. Isolation and partial amino acid sequence of the trypsin inhibitor from the seeds of cucurbita maxima. *Acta Biochim. Pol.* **1980**, *27*, 371–382. [PubMed]
202. Korsinczky, M.L.; Schirra, H.J.; Craik, D.J. Sunflower trypsin inhibitor-1. *Curr. Protein Pept. Sci.* **2004**, *5*, 351–364. [CrossRef] [PubMed]
203. Hass, G.M.; Ryan, C.A. Carboxypeptidase inhibitor from ripened tomatoes - purification and properties. *Phytochemistry* **1980**, *19*, 1329–1333. [CrossRef]
204. Arolas, J.L.; Lorenzo, J.; Rovira, A.; Vendrell, J.; Aviles, F.X.; Ventura, S. Secondary binding site of the potato carboxypeptidase inhibitor. Contribution to its structure, folding, and biological properties. *Biochemistry* **2004**, *43*, 7973–7982. [CrossRef] [PubMed]
205. Marino-Buslje, C.; Venhudova, G.; Molina, M.A.; Oliva, B.; Jorba, X.; Canals, F.; Aviles, F.X.; Querol, E. Contribution of c-tail residues of potato carboxypeptidase inhibitor to the binding to carboxypeptidase a a mutagenesis analysis. *Eur. J. Biochem.* **2000**, *267*, 1502–1509. [CrossRef] [PubMed]
206. Craik, D.J. Plant cyclotides: Circular, knotted peptide toxins. *Toxicon* **2001**, *39*, 1809–1813. [CrossRef]
207. Gould, A.; Ji, Y.; Aboye, T.L.; Camarero, J.A. Cyclotides, a novel ultrastable polypeptide scaffold for drug discovery. *Curr. Pharm. Des.* **2011**, *17*, 4294–4307. [CrossRef] [PubMed]

208. Daly, N.L.; Rosengren, K.J.; Craik, D.J. Discovery, structure and biological activities of cyclotides. *Adv. Drug Deliv. Rev.* **2009**, *61*, 918–930. [CrossRef] [PubMed]
209. Gran, L. On the effect of a polypeptide isolated from "kalata-kalata" (oldenlandia affinis dc) on the oestrogen dominated uterus. *Acta Pharmacol. Toxicol. (Copenh)* **1973**, *33*, 400–408. [CrossRef] [PubMed]
210. Rosengren, K.J.; Daly, N.L.; Plan, M.R.; Waine, C.; Craik, D.J. Twists, knots, and rings in proteins. Structural definition of the cyclotide framework. *J. Biol. Chem.* **2003**, *278*, 8606–8616. [CrossRef] [PubMed]
211. Tam, J.P.; Lu, Y.A.; Yang, J.L.; Chiu, K.W. An unusual structural motif of antimicrobial peptides containing end-to-end macrocycle and cystine-knot disulfides. *Proc. Natl. Acad. Sci. USA* **1999**, *96*, 8913–8918. [CrossRef] [PubMed]
212. Gran, L.; Sletten, K.; Skjeldal, L. Cyclic peptides from oldenlandia affinis dc. Molecular and biological properties. *Chem. Biodivers.* **2008**, *5*, 2014–2022. [CrossRef] [PubMed]
213. Pranting, M.; Loov, C.; Burman, R.; Goransson, U.; Andersson, D.I. The cyclotide cycloviolacin o2 from viola odorata has potent bactericidal activity against gram-negative bacteria. *J. Antimicrob. Chemother.* **2010**, *65*, 1964–1971. [CrossRef] [PubMed]
214. Wong, C.T.; Taichi, M.; Nishio, H.; Nishiuchi, Y.; Tam, J.P. Optimal oxidative folding of the novel antimicrobial cyclotide from hedyotis biflora requires high alcohol concentrations. *Biochemistry* **2011**, *50*, 7275–7283. [CrossRef] [PubMed]
215. Hernandez, J.F.; Gagnon, J.; Chiche, L.; Nguyen, T.M.; Andrieu, J.P.; Heitz, A.; Trinh Hong, T.; Pham, T.T.; Le Nguyen, D. Squash trypsin inhibitors from momordica cochinchinensis exhibit an atypical macrocyclic structure. *Biochemistry* **2000**, *39*, 5722–5730. [CrossRef] [PubMed]
216. Chiche, L.; Heitz, A.; Gelly, J.C.; Gracy, J.; Chau, P.T.; Ha, P.T.; Hernandez, J.F.; Le-Nguyen, D. Squash inhibitors: From structural motifs to macrocyclic knottins. *Curr. Protein Pept. Sci.* **2004**, *5*, 341–349. [CrossRef] [PubMed]
217. Heitz, A.; Hernandez, J.F.; Gagnon, J.; Hong, T.T.; Pham, T.T.; Nguyen, T.M.; Le-Nguyen, D.; Chiche, L. Solution structure of the squash trypsin inhibitor mcoti-ii. A new family for cyclic knottins. *Biochemistry* **2001**, *40*, 7973–7983. [CrossRef] [PubMed]
218. Henriques, S.T.; Craik, D.J. Cyclotides as templates in drug design. *Drug Discov. Today* **2010**, *15*, 57–64. [CrossRef] [PubMed]
219. Shenkarev, Z.O.; Nadezhdin, K.D.; Sobol, V.A.; Sobol, A.G.; Skjeldal, L.; Arseniev, A.S. Conformation and mode of membrane interaction in cyclotides. Spatial structure of kalata b1 bound to a dodecylphosphocholine micelle. *FEBS J.* **2006**, *273*, 2658–2672. [CrossRef] [PubMed]
220. Wang, C.K.; Colgrave, M.L.; Ireland, D.C.; Kaas, Q.; Craik, D.J. Despite a conserved cystine knot motif, different cyclotides have different membrane binding modes. *Biophys. J.* **2009**, *97*, 1471–1481. [CrossRef] [PubMed]
221. Wong, C.T.T.; Rowlands, D.K.; Wong, C.-H.; Lo, T.W.C.; Nguyen, G.K.T.; Li, H.-Y.; Tam, J.P. Orally active peptidic bradykinin b1 receptor antagonists engineered from a cyclotide scaffold for inflammatory pain treatment. *Angew. Chem. Int. Ed.* **2012**, *51*, 5620–5624. [CrossRef] [PubMed]
222. Hemu, X.; Taichi, M.; Qiu, Y.; Liu, D.-X.; Tam, J.P. Biomimetic synthesis of cyclic peptides using novel thioester surrogates. *Pept. Sci.* **2013**, *100*, 492–501. [CrossRef] [PubMed]
223. Qiu, Y.; Hemu, X.; Liu, D.X.; Tam, J.P. Selective bi-directional amide bond cleavage of *N*-methylcysteinyl peptide. *Eur. J. Org. Chem.* **2014**, *2014*, 4370–4380. [CrossRef]
224. Taichi, M.; Hemu, X.; Qiu, Y.; Tam, J.P. A thioethylalkylamido (tea) thioester surrogate in the synthesis of a cyclic peptide via a tandem acyl shift. *Org. Lett.* **2013**, *15*, 2620–2623. [CrossRef] [PubMed]
225. Tam, J.P.; Lu, Y.A. Synthesis of large cyclic cystine-knot peptide by orthogonal coupling strategy using unprotected peptide precursor. *Tetrahedron Lett.* **1997**, *38*, 5599–5602. [CrossRef]
226. Tam, J.P.; Lu, Y.A. A biomimetic strategy in the synthesis and fragmentation of cyclic protein. *Protein Sci.* **1998**, *7*, 1583–1592. [CrossRef] [PubMed]
227. Daly, N.L.; Love, S.; Alewood, P.F.; Craik, D.J. Chemical synthesis and folding pathways of large cyclic polypeptide: Studies of the cystine knot polypeptide kalata b1. *Biochemistry* **1999**, *38*, 10606–10614. [CrossRef] [PubMed]
228. Thongyoo, P.; Roque-Rosell, N.; Leatherbarrow, R.J.; Tate, E.W. Chemical and biomimetic total syntheses of natural and engineered mcoti cyclotides. *Org. Biomol. Chem.* **2008**, *6*, 1462–1470. [CrossRef] [PubMed]

229. Thongyoo, P.; Jaulent, A.M.; Tate, E.W.; Leatherbarrow, R.J. Immobilized protease-assisted synthesis of engineered cysteine-knot microproteins. *ChemBioChem* **2007**, *8*, 1107–1109. [CrossRef] [PubMed]
230. Kimura, R.H.; Tran, A.T.; Camarero, J.A. Biosynthesis of the cyclotide kalata b1 by using protein splicing. *Angew. Chem. Int. Ed.* **2006**, *45*, 973–976. [CrossRef] [PubMed]
231. Austin, J.; Wang, W.; Puttamadappa, S.; Shekhtman, A.; Camarero, J.A. Biosynthesis and biological screening of a genetically encoded library based on the cyclotide mcoti-i. *ChemBioChem* **2009**, *10*, 2663–2670. [CrossRef] [PubMed]
232. Tam, J.P.; Lu, Y.A.; Yu, Q.T. Thia zip reaction for synthesis of large cyclic peptides: Mechanisms and applications. *J. Am. Chem. Soc.* **1999**, *121*, 4316–4324. [CrossRef]
233. Duvick, J.P.; Rood, T.; Rao, A.G.; Marshak, D.R. Purification and characterization of a novel antimicrobial peptide from maize (*Zea mays* L.) kernels. *J. Biol. Chem.* **1992**, *267*, 18814–18820. [PubMed]
234. Marcus, J.P.; Green, J.L.; Goulter, K.C.; Manners, J.M. A family of antimicrobial peptides is produced by processing of a 7s globulin protein in macadamia integrifolia kernels. *Plant J.* **1999**, *19*, 699–710. [CrossRef] [PubMed]
235. Nolde, S.B.; Vassilevski, A.A.; Rogozhin, E.A.; Barinov, N.A.; Balashova, T.A.; Samsonova, O.V.; Baranov, Y.V.; Feofanov, A.V.; Egorov, T.A.; Arseniev, A.S.; *et al.* Disulfide-stabilized helical hairpin structure and activity of a novel antifungal peptide ecamp1 from seeds of barnyard grass (*Echinochloa crus-galli*). *J. Biol. Chem.* **2011**, *286*, 25145–25153. [CrossRef] [PubMed]
236. Utkina, L.L.; Andreev, Y.A.; Rogozhin, E.A.; Korostyleva, T.V.; Slavokhotova, A.A.; Oparin, P.B.; Vassilevski, A.A.; Grishin, E.V.; Egorov, T.A.; Odintsova, T.I. Genes encoding 4-cys antimicrobial peptides in wheat triticum kiharae dorof. Et migush.: Multimodular structural organization, instraspecific variability, distribution and role in defence. *FEBS J.* **2013**, *280*, 3594–3608. [CrossRef] [PubMed]
237. Slavokhotova, A.A.; Rogozhin, E.A.; Musolyamov, A.K.; Andreev, Y.A.; Oparin, P.B.; Berkut, A.A.; Vassilevski, A.A.; Egorov, T.A.; Grishin, E.V.; Odintsova, T.I. Novel antifungal alpha-hairpinin peptide from stellaria media seeds: Structure, biosynthesis, gene structure and evolution. *Plant. Mol. Biol.* **2014**. [CrossRef] [PubMed]
238. Conners, R.; Konarev, A.V.; Forsyth, J.; Lovegrove, A.; Marsh, J.; Joseph-Horne, T.; Shewry, P.; Brady, R.L. An unusual helix-turn-helix protease inhibitory motif in a novel trypsin inhibitor from seeds of veronica (veronica hederifolia l.). *J. Biol. Chem.* **2007**, *282*, 27760–27768. [CrossRef] [PubMed]
239. Oparin, P.B.; Mineev, K.S.; Dunaevsky, Y.E.; Arseniev, A.S.; Belozersky, M.A.; Grishin, E.V.; Egorov, T.A.; Vassilevski, A.A. Buckwheat trypsin inhibitor with helical hairpin structure belongs to a new family of plant defence peptides. *Biochem. J.* **2012**, *446*, 69–77. [CrossRef] [PubMed]
240. Ng, Y.M.; Yang, Y.; Sze, K.H.; Zhang, X.; Zheng, Y.T.; Shaw, P.C. Structural characterization and anti-hiv-1 activities of arginine/glutamate-rich polypeptide luffin p1 from the seeds of sponge gourd (*Luffa cylindrica*). *J. Struct. Biol.* **2011**, *174*, 164–172. [CrossRef] [PubMed]
241. Kader, J.C. Lipid-transfer proteins in plants. *Annu Rev. Plant. Physiol Plant. Mol. Biol* **1996**, *47*, 627–654. [CrossRef] [PubMed]
242. Carvalho Ade, O.; Gomes, V.M. Role of plant lipid transfer proteins in plant cell physiology-a concise review. *Peptides* **2007**, *28*, 1144–1153. [CrossRef] [PubMed]
243. Terras, F.R.G.; Goderis, I.J.; Vanleuven, F.; Vanderleyden, J.; Cammue, B.P.A.; Broekaert, W.F. Invitro antifungal activity of a radish (*Raphanus-sativus* L.) seed protein homologous to nonspecific lipid transfer proteins. *Plant. Physiol.* **1992**, *100*, 1055–1058. [CrossRef] [PubMed]
244. Molina, A.; Segura, A.; Garcia-Olmedo, F. Lipid transfer proteins (nsltps) from barley and maize leaves are potent inhibitors of bacterial and fungal plant pathogens. *FEBS Lett.* **1993**, *316*, 119–122. [CrossRef]
245. Segura, A.; Moreno, M.; Garcia-Olmedo, F. Purification and antipathogenic activity of lipid transfer proteins (ltps) from the leaves of arabidopsis and spinach. *FEBS Lett.* **1993**, *332*, 243–246. [CrossRef]
246. Cammue, B.P.; Thevissen, K.; Hendriks, M.; Eggermont, K.; Goderis, I.J.; Proost, P.; Van Damme, J.; Osborn, R.W.; Guerbette, F.; Kader, J.C.; *et al.* A potent antimicrobial protein from onion seeds showing sequence homology to plant lipid transfer proteins. *Plant Physiol.* **1995**, *109*, 445–455. [CrossRef] [PubMed]
247. Arondel, V.V.; Vergnolle, C.; Cantrel, C.; Kader, J. Lipid transfer proteins are encoded by a small multigene family in arabidopsis thaliana. *Plant Sci.* **2000**, *157*, 1–12. [CrossRef]

248. Douliez, J.P.; Pato, C.; Rabesona, H.; Molle, D.; Marion, D. Disulfide bond assignment, lipid transfer activity and secondary structure of a 7-kda plant lipid transfer protein, ltp2. *Eur. J. Biochem.* **2001**, *268*, 1400–1403. [CrossRef] [PubMed]
249. Pons, J.L.; de Lamotte, F.; Gautier, M.F.; Delsuc, M.A. Refined solution structure of a liganded type 2 wheat nonspecific lipid transfer protein. *J. Biol. Chem.* **2003**, *278*, 14249–14256. [CrossRef] [PubMed]
250. Samuel, D.; Liu, Y.J.; Cheng, C.S.; Lyu, P.C. Solution structure of plant nonspecific lipid transfer protein-2 from rice (*Oryza sativa*). *J. Biol. Chem.* **2002**, *277*, 35267–35273. [CrossRef] [PubMed]
251. Gomar, J.; Sodano, P.; Sy, D.; Shin, D.H.; Lee, J.Y.; Suh, S.W.; Marion, D.; Vovelle, F.; Ptak, M. Comparison of solution and crystal structures of maize nonspecific lipid transfer protein: A model for a potential *in vivo* lipid carrier protein. *Proteins* **1998**, *31*, 160–171. [CrossRef]
252. Tassin, S.; Broekaert, W.F.; Marion, D.; Acland, D.P.; Ptak, M.; Vovelle, F.; Sodano, P. Solution structure of ace-amp1, a potent antimicrobial protein extracted from onion seeds. Structural analogies with plant nonspecific lipid transfer proteins. *Biochemistry* **1998**, *37*, 3623–3637. [CrossRef] [PubMed]
253. Lee, J.Y.; Min, K.; Cha, H.; Shin, D.H.; Hwang, K.Y.; Suh, S.W. Rice non-specific lipid transfer protein: The 1.6 a crystal structure in the unliganded state reveals a small hydrophobic cavity. *J. Mol. Biol.* **1998**, *276*, 437–448. [CrossRef] [PubMed]
254. Han, G.W.; Lee, J.Y.; Song, H.K.; Chang, C.; Min, K.; Moon, J.; Shin, D.H.; Kopka, M.L.; Sawaya, M.R.; Yuan, H.S.; *et al.* Structural basis of non-specific lipid binding in maize lipid-transfer protein complexes revealed by high-resolution x-ray crystallography. *J. Mol. Biol.* **2001**, *308*, 263–278. [CrossRef] [PubMed]
255. Cheng, H.C.; Cheng, P.T.; Peng, P.; Lyu, P.C.; Sun, Y.J. Lipid binding in rice nonspecific lipid transfer protein-1 complexes from *Oryza sativa*. *Protein Sci.* **2004**, *13*, 2304–2315. [CrossRef] [PubMed]
256. Poznanski, J.; Sodano, P.; Suh, S.W.; Lee, J.Y.; Ptak, M.; Vovelle, F. Solution structure of a lipid transfer protein extracted from rice seeds. Comparison with homologous proteins. *Eur. J. Biochem.* **1999**, *259*, 692–708. [CrossRef] [PubMed]
257. Gincel, E.; Simorre, J.P.; Caille, A.; Marion, D.; Ptak, M.; Vovelle, F. Three-dimensional structure in solution of a wheat lipid-transfer protein from multidimensional 1h-nmr data. A new folding for lipid carriers. *Eur. J. Biochem.* **1994**, *226*, 413–422. [CrossRef] [PubMed]
258. Charvolin, D.; Douliez, J.P.; Marion, D.; Cohen-Addad, C.; Pebay-Peyroula, E. The crystal structure of a wheat nonspecific lipid transfer protein (ns-ltp1) complexed with two molecules of phospholipid at 2.1 a resolution. *Eur. J. Biochem.* **1999**, *264*, 562–568. [CrossRef] [PubMed]
259. Lerche, M.H.; Kragelund, B.B.; Bech, L.M.; Poulsen, F.M. Barley lipid-transfer protein complexed with palmitoyl coa: The structure reveals a hydrophobic binding site that can expand to fit both large and small lipid-like ligands. *Structure* **1997**, *5*, 291–306. [CrossRef]
260. Lerche, M.H.; Poulsen, F.M. Solution structure of barley lipid transfer protein complexed with palmitate. Two different binding modes of palmitate in the homologous maize and barley nonspecific lipid transfer proteins. *Protein Sci.* **1998**, *7*, 2490–2498. [CrossRef] [PubMed]
261. Gomar, J.; Petit, M.C.; Sodano, P.; Sy, D.; Marion, D.; Kader, J.C.; Vovelle, F.; Ptak, M. Solution structure and lipid binding of a nonspecific lipid transfer protein extracted from maize seeds. *Protein Sci.* **1996**, *5*, 565–577. [CrossRef] [PubMed]
262. Castro, M.S.; Gerhardt, I.R.; Orru, S.; Pucci, P.; Bloch, C., Jr. Purification and characterization of a small (7.3 kda) putative lipid transfer protein from maize seeds. *J. Chromatogr. B Analyt. Technol. Biomed. Life Sci.* **2003**, *794*, 109–114. [CrossRef]
263. Gizatullina, A.K.; Finkina, E.I.; Mineev, K.S.; Melnikova, D.N.; Bogdanov, I.V.; Telezhinskaya, I.N.; Balandin, S.V.; Shenkarev, Z.O.; Arseniev, A.S.; Ovchinnikova, T.V. Recombinant production and solution structure of lipid transfer protein from lentil lens culinaris. *Biochem. Biophys. Res. Commun.* **2013**, *439*, 427–432. [CrossRef] [PubMed]
264. Lin, K.F.; Liu, Y.N.; Hsu, S.T.; Samuel, D.; Cheng, C.S.; Bonvin, A.M.; Lyu, P.C. Characterization and structural analyses of nonspecific lipid transfer protein 1 from mung bean. *Biochemistry* **2005**, *44*, 5703–5712. [CrossRef] [PubMed]
265. Da Silva, P.; Landon, C.; Industri, B.; Marais, A.; Marion, D.; Ponchet, M.; Vovelle, F. Solution structure of a tobacco lipid transfer protein exhibiting new biophysical and biological features. *Proteins* **2005**, *59*, 356–367. [CrossRef] [PubMed]

266. Cheng, C.S.; Chen, M.N.; Lai, Y.T.; Chen, T.; Lin, K.F.; Liu, Y.J.; Lyu, P.C. Mutagenesis study of rice nonspecific lipid transfer protein 2 reveals residues that contribute to structure and ligand binding. *Proteins* **2008**, *70*, 695–706. [CrossRef] [PubMed]
267. Cheng, C.S.; Samuel, D.; Liu, Y.J.; Shyu, J.C.; Lai, S.M.; Lin, K.F.; Lyu, P.C. Binding mechanism of nonspecific lipid transfer proteins and their role in plant defense. *Biochemistry* **2004**, *43*, 13628–13636. [CrossRef] [PubMed]
268. Lin, P.; Xia, L.; Wong, J.H.; Ng, T.B.; Ye, X.; Wang, S.; Shi, X. Lipid transfer proteins from brassica campestris and mung bean surpass mung bean chitinase in exploitability. *J. Pept. Sci.* **2007**, *13*, 642–648. [CrossRef] [PubMed]
269. Molina, A.; Garcia-Olmedo, F. Enhanced tolerance to bacterial pathogens caused by the transgenic expression of barley lipid transfer protein ltp2. *Plant J.* **1997**, *12*, 669–675. [CrossRef] [PubMed]
270. Lascombe, M.B.; Bakan, B.; Buhot, N.; Marion, D.; Blein, J.P.; Larue, V.; Lamb, C.; Prange, T. The structure of "defective in induced resistance" protein of arabidopsis thaliana, dir1, reveals a new type of lipid transfer protein. *Protein Sci.* **2008**, *17*, 1522–1530. [CrossRef] [PubMed]
271. Yeats, T.H.; Rose, J.K. The biochemistry and biology of extracellular plant lipid-transfer proteins (ltps). *Protein Sci.* **2008**, *17*, 191–198. [CrossRef] [PubMed]
272. Kader, J.C. Proteins and intracellular exchange of lipids.1. Stimulation of phospholipid exchange between mitochondria and microsomal fractions by proteins isolated from potato-tuber. *Biochem. Biophys. Acta* **1975**, *380*, 31–44. [CrossRef]
273. Kader, J.C.; Julienne, M.; Vergnolle, C. Purification and characterization of a spinach-leaf protein capable of transferring phospholipids from liposomes to mitochondria or chloroplasts. *Eur. J. Biochem.* **1984**, *139*, 411–416. [CrossRef] [PubMed]
274. Thoma, S.; Kaneko, Y.; Somerville, C. A non-specific lipid transfer protein from arabidopsis is a cell wall protein. *Plant J.* **1993**, *3*, 427–436. [CrossRef] [PubMed]
275. Pyee, J.; Yu, H.S.; Kolattukudy, P.E. Identification of a lipid transfer protein as the major protein in the surface wax of broccoli (*Brassica oleracea*) leaves. *Archiv. Biochem. Biophys.* **1994**, *311*, 460–468. [CrossRef]
276. Regente, M.C.; Giudici, A.M.; Villalain, J.; de la Canal, L. The cytotoxic properties of a plant lipid transfer protein involve membrane permeabilization of target cells. *Lett. Appl. Microbiol.* **2005**, *40*, 183–189. [CrossRef] [PubMed]
277. Segura, A.; Moreno, M.; Madueno, F.; Molina, A.; Garcia-Olmedo, F. Snakin-1, a peptide from potato that is active against plant pathogens. *Mol. Plant Microbe Interact.* **1999**, *12*, 16–23. [CrossRef] [PubMed]
278. Berrocal-Lobo, M.; Segura, A.; Moreno, M.; Lopez, G.; Garcia-Olmedo, F.; Molina, A. Snakin-2, an antimicrobial peptide from potato whose gene is locally induced by wounding and responds to pathogen infection. *Plant Physiol.* **2002**, *128*, 951–961. [CrossRef] [PubMed]
279. Porto, W.F.; Franco, O.L. Theoretical structural insights into the snakin/gasa family. *Peptides* **2013**, *44*, 163–167. [CrossRef] [PubMed]
280. Bindschedler, L.V.; Whitelegge, J.P.; Millar, D.J.; Bolwell, G.P. A two component chitin-binding protein from french bean – association of a proline-rich protein with a cysteine-rich polypeptide. *FEBS Lett.* **2006**, *580*, 1541–1546. [CrossRef] [PubMed]
281. Daneshmand, F.; Zare-Zardini, H.; Ebrahimi, L. Investigation of the antimicrobial activities of snakin-z, a new cationic peptide derived from zizyphus jujuba fruits. *Nat. Prod. Res.* **2013**, *27*, 2292–2296. [CrossRef] [PubMed]
282. Mandal, S.M.; Porto, W.F.; Dey, P.; Maiti, M.K.; Ghosh, A.K.; Franco, O.L. The attack of the phytopathogens and the trumpet solo: Identification of a novel plant antifungal peptide with distinct fold and disulfide bond pattern. *Biochimie* **2013**, *2013*, 1939–1948. [CrossRef] [PubMed]
283. Tailor, R.H.; Acland, D.P.; Attenborough, S.; Cammue, B.P.; Evans, I.J.; Osborn, R.W.; Ray, J.A.; Rees, S.B.; Broekaert, W.F. A novel family of small cysteine-rich antimicrobial peptides from seed of impatiens balsamina is derived from a single precursor protein. *J. Biol. Chem.* **1997**, *272*, 24480–24487. [CrossRef] [PubMed]
284. Thevissen, K.; Francois, I.E.; Sijtsma, L.; van Amerongen, A.; Schaaper, W.M.; Meloen, R.; Posthuma-Trumpie, T.; Broekaert, W.F.; Cammue, B.P. Antifungal activity of synthetic peptides derived from impatiens balsamina antimicrobial peptides ib-amp1 and ib-amp4. *Peptides* **2005**, *26*, 1113–1119. [CrossRef] [PubMed]

285. Patel, S.U.; Osborn, R.; Rees, S.; Thornton, J.M. Structural studies of impatiens balsamina antimicrobial protein (ib-amp1). *Biochemistry* **1998**, *37*, 983–990. [CrossRef] [PubMed]
286. Wang, P.; Bang, J.K.; Kim, H.J.; Kim, J.K.; Kim, Y.; Shin, S.Y. Antimicrobial specificity and mechanism of action of disulfide-removed linear analogs of the plant-derived cys-rich antimicrobial peptide ib-amp1. *Peptides* **2009**, *30*, 2144–2149. [CrossRef] [PubMed]
287. Fujimura, M.; Ideguchi, M.; Minami, Y.; Watanabe, K.; Tadera, K. Amino acid sequence and antimicrobial activity of chitin-binding peptides, pp-amp 1 and pp-amp 2, from japanese bamboo shoots (phyllostachys pubescens). *Biosci. Biotechnol. Biochem.* **2005**, *69*, 642–645. [CrossRef] [PubMed]
288. Astafieva, A.A.; Rogozhin, E.A.; Odintsova, T.I.; Khadeeva, N.V.; Grishin, E.V.; Egorov Ts, A. Discovery of novel antimicrobial peptides with unusual cysteine motifs in dandelion taraxacum officinale wigg. Flowers. *Peptides* **2012**, *36*, 266–271. [CrossRef] [PubMed]
289. Astafieva, A.A.; Rogozhin, E.A.; Andreev, Y.A.; Odintsova, T.I.; Kozlov, S.A.; Grishin, E.V.; Egorov, T.A. A novel cysteine-rich antifungal peptide toamp4 from taraxacum officinale wigg. Flowers. *Plant Physiol. Biochem.* **2013**, *70*, 93–99. [CrossRef] [PubMed]
290. McManus, A.M.; Nielsen, K.J.; Marcus, J.P.; Harrison, S.J.; Green, J.L.; Manners, J.M.; Craik, D.J. Miamp1, a novel protein from macadamia integrifolia adopts a greek key beta-barrel fold unique amongst plant antimicrobial proteins. *J. Mol. Biol.* **1999**, *293*, 629–638. [CrossRef] [PubMed]
291. Silva, O.N.; Porto, W.F.; Migliolo, L.; Mandal, S.M.; Gomes, D.G.; Holanda, H.H.; Silva, R.S.; Dias, S.C.; Costa, M.P.; Costa, C.R.; *et al.* Cn-amp1: A new promiscuous peptide with potential for microbial infections treatment. *Biopolymers* **2012**, *98*, 322–331. [CrossRef] [PubMed]
292. Mandal, S.M.; Migliolo, L.; Das, S.; Mandal, M.; Franco, O.L.; Hazra, T.K. Identification and characterization of a bactericidal and proapoptotic peptide from cycas revoluta seeds with DNA binding properties. *J. Cell. Biochem.* **2012**, *113*, 184–193. [CrossRef] [PubMed]
293. Pelegrini, P.B.; Murad, A.M.; Silva, L.P.; Dos Santos, R.C.; Costa, F.T.; Tagliari, P.D.; Bloch, C., Jr.; Noronha, E.F.; Miller, R.N.; Franco, O.L. Identification of a novel storage glycine-rich peptide from guava (psidium guajava) seeds with activity against gram-negative bacteria. *Peptides* **2008**, *29*, 1271–1279. [CrossRef] [PubMed]
294. Tavares, L.S.; Rettore, J.V.; Freitas, R.M.; Porto, W.F.; Duque, A.P.; Singulani Jde, L.; Silva, O.N.; Detoni Mde, L.; Vasconcelos, E.G.; Dias, S.C.; *et al.* Antimicrobial activity of recombinant pg-amp1, a glycine-rich peptide from guava seeds. *Peptides* **2012**, *37*, 294–300. [CrossRef] [PubMed]
295. Park, C.J.; Park, C.B.; Hong, S.S.; Lee, H.S.; Lee, S.Y.; Kim, S.C. Characterization and cdna cloning of two glycine- and histidine-rich antimicrobial peptides from the roots of shepherd's purse, capsella bursa-pastoris. *Plant. Mol. Biol.* **2000**, *44*, 187–197. [CrossRef] [PubMed]
296. Rahnamaeian, M. Antimicrobial peptides: Modes of mechanism, modulation of defense responses. *Plant Signal. Behav.* **2011**, *6*, 1325–1332. [CrossRef] [PubMed]
297. Barbosa Pelegrini, P.; Del Sarto, R.P.; Silva, O.N.; Franco, O.L.; Grossi-de-Sa, M.F. Antibacterial peptides from plants: What they are and how they probably work. *Biochem. Res. Int.* **2011**, *2011*, 250349. [CrossRef] [PubMed]
298. Kagan, B.L.; Selsted, M.E.; Ganz, T.; Lehrer, R.I. Antimicrobial defensin peptides form voltage-dependent ion-permeable channels in planar lipid bilayer membranes. *Proc. Natl. Acad. Sci. USA* **1990**, *87*, 210–214. [CrossRef] [PubMed]
299. Miyazaki, Y.; Aoki, M.; Yano, Y.; Matsuzaki, K. Interaction of antimicrobial peptide magainin 2 with gangliosides as a target for human cell binding. *Biochemistry* **2012**, *51*, 10229–10235. [CrossRef] [PubMed]
300. Sarika; Iquebal, M.A.; Rai, A. Biotic stress resistance in agriculture through antimicrobial peptides. *Peptides* **2012**, *36*, 322–330. [CrossRef] [PubMed]
301. Montesinos, E. Antimicrobial peptides and plant disease control. *FEMS Microbiol. Lett.* **2007**, *270*, 1–11. [CrossRef] [PubMed]
302. Jagadish, K.; Camarero, J.A. Cyclotides, a promising molecular scaffold for peptide-based therapeutics. *Biopolymers* **2010**, *94*, 611–616. [CrossRef] [PubMed]
303. Yu, Q.; Lehrer, R.I.; Tam, J.P. Engineered salt-insensitive alpha-defensins with end-to-end circularized structures. *J. Biol. Chem.* **2000**, *275*, 3943–3949. [CrossRef] [PubMed]
304. Chan, L.Y.; Gunasekera, S.; Henriques, S.T.; Worth, N.F.; Le, S.J.; Clark, R.J.; Campbell, J.H.; Craik, D.J.; Daly, N.L. Engineering pro-angiogenic peptides using stable, disulfide-rich cyclic scaffolds. *Blood* **2011**, *118*, 6709–6717. [CrossRef] [PubMed]

305. Eliasen, R.; Daly, N.L.; Wulff, B.S.; Andresen, T.L.; Conde-Frieboes, K.W.; Craik, D.J. Design, synthesis, structural and functional characterization of novel melanocortin agonists based on the cyclotide kalata b1. *J. Biol. Chem.* **2012**, *287*, 40493–40501. [CrossRef] [PubMed]
306. Abdallah, N.A.; Shah, D.; Abbas, D.; Madkour, M. Stable integration and expression of a plant defensin in tomato confers resistance to fusarium wilt. *GM Crops* **2010**, *1*, 344–350. [CrossRef] [PubMed]

9

Ground Calcium Carbonate as a Low Cost and Biosafety Excipient for Solubility and Dissolution Improvement of Praziquantel

Ana Borrego-Sánchez [1,2,*], Rita Sánchez-Espejo [1], Beatrice Albertini [3], Nadia Passerini [3], Pilar Cerezo [2], César Viseras [1,2] and C. Ignacio Sainz-Díaz [1]

1 Instituto Andaluz de Ciencias de la Tierra (CSIC-University of Granada), Av. de las Palmeras 4, 18100 Granada, Spain; ritaespejo@hotmail.com (R.S.-E.); cviseras@ugr.es (C.V.); ignacio.sainz@iact.ugr-csic.es (C.I.S.-D.)

2 Department of Pharmacy and Pharmaceutical Technology, Faculty of Pharmacy, University of Granada, Campus de Cartuja s/n, 18071 Granada, Spain; mcerezo@ugr.es

3 Department of Pharmacy and BioTechnology, University of Bologna, Via S. Donato 19/2, 40127 Bologna, Italy; beatrice.albertini@unibo.it (B.A.); nadia.passerini@unibo.it (N.P.)

* Correspondence: anaborrego@iact.ugr-csic.es;

Abstract: Calcium carbonate is an abundant mineral with several advantages to be a successful carrier to improve oral bioavailability of poorly water-soluble drugs, such as praziquantel. Praziquantel is an antiparasitic drug classified in group II of the Biopharmaceutical Classification System hence characterized by high-permeability and low-solubility. Therefore, the dissolution rate is the limiting factor for the gastrointestinal absorption that contributes to the low bioavailability. Consequently, the therapeutic dose of the praziquantel must be high and big tablets and capsules are required, which are difficult to swallow, especially for pediatric and elderly patients. Mixtures of praziquantel and calcium carbonate using solid-solid physical mixtures and solid dispersions were prepared and characterized using several techniques (X-ray diffraction differential scanning calorimetry, thermogravimetric analysis, scanning electron microscopy, laser diffraction, Fourier transform infrared and Raman spectroscopies). Solubility of these formulations evidenced that the solubility of praziquantel-calcium carbonate interaction product increased in physiological media. *In vitro* dissolution tests showed that the interaction product increased the dissolution rate of the drug in acidic medium. Theoretical models were studied to understand this experimental behavior. Cytotoxicity and cell cycle studies were performed, showing that praziquantel-calcium carbonate physical mixture and interaction product were biocompatible with the HTC116 cells, because it did not produce a decrease in cell viability or alterations in the cell cycle.

Keywords: praziquantel; calcium carbonate; schistosomiasis; bioavailability; solubility; cytotoxicity

1. Introduction

Calcium carbonate, $CaCO_3$, being a low cost material, with high surface area, excellent safety, biocompatibility and biodegradability, is a well-documented excipient in pharmaceutical solid dosage forms, mainly used as diluent [1]. Recently, it has also been demonstrated that calcium carbonate can successfully act as hydrophilic porous carrier to improve the oral bioavailability of low water soluble drugs [2–5]. Functionalization with hydroxypropyl-β-cyclodextrin [6], enzymatic macromolecules [7], or incorporation in polymeric hydrogels [8–11] can further enhance the ability of calcium carbonate to improve oral delivery of several biomolecules, including proteins [12] and anti-cancer drugs [13]. As recently reviewed, most of the successfully designed calcium carbonate carriers have been prepared by emulsion techniques or chemical precipitation of the carbonate micro/nanoparticles [14]. However, precipitation of calcium carbonate micro/nanoparticles is difficult to reproduce and scale up of the procedure is most of times challenging, avoiding the clinical use of these carriers. Moreover, detailed understanding of biosafety and *in vivo* degradation of the new calcium carbonate particles would require preclinical studies. An interesting alternative is to overcome these challenges by using normalized pharmaceutical excipients grades of calcium carbonate as drug delivery carriers [1].

Praziquantel (PZQ) is the drug of choice in the treatment of schistosomiasis [15], being included in the WHO Model List of Essential Drug for the treatment of adults and children [16]. Schistosomiasis affects approximately 210 million people, causing 200,000 deaths every year. Moreover, it is widely extended, mainly in 78 developing countries in the tropics and subtropics, although at least 92% of people who need treatment for schistosomiasis live in Africa and, is the second of the most prevalent disease (after malaria) affecting African children. PZQ is classified in group II of the Biopharmaceutical Classification System (BCS) and hence characterized by high permeability and low solubility [17]. Therefore, the dissolution rate is the limiting factor for the gastrointestinal absorption that contributes to the low oral bioavailability. Moreover, absorbed amounts of PZQ suffer an extensive first-pass metabolism [18], leading to administration of high-dosed dosage forms, which are difficult to swallow, especially for pediatric patients [19].

Enhancing the water solubility and the dissolution rate is critical to increase the oral bioavailability of PZQ. Several studies and strategies have been carried out to improve PZQ water solubility, such as incorporation into liposome vectors [20], preparation of solid dispersions of the drug with different excipients such as clay minerals [21], β-cyclodextrins [22–24], polyvinyl-pyrrolidone [25–27], polyethylene glycols [28–30], sodium starch glycolate [31] and preparation of dispersible granules [14]. In addition, other techniques have been used to increase the solubility of PZQ such as co-grinding with several excipients [32], melt granulation and ultrasonic spray congealing [27], and the transition in a new crystalline polymorph by milling [19]. More recently, our previous paper evidenced conformational changes of PZQ in association with calcium carbonate after a solvent evaporation process [33]. This interaction product revealed the formation of modifications of the pristine racemic drug attributable to either polymorph B [19] or disordered pseudoracemate solid phases [33].

Given these premises, the first aim of this work was to verify if PZQ solid state modification within calcium carbonate solid dispersion is due to the solvent evaporation process or to drug-carrier interactions that would happen during a mere blending procedure. Thus, the physico-chemical properties of the physical mixture were compared to those of the interaction product. Further, we explored the possibilities of calcium carbonate/PZQ systems for the improvement of biopharmaceutical properties of the drug. In particular, solubility and dissolution profiles of PZQ from interaction product were compared to the corresponding physical mixture, and the results explained by using theoretical modeling. In addition, we investigated the *in vitro* cytotoxicity and cell cycle studies of calcium carbonate/PZQ systems.

2. Materials and Methods

2.1. Materials

PZQ drug was kindly donated by Fatro S.p.A. (Bologna, Italy). Ground Calcium Carbonate Calcitec Pure PH V/40S (GCC) was purchased from Mineraria Sacilese (Sacile, Italy). This kind of calcium carbonate is used in the pharmaceutical industry and was accepted in the latest edition of the European and United States Pharmacopoeias. The GCC finds also employment in the food industry and in industries where is requested a low content of heavy metals. Ethanol of 96% of purity was used as solvent.

2.2. *Preparation of the PZQ and GCC Physical Mixture*

Physical mixtures (PM) of PZQ and GCC (1:5 *w/w*) were prepared blending both solids in an agate mortar of 100 mm of diameter at room temperature for 5 min.

2.3. *Preparation of the PZQ and GCC Interaction Product (IP)*

GCC was dispersed in 1 L of ethanolic solution of PZQ under magnetic stirring at room temperature for 24 h, so drug/GCC ratio was 1:5 *w/w* in order to ensure the complete interaction between PZQ and GCC. After 24 h, the solvent was evaporated with rotary evaporator (Rotary evaporator Buchi® R II, Flawil, Switzerland) at 40 °C and reduced pressure. The solid residue was dried in a desiccator and then it was pulverized.

2.4. *Solid State Characterization of Calcium Carbonate/Praziquantel Systems*

2.4.1. X-ray Diffraction (XRD)

An X-Pert Pro® diffractometer (Marvel Panalytical, Madrid, Spain) with the CuKα radiation was used for performing powder X-ray diffraction. The powder samples were scanned in the range of 4°–70° of the 2θ angle, steps were of 0.008 of 2θ and the counting time was of 10.16 sec/step. The diffraction results were analyzed with the XPOWDER® software version 2004 [34].

2.4.2. Thermal Analysis

Differential scanning calorimetric analysis (DSC) and thermogravimetric analysis (TGA) were performed with a mod. TGA/DSC1 calorimeter (Mettler Toledo, Barcelona, Spain) equipped with a sensor and FRS5 microbalance (precision 0.1 μg) and FP89 software package. Samples were heated in air atmosphere at 5 °C/min in the in the 30–200 °C temperature range for DSC and 30–420 °C temperature range for TGA.

2.4.3. Scanning Electron Microscope (SEM)

Microphotographs of the samples were performed using a Hitachi S-510 scanning electron microscope (voltage 25 kV, secondary electron images) (Hitachi Scientific Instruments Ltd., Tokyo, Japan). The samples were mounted on adhesive carbon paper, fixed with colloidal gold and metallized with gold in two orientations (20–30°). The images were captured digitally using the program attached to the microscope (ScanVision, Version 1.2).

2.4.4. Particle Size Analysis

The particle size distribution of the solid sample materials suspended in liquid medium was analyzed with Laser Light Diffraction technology. The equipment used was a Mastersizer 2000LF from Malvern Panalytical Instruments (Madrid, Spain) consisting of HYDRO MU Malvern manual liquid sample dispersion unit and Malvern HYDRO 2000Up minimum volume liquid sample dispersion unit.

2.4.5. Fourier Transform Infrared and Raman Spectroscopies

Fourier Transform Infrared Spectroscopy (FTIR) spectra were recorded with a 6200 spectrophotometer (JASCO, Pfungstadt, Germany) in the range 4000–600 cm^{-1} with a 0.5 cm^{-1} resolution and a well-plate sampler along with the Spectra Manager II software.

Raman spectra were recorded using a JASCO NRS-5100 Micro-Raman dispersive spectrophotometer in the range 3500–800 cm^{-1} with a 6.48 cm^{-1} resolution, with laser light source VIS-NIR with red diode at 785 nm with 500 mW of power (Torsana Starbright) refrigerated by air and the KnowItAll JASCO for Raman software.

2.5. Solubility Studies

The solubility of PZQ as well as the physical mixture PM PZQ-GCC and the interaction product IP PZQ-GCC were studied separately in two media: an acidic medium of HCl 0.001 M and a simulated intestinal fluid (SIF) without enzymes with a buffer at pH 6.8. The solubility of PZQ was calculated by placing a supersaturated solution of the pristine drug, specifically 30 mg in 10 mL in each of the media. The supersaturated solution was stirred in a thermostatic bath for 72 h at 37 °C. After 72 h, it was centrifuged, and the supernatant was filtered and measured on high-performance liquid chromatography (HPLC). Obtaining by means of the HPLC the amount of dissolved drug that corresponds to its solubility. This experiment was repeated 6 times. In the same way this procedure was applied for the PM and the IP PZQ-GCC.

2.6. Dissolution Studies

PZQ-GCC physical mixture or PZQ-GCC interaction product (210 mg) were encapsulated in double zero (00) gelatin capsules, corresponding to 35 mg of PZQ and 175 mg of GCC in each capsule. As well as, 35 mg of PZQ were encapsulated as reference. The obtained capsules were subjected to sink conditions dissolution tests using the official Pharmacopoeia USP apparatus 2 for the dissolution test of oral solid dosage forms (Sotax AT7, S). This apparatus is equipped with a rotation system type palettes and sinkers, piston pump for the automatic sampling at scheduled times and collector of fractions. The measurements were performed at 37 °C and 150 rpm in 1 L of medium. Two separate dissolution media were studied: an acidic medium of HCl 0.001 M (simulated stomach) and a SIF medium without enzymes with a buffer at pH 6.8 (simulated intestine). Aliquots of 5 mL were collected from the dissolution test, filtered through 0.45 μm Millipore® (S) membranes and analyzed by HPLC for drug content. Volumes of 5 mL of fresh dissolution medium were replaced after each sampling to maintain the volume constant. At least three replicates for each sample were assayed.

2.7. HPLC Analysis

Drug analysis was performed using a 1260 Infinity II Agilent HPLC system (Santa Clara, CA, USA) equipped with quaternary pump, autosampler, column oven and UV-VIS diode-array spectrophotometer. The stationary phase was a Kromasil® C18 column, 5 μm, 250 × 4.6 mm (Teknokroma, Barcelona, Spain) and the mobile phase was a mixture of H_2O and CH_3CN (35:65 *v/v*). The flow rate was set at 0.8 mL/min with an injection volume of 10 μL. A spectrophotometer detector at a 225 nm wavelength was used and the run time for each analysis was 5 min. Data were recorded and analyzed by using software LC Open LAB HPLC 1260 (Agilent). The response of the analytical method was linear in the concentration range 5–100 mg/L of PZQ in both media, resulting in correlation coefficients of 1 (both in HCl 0.001 M and SIF).

2.8. Computational Methods

The molecular model of PZQ was extracted from previous calculations [35] and the rest of components were placed by hand. The Compass force field (FF) [36] based on empirical interatomic potentials was used within the Discover program of the Materials Studio package [37]. This FF was used previously to describe PZQ molecules and crystal structure with satisfactory results [35,38]. An atomic interactions cut-off of 18.5 Å was used for calculating Van der Waals and Coulomb interactions.

2.9. Cell Culture

Cell viability tests and study the cell cycle profiles were performed for observing a possible production of cell death in a tumor line of cells derived from colorectal carcinoma, called HCT116. This tumor line of HCT116 colorectal carcinoma cells were cultured in Dulbecco's Modified Eagle's Medium (DMEM) (Gibco Invitrogen, Dublin, Ireland) supplemented 10% with decomplemented Heat-Inactivated Fetal Bovine Serum (FBS) (Gibco Invitrogen), with glutamax (BioWhittaker, Cologne,

Germany) at 1% and with Penicillin/Streptomycin (BioWhittaker) at 1%. The cell culture was kept in an incubator at 37 °C and 5% of CO_2.

2.10. Cytotoxicity Studies

Firstly, PZQ and GCC samples were prepared relying on the administered drug amount in animals as antiparasitic. In such way, the amount of the mineral was five times more than that of PZQ. To do this, we prepared an intermediate dilution in dimethylsulfoxide (DMSO) at a concentration of 100 mM and then another dilution at 10 mM. The physical mixture and the interaction product PZQ-GCC were studied using the same procedure.

To perform the proliferation assays by Alamar Blue, about 10,000–20,000 cells/well of HCT116 were seeded in 96-well plates, in a final volume of 200 µL of DMEM medium using several concentrations (100 µM, 20 µM, 4 µM, 800 nM, 160 nM, 32 nM and 6.4 nM) for each sample studied (PZQ, GCC, PM and IP PZQ-GCC). Cells were incubated at 37 °C, 5% CO_2 for 48 h. After the incubation time, 10 µL per well of the PrestoBlue cell Viability Reagent (Invitrogen, Thermo Fisher Scientific, Carlsbad, CA, USA) was added, incubating for 15 min. After this period, fluorescence was measured at 535–90 nm in a Tecan reader (Männedorf, Switzerland). This reagent is based on resazurin compound, which works as an indicator of viability when it is reduced by living cells and presents a colour change from blue (dead cells) to pink (living cells).

2.11. Cell Cycle Studies

The cells were cultured in 24 well plates at a concentration of 250,000 cells/well in 500 µL and treated with the previously selected PZQ, GCC, PM and IP PZQ-GCC samples, at increasing concentrations of 0.8, 4, 20 and 100 µM for 48 h. Dead cells (apoptotic and necrotic) were detected based on staining with propidium iodide following the protocol described [39]. Briefly, the cells after the corresponding treatments were collected and washed with 2 mL of phosphate buffered saline (PBS) at 4 °C and fixed with 100 µL of PBS and 900 µL of 70% ethanol on ice for 5 min. After washing with PBS, they were resuspended in 250 µL of PBS and another 250 µL of a DNA extraction solution (0.2 M Na_2HPO_4, 0.1M C6H8O7, pH 7.8) and incubated at 37 °C for 10 min. The supernatant was removed and 200 µL of the staining solution was added (8 µL propidium iodide (1 mg/mL) and 2 µL RNAse 100 (µg/mL)), incubating the samples for 10 min at 37 °C in the dark. Fluorescence was measured in the FL2 detector of the FACScalibur cytometer (Becton Dickinson & Co., Franklin Lakes, NJ, USA) and the analysis of the sub-G1 population (population of dead cells: necrotic and apoptotic) was done using the BD CellQuest software v1.0.2 (BD, Biosciences).

3. Results and Discussion

3.1. Solid State Characterization of Calcium Carbonate/Praziquantel Systems

PZQ and GCC (1:5) solid dispersions obtained by solvent evaporation evidenced conformational changes of the pristine drug solid state [33]. Recently, a number of papers [19,32,40] have elucidated that the mechanochemical activation of PZQ, via neat grinding or comilling PZQ with different polymers (Povidone, Copovidone, Crospovidone and Sodium Starch Glycolate) enabled the transformation of the original PZQ polymorphic form into a new polymorphic variety of racemic PZQ or into a drug amorphous state.

In this study, the properties of PZQ-GCC physical mixture (produced by blending) were compared to those of the PZQ-GCC interaction product (obtained by solvent evaporation). A solid state characterization of the samples studied was performed by X-ray diffraction (Figure S1), differential scanning calorimetric analysis (Figure S2), thermogravimetric analysis (Figure S3), scanning electron microscope (Figure S4), Fourier Transform Infrared and Raman Spectroscopies (Figure S5) and particle size analysis. The results demonstrated that PZQ-GCC physical mixture did not show any chemical-physical change with respect to the pure drug. On the contrary, in the PZQ-GCC interaction product multiple changes were observed, as already described in a previous work [33]. The detailed results and analyses of the solid state characterization of the samples studied (PZQ, GCC, PM and IP) are provided in the Supplementary Material.

3.2. Solubility Studies

The solubility tests showed that the IP PZQ-GCC increased the solubility of the pure drug from 0.50 mg/mL to 1.42 mg/mL in an acid aqueous medium with 0.001 M HCl (pH = 3), due to its interaction with the GCC and the solubility of the GCC in acidic medium. On the contrary, the PM PZQ-GCC showed a small and unimportant increase in the solubility of the drug (Table 1). The results in a SIF medium (pH = 6.8) revealed that the IP PZQ-GCC increased the solubility of PZQ from 0.45 mg/mL to 0.73 mg/mL; while the PM showed a slight increase in the solubility of PZQ from 0.45 mg/mL to 0.50 mg/mL, which was not considered notable. Therefore, the solubility of the IP PZQ-GCC improves in acid and SIF media with respect to the PZQ and PM. This increase is much higher at pH 3 (Table 1).

Table 1. Solubility values of praziquantel (PZQ), physical mixture (PM) of PZQ-GCC and interaction product (IP) of PZQ-GCC in acid and simulated intestinal fluid (SIF) media (mean values ± standard deviation; $n = 0.07$).

Sample	HCl 0.001 M Medium, pH = 3	SIF Medium, pH = 6.8
PZQ	0.50 mg/mL	0.45 mg/mL
PM PZQ-GCC	0.52 mg/mL	0.50 mg/mL
IP PZQ-GCC	1.42 mg/mL	0.73 mg/mL

3.3. Dissolution Studies

In order to explore the *in vitro* bioavailability of PZQ, dissolution tests in both media simulating the gastric and the intestinal fluids, were performed for the pristine drug and the combinations of PZQ with GCC (IP and PM) (Figure 1).

PZQ-GCC physical mixture presented a similar behavior to the pristine PZQ in both dissolution media (Figure 1a,b), while the IP showed a completely different behavior at pH 3 with respect to pH 6.8. Interaction product PZQ-GCC showed an increase in the dissolution rate in acid medium (Figure 1a) and a strong decrease in SIF (Figure 1b). These results were concordant with solubility tests results, where the solubility of IP PZQ-GCC is higher in acid medium than in SIF. This behaviour may be correlated to the different solubility of GCC at acidic and neutral pH and to structural changes observed in IP: as GCC is soluble at low pH, its interaction at molecular level with water and PZQ favoured the dissolution and solubility of the drug. Likewise, the PZQ-GCC interaction at pH 6.8, where the carbonate is completely insoluble, negatively affected the solubilisation of the PZQ molecules.

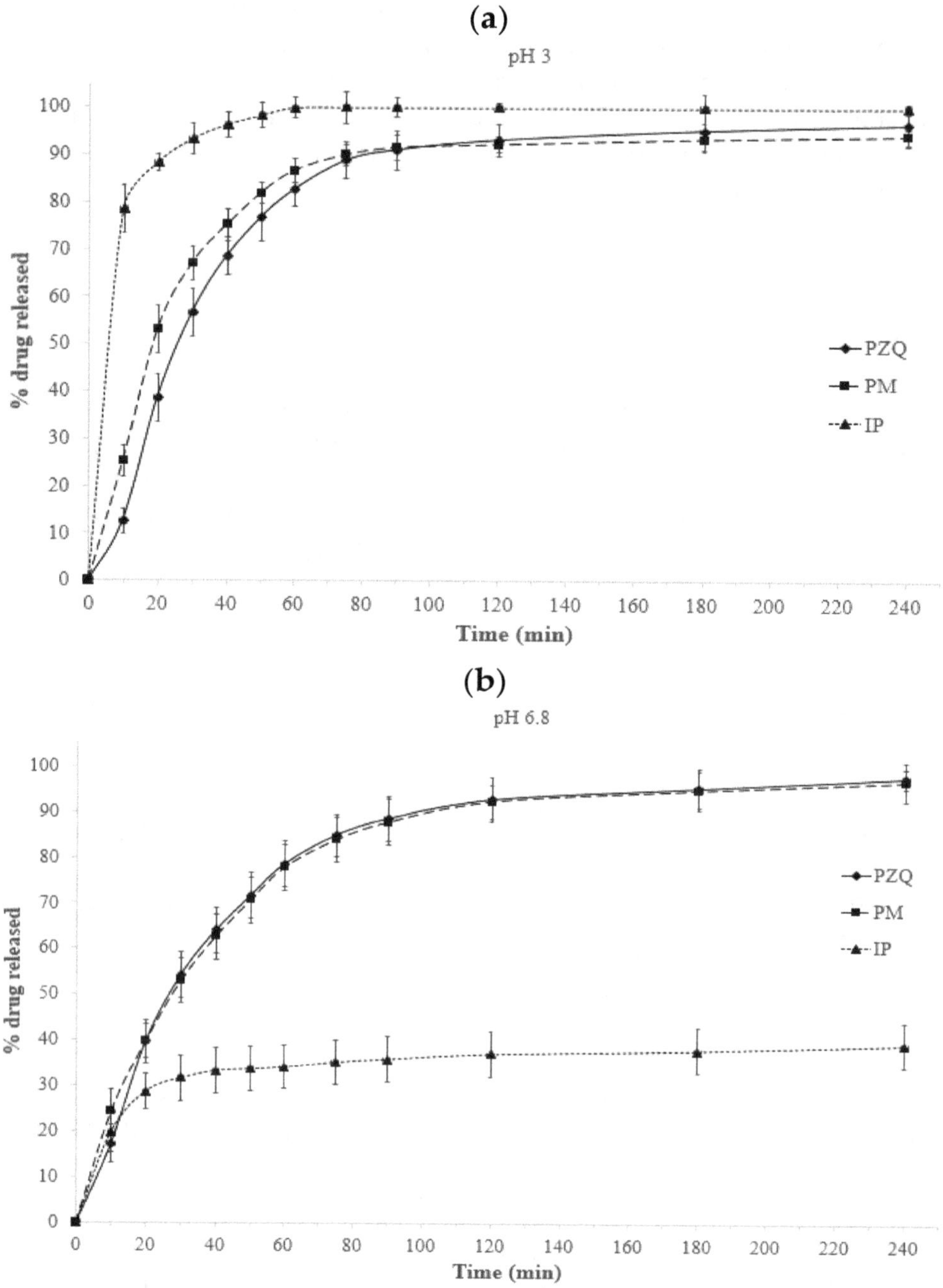

Figure 1. Drug release (% *w/w*) profiles from the PZQ and the PM in 0.001 M HCl at pH = 3 (**a**) and in a SIF medium at pH = 6.8 (**b**) in sink conditions; (mean values ± standard deviation; $n = 5$).

3.4. Modeling Approach

In order to explain the dissolution behavior of the PZQ-GCC systems, small models of PZQ molecules with the GCC and water molecules were created (Figure 2). In the PM, the carbonyl groups of PZQ are at the same side of the molecule as a *syn* conformer, whereas in IP the proportion of the *anti* conformer is higher [38]. The geometry of these models was optimized with Compass FF calculations, using the SPC water model (Figure 2c,d). In both models the carbonate anion is coordinated with the Ca^{2+} cation d(Ca ... OCO) = 1.88–1.91 Å and at least one water molecule is between the Ca^{2+} cation and a carbonyl group forming a hydrogen bond with the corresponding carbonyl group d(HOH ... O=C) = 1.84–1.88 Å. In the *syn* conformer, both water molecules are coordinating the Ca^{2+} cation and the water H atoms d(HOH ... Ca) = 2.27 Å (Figure 2c).

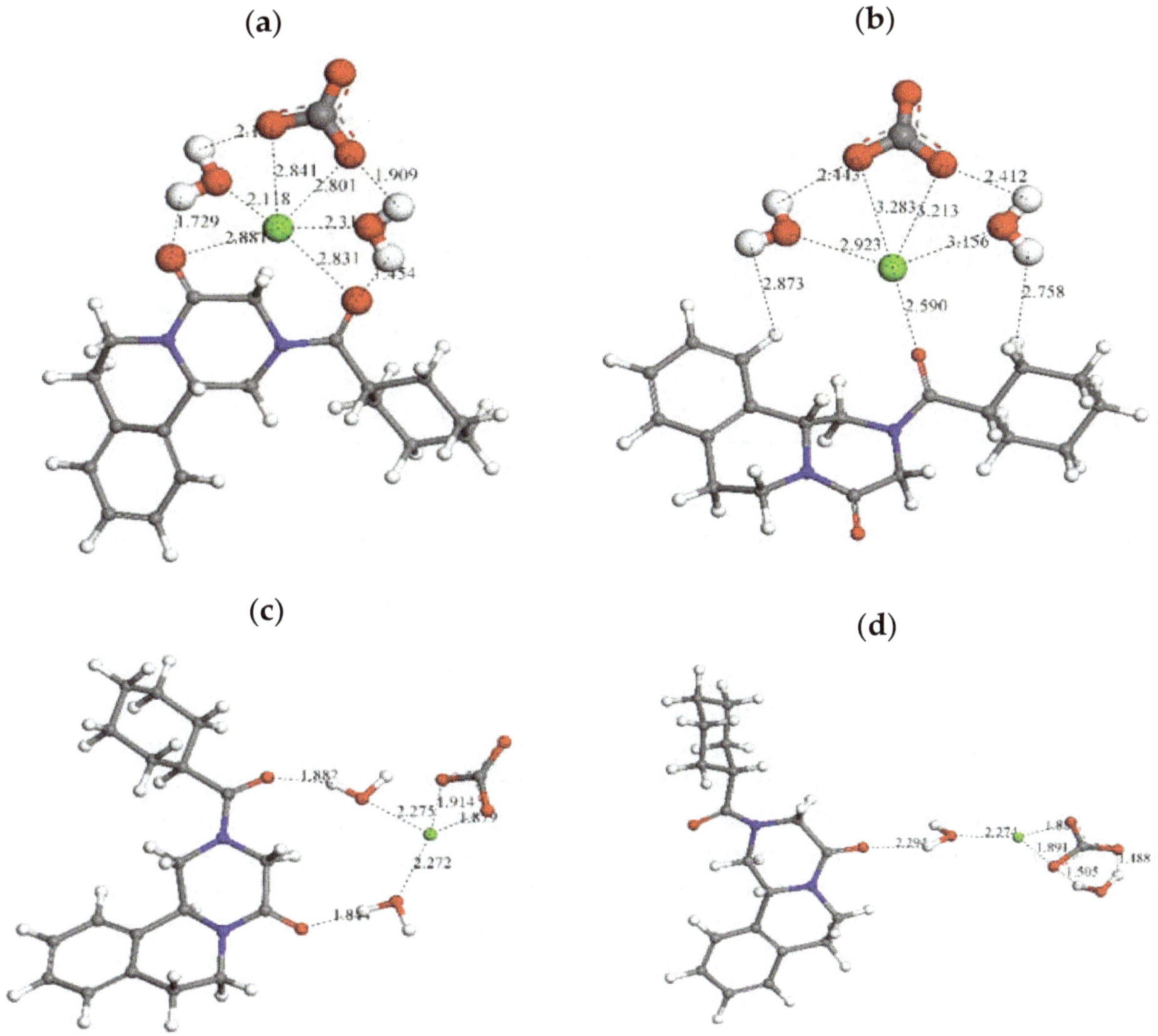

Figure 2. Possible complexes of PZQ molecule conformer *syn* (**a**) and *anti* (**b**) with hydrated Ca^{2+} carbonates clusters, and optimized complexes of *syn* (**c**) and *anti* (**d**) PZQ (non-bonding distances are included in Å). The C, Ca, H, N, and O atoms are in grey, green, white, blue, and red color.

In the *anti* conformer, one water molecule is coordinating the Ca^{2+} cation, d(O … Ca) = 2.27 Å, and one carbonyl O atom d(CO … H) = 2.22 Å leaving the another carbonyl group free in the opposite side of the molecule to form an additional carbonate complex. The conformer *syn* can form only one complex with the hydrated Ca^{2+} cation (Figure 2). This could explain the higher dissolution process of the *anti* form of PZQ and hence the higher solubility of IP PZQ-GCC.

3.5. Cytotoxicity Studies

In vitro cytotoxicity tests in the HCT116 cell line showed that all the PZQ and GCC pure concentrations (6.4 nM–100 µM) tested provided viability values slightly lower than the untreated cells (control). Therefore, PZQ and GCC pure samples can be considered biocompatible toward HCT116 cell lines (Figure 3). In the IP and PM PZQ-GCC products similar results were found, whose biocompatibility across the range of concentrations was evaluated and a trend similar to the control was observed and slightly positive with respect to the pure samples (PZQ and GCC) in cell growth. Therefore, it is notable that IP and PM PZQ-GCC products have a biocompatible behaviour, so the interaction between PZQ and GCC had a positive effect in the cell viability (Figure 3).

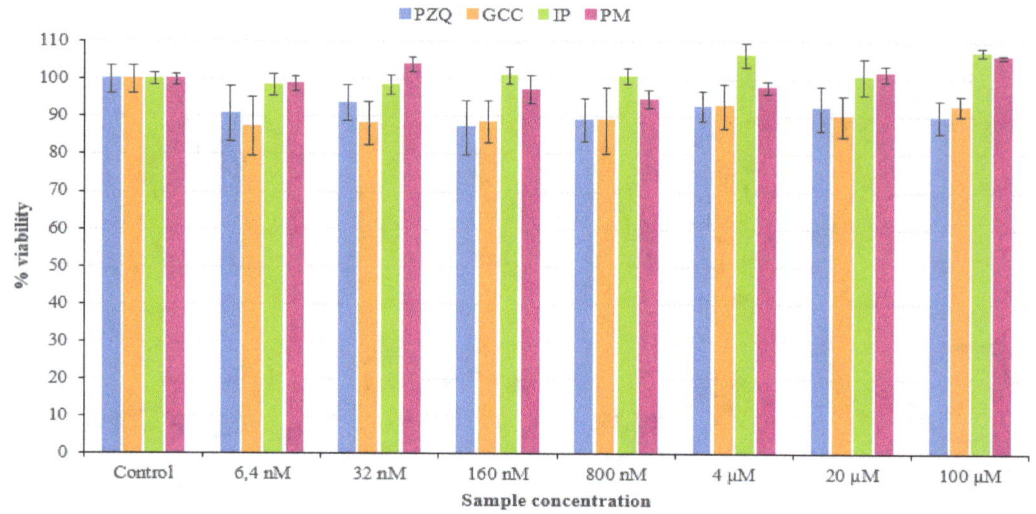

Figure 3. Cell viability from the studied samples after 48 h of treatment. (Control: untreated cells in complete medium; mean values ± standard error; $n = 8$).

3.6. Cell Cycle Studies

A study of the cell cycle by means of propidium iodide was carried out to study the cell cycle corresponding to the Sub-G1 phase of the cells in contact with our samples (Figure 4). Once observed through cytotoxicity studies that the samples tested did not cause cell death, a cell cycle study was carried out to check whether the compounds affected any phase of the cell cycle despite not affecting proliferation. In the upper part of the figure the control tests can be observed: an example of the cell cycle of healthy untreated cells, an example of cells treated with DMSO, where it is observed that DMSO does not affect the cell and also an example of cells treated with etoposide, an antineoplastic drug that damages cells. In this last example, the cell cycle of the control cells is severely affected and induces death to 64.3% of the cell population.

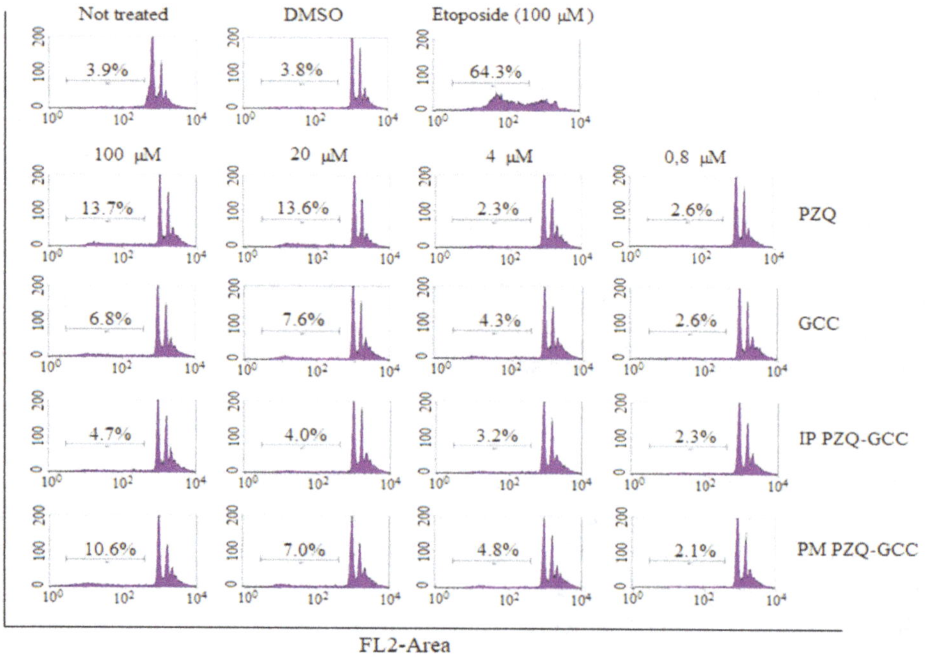

Figure 4. Cell cycle of the HCT116 line treated with the sample studies. The percentages indicate the number of cells in Sub-G1 (apoptotic or necrotic).

The studied samples showed that they do not affect in any case the cellular cycle of the cells, only in some cases at high concentrations can the cell death increase slightly, although not in a noteworthy way (Figure 4).

4. Conclusions

Interaction products obtained with PZQ and GCC increased the solubility of PZQ in physiological media, particularly in acid medium. *In vitro* dissolution tests evidenced that the interaction product increased the dissolution rate of the drug in acidic medium. *In vitro* cytotoxicity and cell cycle studies were performed, showing neither the PZQ-GCC physical mixture nor the interaction product produced cellular damage in any of the studied concentrations. Therefore, the samples studied did not produce cell death or alteration in the cell cycle and were biocompatible with the HTC116 cells.

As a general conclusion, the use of low cost GCCimprove solubility and dissolution rates of PZQ, without producing cytotoxicity or alterations in the cell cycle of HTC116 cells. This allows exploring the use of GCC as an interesting technological strategy for a drug administration in a more effective biopharmaceutical and clinical way ofPZQ. Also providing the great advantage that the design and development of the PZQ-GCC new formulations would not increase the final cost of the drug, overcoming a great challenge due to the population which the treatment is destined and the high prevalent of the neglected tropical disease.

Author Contributions: Conceptualization, B.A., N.P., C.V. and C.I.S.-D.; methodology, A.B.-S., C.V. and C.I.S.-D.; software, A.B.-S. and C.I.S.-D.; formal analysis, A.B.-S. and R.S.-E.; investigation, A.B.-S. and R.S.-E.; resources, P.C., C.V. and C.I.S.-D.; writing—original draft preparation, A.B.-S.; writing—review and editing, A.B.-S., B.A., N.P., P.C., R.S.-E., C.V. and C.I.S.-D.; supervision, A.B.-S., C.V. and C.I.S.-D.; project administration, A.B.-S.; funding acquisition, P.C., C.V. and C.I.S.-D.

Acknowledgments: The authors are thankful to Fatro S.p.A. for donating the praziquantel drug and to Xtrem Biotech, specially Ignacio Molina and Sara Torres, for their contributions with the cytotoxicity and cell cycle experiments. We also acknowledge for financial support the MINECO, for projects FIS2016-77692-C2-2-P and CGL2016-80833-R, and the Andalusian government, for project RNM1897.

References

1. Rowe, R.C.; Sheskey, P.J.; Weller, P.J. Calcium Carbonate. In *Handbook of Pharmaceutical Excipients*, 6th ed.; Pharmaceutical Press: London, UK, 2009.
2. Ueno, Y.; Futagawa, H.; Takagi, Y.; Ueno, A.; Mizushima, Y. Drug-incorporating calcium carbonate nanoparticles for a new delivery system. *J. Control. Release* **2005**, *103*, 93–98. [CrossRef] [PubMed]
3. Preisig, D.; Haid, D.; Varum, F.J.; Bravo, R.; Alles, R.; Huwyler, J.; Puchkov, M. Drug loading into porous calcium carbonate microparticles by solvent evaporation. *Eur. J. Pharm. Biopharm.* **2014**, *87*, 548–558. [CrossRef] [PubMed]
4. Manzine Costa, L.M.; Molina de Olyveira, G.; Salomão, R. Precipitated Calcium Carbonate Nano-Microparticles: Applications in Drug Delivery. *Adv. Tissue Eng. Regen. Med.* **2017**, *3*, 2.
5. Dizaj, S.M.; Barzegar-Jalali, M.; Zarrintan, M.H.; Adibkia, K.; Lotfipour, F. Calcium carbonate nanoparticles as cancer drug delivery system. *Expert Opin. Drug Deliv.* **2015**, *12*, 1649–1660. [CrossRef]
6. Zhang, L.; Zhu, W.; Lin, Q.; Han, J.; Jiang, L.; Zhang, Y. Hydroxypropyl-β-cyclodextrin functionalized calcium carbonate microparticles as a potential carrier for enhancing oral delivery of water-insoluble drugs. *Int. J. Nanomed.* **2015**, *10*, 3291–3302. [CrossRef]

7. Islan, G.A.; Cacicedo, M.L.; Bosio, V.E.; Castro, G.R. Development and characterization of new enzymatic modified hybrid calcium carbonate microparticles to obtain nano-architectured surfaces for enhanced drug loading. *J. Colloid Interface Sci.* **2015**, *439*, 76–87. [CrossRef]
8. Wang, J.; Chen, J.-S.; Zong, J.-Y.; Zhao, D.; Li, F.; Zhuo, R.-X.; Cheng, S.-X. Calcium Carbonate/Carboxymethyl Chitosan Hybrid Microspheres and Nanospheres for Drug Delivery. *J. Phys. Chem. C* **2010**, *114*, 18940–18945. [CrossRef]
9. Wang, C.; Liu, H.; Gao, Q.; Liu, X.; Tong, Z. Alginate-calcium carbonate porous microparticle hybrid hydrogels with versatile drug loading capabilities and variable mechanical strengths. *Carbohydr. Polym.* **2008**, *71*, 476–480. [CrossRef]
10. Wang, J.; Kong, Y.; Liu, F.; Shou, D.; Tao, Y.; Qin, Y. Construction of pH-responsive drug delivery platform with calcium carbonate microspheres induced by chitosan gels. *Ceram. Int.* **2018**, *44*, 7902–7907. [CrossRef]
11. Vergaro, V.; Papadia, P.; Leporatti, S.; De Pascali, S.A.; Fanizzi, F.P.; Ciccarella, G. Synthesis of biocompatible polymeric nano-capsules based on calcium carbonate: A potential cisplatin delivery system. *J. Inorg. Biochem.* **2015**, *153*, 284–292. [CrossRef]
12. Roth, R.; Schoelkopf, J.; Huwyler, J.; Puchkov, M. Functionalized calcium carbonate microparticles for the delivery of proteins. *Eur. J. Pharm. Biopharm.* **2018**, *122*, 96–103. [CrossRef] [PubMed]
13. Svenskaya, Y.; Parakhonskiy, B.; Haase, A.; Atkin, V.; Lukyanets, E.; Gorin, D.; Antolini, R. Anticancer drug delivery system based on calcium carbonate particles loaded with a photosensitizer. *Biophys. Chem.* **2013**, *182*, 11–15. [CrossRef] [PubMed]
14. Trofimov, A.D.; Ivanova, A.A.; Zyuzin, M.V.; Timin, A.S. Porous Inorganic carriers Based on Silica, Calcium Carbonate and Calcium Phosphate for Controlled/Modulated Drug Delivery: Fresh Outlook and Future Perspectives. *Pharmaceutics* **2018**, *10*, 167. [CrossRef] [PubMed]
15. Trastullo, R.; Dolci, L.S.; Passerini, N.; Albertini, B. Development of flexible and dispersible oral formulations containing praziquantel for potential schistosomiasis treatment of pre-school age children. *Int. J. Pharm.* **2015**, *495*, 536–550. [CrossRef] [PubMed]
16. WHO, World Health Organization. Schistosomiasis. Available online: http://www.who.int/es/news-room/fact-sheets/detail/schistosomiasis (accessed on 12 October 2019).
17. Lindenberg, M.; Kopp, S.; Dressman, J.B. Classification of orally administered drugs on the World Health Organization Model list of Essential Medicines according to the biopharmaceutics classification system. *Eur. J. Pharm. Biopharm.* **2004**, *58*, 265–278. [CrossRef]
18. El-Subbagh, H.I.; Al-Badr, A.A. Praziquantel. In *Analytical Profiles of Drug Substances and Excipients*; Academic Press Inc.: New York, NY, USA, 1998; Volume 25, pp. 463–500.
19. Zanolla, D.; Perissutti, B.; Passerini, N.; Chierotti, M.R.; Hasa, D.; Voinovich, D.; Gigli, L.; Demitri, N.; Geremia, S.; Keiser, J.; et al. A new soluble and bioactive polymorph of praziquantel. *Eur. J. Pharm. Biopharm.* **2018**, *127*, 19–28. [CrossRef]
20. Mourao, S.C.; Costa, P.I.; Salgado, H.R.N.; Gremiao, M.P.D. Improvement of antischistosomal activity of praziquantel by incorporation into phosphatidylcholine-containing liposomes. *Int. J. Pharm.* **2005**, *295*, 157–162. [CrossRef]
21. Borrego-Sánchez, A.; Carazo, E.; Aguzzi, C.; Viseras, C.; Sainz-Díaz, C.I. Biopharmaceutical improvement of praziquantel by interaction with montmorillonite and sepiolite. *Appl. Clay Sci.* **2018**, *160*, 173–179. [CrossRef]
22. Rodrigues, S.G.; Chaves, I.S.; Melo, N.F.S.; de Jesus, M.B.; Fraceto, L.F.; Fernandes, S.A.; de Paula, E.; de Freitas, M.P.; Pinto, L.M.A. Computational analysis and physico-chemical characterization of an inclusion compound between praziquantel and methyl-β-cyclodextrin for use as an alternative in the treatment of schistosomiasis. *J. Incl. Phenom. Macrocycl. Chem.* **2011**, *70*, 19–28. [CrossRef]
23. Maragos, S.; Archontaki, H.; Macheras, P.; Valsami, G. Effect of Cyclodextrin Complexation on the Aqueous Solubility and Solubility/Dose Ratio of Praziquantel. *AAPS Pharm. Sci. Tech.* **2009**, *10*, 1444. [CrossRef]
24. Becket, G.; Schep, L.J.; Tan, M.Y. Improvement of the in vitro dissolution of praziquantel by complexation with α-, β-, and γ-cyclodextrins. *Int. J. Pharm.* **1999**, *179*, 65–71. [CrossRef]
25. De la Torre, P.; Torrado, S.; Torrado, S. Preparation, Dissolution and Characterization of Praziquantel Solid Dispersions. *Chem. Pharm. Bull.* **1999**, *47*, 1629–1633. [CrossRef]
26. El-Arini, S.K.; Leuenberger, H. Dissolution properties of praziquantel-PVP systems. *Pharm. Acta Helv.* **1998**, *73*, 89–94. [CrossRef]

27. Costa, E.D.; Priotti, J.; Orlandi, S.; Leonardi, D.; Lamas, M.C.; Nunes, T.G.; Diogo, H.P.; Salomon, C.J.; Ferreira, M.J. Unexpected solvent impact in the crystallinity of praziquantel/poly(vinylpyrrolidone) formulations. A solubility, DSC and solid-state NMR study. *Int. J. Pharm.* **2016**, *511*, 983–993. [CrossRef]
28. Passerini, N.; Albertini, B.; Perissutti, B.; Rodriguez, L. Evaluation of melt granulation and ultrasonic spray congealing as techniques to enhance the dissolution of praziquantel. *Int. J. Pharm.* **2006**, *318*, 92–102. [CrossRef]
29. Liu, Y.; Wang, T.; Ding, W.; Dong, C.; Wang, X.; Chen, J.; Li, Y. Dissolution and oral bioavailability enhancement of praziquantel by solid dispersions. *Drug Deliv. Transl. Res.* **2018**, *8*, 580–590. [CrossRef]
30. Cheng, L.; Lei, L.; Guo, S. In vitro and in vivo evaluation of praziquantel loaded implants based on PEG/PCL blends. *Int. J. Pharm.* **2010**, *387*, 129–138. [CrossRef]
31. Chaud, M.V.; Lima, A.C.; Vila, M.M.D.C.; Paganelli, M.O.; Paula, F.C.; Pedreiro, L.N.; Gremião, M.P.D. Development and evaluation of praziquantel solid dispersions in sodium starch glycolate. *Trop. J. Pharm. Res.* **2013**, *12*, 163–168. [CrossRef]
32. Perissutti, B.; Passerini, N.; Trastullo, R.; Keiser, J.; Zanolla, D.; Zingone, G.; Voinovich, D.; Albertini, B. An explorative analysis of process and formulation variables affecting comilling in a vibrational mill: The case of praziquantel. *Int. J. Pharm.* **2017**, *533*, 402–412. [CrossRef]
33. Borrego-Sánchez, A.; Carazo, E.; Albertini, B.; Passerini, N.; Perissutti, B.; Cerezo, P.; Viseras, C.; Aguzzi, C.; Sainz-Díaz, C.I. Conformational polymorphic changes in the crystal structure of the chiral antiparasitic drug praziquantel and interactions with calcium carbonate. *Eur. J. Pharm. Biopharm.* **2018**, *132*, 180–191. [CrossRef]
34. Martín-Ramos, J.D. XPowder software. 2005. Available online: http://www.xpowder.com (accessed on 12 October 2019).
35. Borrego-Sánchez, A.; Viseras, C.; Aguzzi, C.; Sainz-Díaz, C.I. Molecular and crystal structure of praziquantel. Spectroscopic properties and crystal polymorphism. *Eur. J. Pharm. Sci.* **2016**, *92*, 266–275. [CrossRef] [PubMed]
36. Sun, H. COMPASS: An ab Initio Force-Field Optimized for Condensed-Phase Applications-Overview with Details on Alkane and Benzene Compounds. *J. Phys. Chem. B* **1998**, *102*, 7338–7364. [CrossRef]
37. *Accelrys Materials Studio*, version v 6.0; Accelrys Inc.: San Diego, CA, USA, 2012.
38. Borrego-Sánchez, A.; Hernández-Laguna, A.; Sainz-Díaz, C.I. Molecular modeling and infrared and Raman spectroscopy of the crystal structure of the chiral anti-parasitic drug praziquantel. *J. Mol. Model.* **2017**, *23*, 106. [CrossRef] [PubMed]
39. Gong, J.P.; Traganos, F.; Darzynkiewicz, Z. A selective procedure for DNA extraction from apoptotic cells applicable for gel electrophoresis and flow cytometry. *Anal. Biochem.* **1994**, *218*, 314–319. [CrossRef] [PubMed]
40. Zanolla, D.; Perissutti, B.; Passerini, N.; Invernizzi, S.; Voinovich, D.; Bertoni, S.; Melegari, C.; Millotti, G.; Albertini, B. Milling and comilling Praziquantel at cryogenic and room temperatures: Assessment of the process-induced effects on drug properties. *J. Pharm. Biomed. Anal.* **2018**, *153*, 82–89. [CrossRef] [PubMed]

10

Designing Fast-Dissolving Orodispersible Films of Amphotericin B for Oropharyngeal Candidiasis

Dolores R. Serrano [1,2], Raquel Fernandez-Garcia [1], Marta Mele [3], Anne Marie Healy [4] and Aikaterini Lalatsa [3,*]

1 Department of Pharmaceutics and Food Technology, School of Pharmacy, Universidad Complutense de Madrid, Plaza Ramon y Cajal s/n, 28040 Madrid, Spain
2 Instituto Universitario de Farmacia Industrial (IUFI), School of Pharmacy, Universidad Complutense de Madrid, Avenida Complutense, 28040 Madrid, Spain
3 School of Pharmacy and Biomedical Sciences, University of Portsmouth, St. Michael's Building, White Swan Road, Portsmouth PO1 2DT, UK
4 Synthesis and Solid State Pharmaceutical Centre, School of Pharmacy and Pharmaceutical Sciences, Trinity College Dublin, Dublin 2, Ireland
* Correspondence: katerina.lalatsa@port.ac.uk;

Abstract: Amphotericin B possesses high activity against *Candida* spp. with low risk of resistance. However, Amphotericin B's high molecular weight compared to other antifungal drugs, such as miconazole and clotrimazole, and poor water solubility hampers its efficacy at the physiological conditions of the oropharyngeal cavity (saliva pH, limited volume for dissolution) and thereby limits its clinical use in oropharyngeal candidiasis. We have prepared fast-dissolving orodispersible films with high loading (1% *w/w*) using solvent casting that enables amphotericin B to remain solubilised in saliva in equilibrium between the monomeric and dimeric states, and able to produce a local antifungal effect. Optimisation of the amphotericin B-loaded orodispersible films was achieved by quality by design studies combining dextran and/or maltodextrin as dextrose-derived-polymer film formers with cellulose-derived film formers (hydroxypropylmethyl/hydroxypropyl cellulose in a 1:4 weight ratio), sorbitol for taste masking, microcrystalline cellulose (Avicel 200) or microcrystalline cellulose-carboxymethylcellulose sodium (Avicel CL-611) for enhancing the mechanical strength of the film, and polyethylene glycol 400 and glycerol (1:1 *w/w*) as plasticizers. The optimised amphotericin B orodispersible films (containing 1% AmB, 25% dextran, 25% maltodextrin, 5% sorbitol, 10% Avicel 200, 10% polyethylene glycol 400, 10% glycerol, 3% hydroxypropylmethyl cellulose acetate succinate, 12% hydroxypropyl cellulose) possessed a fast disintegration time (60 ± 3 s), quick release in artificial saliva (>80% in 10 min), high burst strength (2190 mN mm) and high efficacy against several *Candida* spp. (*C. albicans*, *C. parapsilosis* and *C. krusei*) (>15 mm inhibition halo). Amphotericin B orodispersible films are stable for two weeks at room temperature (25 °C) and up to 1 year in the fridge. Although further toxicological and in vivo efficacy studies are required, this novel Amphotericin B orodispersible films is a promising, physicochemically stable formulation with potential wide application in clinical practice, especially for immunocompromised patients suffering from oropharyngeal candidiasis.

Keywords: orodispersible films; fast-dissolving films; micelles; amphotericin B; fungal infections

---

1. Introduction

Fungal infections of the oral cavity are opportunistic, usually caused by *Candida albicans*, and occur more frequently in patients that are immunocompromised (e.g., HIV, cancer patients), diabetics or having predisposing factors such as antibiotic and corticosteroid therapy, poor buccal hygiene and ill-fitted dentures. Local therapy of oral and pharyngeal candidiasis is desirable as it avoids adverse effects linked to systemic antifungal use [1]. A major challenge to effective local treatments remains the low volume for dissolution and need for rapid permeability of the oropharyngeal cavity in order to deliver adequate drug concentrations for local action. The majority of formulations rely on oral suspensions due to the poor aqueous solubility of most antifungals that are swished around in the mouth for a few seconds, gargled, and swallowed or spat out. This short contact time with the oral mucosa requires a readily available and solubilised drug to exert an antifungal effect.

Amphotericin B (AmB) is a broad spectrum antifungal effective in the nanomolar range (IC_{50} of 0.25–1 μg mL^{-1}). Compared to azoles, there is a low frequency of *C. albicans* strains that are resistant to AmB [2]. The poor aqueous solubility of AmB (BCS Class IV) makes it difficult to solubilise in an adequate concentration in the small volume of saliva that is available in the oral cavity (1 mL) [3]. AmB is only commercialised as lyophilised formulations (micellar or lipidic nanoparticulate formulations) that are stable after reconstitution in aqueous media for a duration shorter than 24 h even when refrigerated [4,5] resulting in wastage, while poor patient compliance is an issue as formulations are not palatable. Taste masked orodispersable films (ODFs) can be potential solid dosage forms to deliver AmB in safe and efficient systems for the treatment of oropharyngeal fungal infections. Compared to other solid formulations, such as tablets and capsules, ODFs benefit from better patient compliance due to the ease of administration to dysphagic, paediatric and geriatric patients, without the need for water, and a rapid onset of action [6,7]. ODFs have shown better performance than semisolid formulations such as gels, because they can be easily transported, allow for accurate dosing and possess superior chemical and physical stability when packed appropriately, which can be important for unstable drugs in aqueous media such as AmB [8,9]. From an industrial and clinical point of view, ODFs would be more cost-effective formulations compared to parenteral AmB formulations, as they do not require sterilisation and lyophilisation, avoiding wastage.

The hypothesis underpinning this work is that AmB-loaded ODFs prepared using GRAS (Generally Regarded as Safe) excipients would enhance the current therapies available for the treatment of fungal infections in the oral and pharyngeal cavities. However, to the best of our knowledge, this has not been achieved to date due to the physicochemical challenges when formulating this drug. Here, we present an optimised fast disintegrating ODF of AmB with improved stability, loaded with high amounts of drug and designed to ensure AmB solubility in small volumes of saliva, while being taste masked and locally effective. To ensure AmB solubility at the physiological pH of the oropharyngeal cavity, we entrapped AmB in sodium deoxycholate micelles that were then embedded within the ODF. Sodium deoxycholate was selected as it interacts with AmB forming micelles, while it accumulates in buccal tissue after penetration without causing a loss of superficial cell layers and interacts with the intercellular or membrane lipids increasing the permeability of drugs through the epithelium [10]. Design of experiment (DoE) studies enabled us to identify the optimal drug:excipient ratio needed to ensure high drug loading (1% AmB) that is critical in achieving local concentrations well above the IC_{50} against *Candida albicans*. The optimised ODF were fully characterised and their *in vitro* antifungal activity evaluated.

2. Materials and Methods

2.1. Materials

AmB was purchased from Azelis (Barcelona, Spain). Hydroxypropylmethyl cellulose acetate succinate (HPMC AS 912, Affinisol™), maltodextrin (Glucidex 12D) and sorbitol were a gift from DowPharma (Dewsbury, UK) and Roquette (Valencia, Spain). Microcrystalline cellulose (Avicel 200) and microcrystalline cellulose and sodium carboxymethylcellulose (Avicel CL-611) were kindly donated by FMC (Cork, Ireland), while hydroxypropyl cellulose (HPC, Klucel HXF) was a gift from Ashland (Barcelona, Spain). Dextrose and dextran from Leuconostoc mesenteroides (16 KDa) were purchased from Sigma (Madrid, Spain). Humidity capsules and stability chambers were purchased from Amebis Limited (Dunshaughlin, Ireland). All other chemicals and solvents were at least of ACS reagent grade and were used without further purification.

2.2. *Quality by Design (QbD) Optimisation of ODF*

Several critical quality attributes (CQAs) such as disintegration time in artificial saliva and the physical characteristics of the ODF (burst strength, flexibility, tackiness) were identified as key factors in order to meet the Target Product Profile (TPP) (Tables S1 and S2 in Supplementary Materials). A Taguchi design (L8 = 2^7) was carried out using Design Expert software 8.04 (Stat-Ease, Minneapolis, MN, USA). Seven formulation variables (factors) and two levels of each factor affecting the film formation were investigated (Table 1). Disintegration time, burst strength and appearance were evaluated as responses (Table 2).

Table 1. Formulation and process variables with their respective high and low levels included in the Taguchi screening design.

Variables	**Levels**	
	Low (−1)	**High (+1)**
Type of dextrose-derived-polymer film former	Maltodextrin	Dextran
Taste masking agent (5%)	Sorbitol	Dextrose
Type of binder/suspending agent	Avicel 200	Avicel CL-611
Amount of Avicel polymers (%)	0	25
Amount of total plasticisers (PEG 400:glycerol, 1:1 *w/w*) (%)	5	20
Methanol	Low (1–2 mL)	High (>3 mL)
Amount of cellulose-derived film formers (HPMC 912 and HPC in a 1:4 weight ratio) (%)	0	15

2.2.1. ODF Manufacture and Response Evaluation

Eight formulations of AmB-loaded ODFs (3 g each) (Table 2) were prepared as follows: dextrose-derived-polymer film former, Avicel 200 or Avicel CL-611, taste masking agent (5%) and plasticisers were weighed and mixed in a mortar and pestle. To this mixture, 3 mL of freshly prepared AmB-loaded micelles (30 mg of AmB and 24.6 mg of sodium deoxycholate [11]) was added and manually mixed until a homogenous mixture was formed. The cellulose-derived film formers were then added, if required, and mixed. Methanol was added to reduce the viscosity of the mixture to a pourable homogenous suspension that was immediately cast onto a release liner (Primeliner 36 μm 1S, Loparex BV, Apeldoorn, The Netherlands) using a coating knife (Multicator 411, Erichsen, Hemer, Germany) and film applicator (Erichsen Coatmaster 510 film applicator, Erichsen, Hemer, Germany), at a speed of 10 mm s^{-1} under vacuum (air pressure 60 Pa), to form a wet film with a thickness of 1000 μm. The film was allowed to dry under vacuum for 4–5 h. Once the films were dried, they were carefully removed from the release liner and properties of the film were evaluated (Table 2).

Table 2. Design matrix of AmB-loaded orodispersable films (ODFs) prepared as per the Taguchi design. The overall appearance of the film was evaluated as the sum of the folding endurance, adhesion and homogeneity. Regarding the folding endurance, a value of 1 was assigned for films with good/flexibility able to fold 180 degrees without breaking above 50 folds, 2 as medium flexibility films (25–50 times) and 3 as poor flexibility films, which break easily when folded more than 25 times. Adhesion of the dried film to the release liner was also taken into account, assigning a number from 1 to 3—with 1 allowing intact removal of the film and 3 complete breakage of the film upon removal. The homogeneity was ranked taking into consideration the value of 1 for films that exhibit a smooth surface with no cracks, 2 for films with some irregular surfaces and 3 for non-homogeneous films with lumps and/or cracks on the surface.

Run	Type of Dextrose-Derived- Polymer Film Former	Taste Masking Excipient	Type of Avicel	Amount of Avicel (%)	Amount of Total Plasticisers (%)	Amount of Methanol	Amount of Cellulose-Derived Film Formers (%)	Disintegration Time (Seconds)	Flexibi-lity	Adhesion	Appea-rance	Burst Strength (Mn mm)
1	Dextran	Sorbitol	200	25	5	1	15	270	2	1	4	1300.9
2	Maltodextrin	Dextrose	200	25	20	2	15	90	1	1	3	2468
3	Maltodextrin	Dextrose	200	0	5	1	0	60	2	3	6	0
4	Dextran	Dextrose	CL611	25	5	2	0	360	3	2	8	0
5	Maltodextrin	Sorbitol	CL611	25	20	1	0	165	2	3	6	0
6	Maltodextrin	Sorbitol	CL611	0	5	2	15	150	2	1	4	1061
7	Dextran	Sorbitol	200	0	20	2	0	15	3	1	7	0
8	Dextran	Dextrose	CL611	0	5	1	15	240	3	2	8	0

Disintegration times of ODFs (1 × 1 cm) were measured in 3 mL of artificial saliva prepared as previously described: 14.4 mM sodium chloride, 16.1 mM mg potassium chloride, 1.31 mM calcium chloride dihydrate, 0.54 mM magnesium chloride hexahydrate, 1.96 mM dibasic potassium phosphate adjusted to pH 5.7 ± 0.01 [12] under gently shaking (30 slow 90° inversions of the vial per min). The mechanical properties (burst strength) of ODFs were evaluated using a texture analyser (Texture Analyser TA-XTplus, Stable Microsystems, Godalming, UK) attached to a film support rig (HDP/FSR, Stable Microsystems) [13]. For burst strength, the force required to rupture or break films was measured using a 5 mm spherical stainless-steel ball probe with probe adapter which was connected to the load cell. A film (35 × 15 mm) was placed in a film supporting rig and the moving probe reached the surface of the film with a pre-test speed of 2 mm s^{-1}, test speed of 1 mm s^{-1} and post-test speed of 10 mm s^{-1}. The force applied had a trigger load of 4.9 N and the force maximum (mN), travel distance (mm) and area under the curve (mN mm) were measured. Finally, the overall appearance of the films was evaluated as the sum of folding endurance, adhesion of the dried film to the release liner and homogeneity. Folding endurance was manually measured by counting the number of times the film could be folded at a 180° angle to the plane without breaking. A value of 1 was assigned for films with good/flexibility able to fold 180 degrees without breaking above 50 folds, 2 as medium flexibility films (25–50 times) and 3 as poor flexibility films, which break easily when folded more than 25 times. Adhesion of the dried film to the release liner was also taken into account, assigning a number from 1 to 3, with 1 indicating intact removal of the film and 3 complete breakage of the film upon removal. The homogeneity was also visually inspected, assigning 1 for films that exhibit a smooth surface with no cracks, 2 for films with some irregular surfaces and 3 for non-homogeneous films with lumps and/or cracks on the surface.

2.2.2. ODF Optimisation

Mathematical modelling was carried out by multiple linear regression analysis (MLRA). Only the statistically significant coefficients ($p < 0.05$) were considered in framing the polynomial equations, and the model was evaluated by analysing the p-value, coefficient of correlation (R^2) and predicted residual sum of squares (PRESS) [14]. Films were optimised in order to minimise the disintegration time and improve overall appearance and mechanical strength.

2.3. Full Physicochemical Characterisation of Optimised ODF

A full evaluation was performed including particle size and zeta potential (after disintegration in artificial saliva), powder X-ray Diffraction (PXRD), Fourier Transformed Infrared (FT-IR), Dynamic Vapour Sorption (DVS), Scanning Electron Microscopy (SEM) and surface area [11,14,15]. Briefly, particle size and zeta potential were measured in a Zetatrac after dilution (1 to 100) with artificial saliva. XRD measurements ($n = 3$) from 5° to 40° (2 theta) and a step scan rate 0.05° per second were performed in a Miniflex II Rigaku diffractometer with Ni-filtered Cu Kα radiation (1.54 Å) using a tube voltage and tube current of 30 kV and 25 mA respectively. FT-IR spectra were scanned in the range of 650–4000 cm^{-1} with a resolution of 4 cm^{-1} on a PerkinElmer Spectrum 1 FT-IR Spectrometer equipped with a UATR and a diamond/ZnSe crystal accessory. Baseline correction and data normalization were performed using Spekwin32 version 1.71.6.1. Water sorption kinetic profiles were obtained using a DVS (Advantage, Surface Measurement Systems, Alperton, UK) at 25.0 ± 0.1 °C. Samples (10–20 mg) were dried at 0% relative humidity (RH) for 1 h followed by step changes of 10% RH up to 90% RH, and the reverse for desorption. SEM was carried out in a Zeiss Supra Variable Pressure Field Emission Scanning Electron Microscope (Oberkochen, Germany) equipped with a secondary electron detector at 15 kV. Surface area was determined by the Brunauer, Emmett, Teller (BET) isotherm method using N2 adsorption with 6 points in the relative pressure range of 0.05–0.3 in a Micromeritics Gemini VI surface area analyser (Particular Sciences Ltd., Dublin, Ireland).

2.4. Content Uniformity

ODF (1 × 1 cm) were weighed and disintegrated in 3 mL of deionised water prior to being diluted (1 to 2) with methanol to ensure full drug solubilisation. Samples were centrifuged to precipitate undissolved excipients (5000 rpm for 10 min) and AmB dissolved in the supernatant was quantified using a validated HPLC method [16]. Experiments were performed using films from ten different sections of the cast ODF (15 × 10 cm).

2.5. Release Studies in Artificial Saliva

ODF (1 × 1 cm) were dissolved in 10 mL of artificial saliva at 37 °C under slow magnetic stirring (50 rpm). Samples (1 mL) were obtained at 1, 2, 4, 6, 8, 10, 15 and 30 min and media were replaced with fresh artificial saliva. Withdrawn samples (0.1 mL) were mixed with methanol (0.1 mL), vortex and centrifuged (5000 rpm, 10 min) for HPLC analysis to determine the percentage of drug released. The remaining sample volume was centrifuged (500 rpm, 1 min) to precipitate undissolved excipients such as microcrystalline cellulose. The particle size of the supernatant was measured using a Malvern Zetasizer (Malvern Nano Zs, Malvern Instruments, Malvern, UK). Additionally, the supernatant was analysed by UV (300–450 nm, Multiskan GO, Thermo Scientific, Basingstoke, UK) to determine the aggregation state of the AmB [17]. The ratio of the absorbance at 332 nm corresponding to dimeric AmB versus the absorbance at 408 nm that corresponds to the monomeric state was plotted to demonstrate the prevalence of the dimeric aggregation state of AmB.

2.6. In Vitro Antifungal Assays

In vitro antifungal activity was tested based on the agar diffusion assay as described by Ruiz et al. [1] according to the National Committee for Clinical Laboratory Standards (NCCLS) Method for antifungal disk diffusion susceptibility testing of yeast, standard M44-A2 [18]. In vitro activity was tested on three different *Candida* spp. (*C. albicans* CECT 1394, *C. parapsilosis* 57744 and *C. krusei* 52009 which was kindly provided by Dr. Pérez (CAQYM, University of Alcala de Henares, Alcalá de Henares, Spain) [1]. Strains were cultured in Sabouraud dextrose agar for 72 h to ensure viability and absence of contamination at 35 °C (±2 °C). Antifungal tests were carried out in Müeller Hinton agar (MHA) supplemented with glucose (2% *w/v*) and methylene blue (0.5 mg/mL). Inoculum was prepared by picking a few distinct colonies, which were suspended in 3 mL of sterile saline (0.9%). The resulting suspension was vortexed and its turbidity was adjusted with a spectrophotometer by adding sufficient sterile saline or more colonies to adjust the transmittance to that produced by a 0.5 McFarland standard at 530 nm wavelength, resulting in a yeast stock suspension of 1×10^6 cells per mL. Yeast suspension was inoculated to the MHA (200 mL) and was casted in disposable sterile petri dishes (instead of spreading it on the surface of the plate as specified in M44-A2). Once solidified, AmB ODFs (circles with a 6 mm diameter) were tested. Four disks were placed in each plate. AmB ODF in vitro activity was compared to commercially available AmB Neo-Sensitabs tablets (10 µg, 6 mm tablets from Rosco diagnostic A/S, Taastrup, Denmark) and AmB impregnated on inoculation 6 mm paper disks (10 µg/20 µL of DMSO) with appropriate DMSO controls. Once the disks were placed on the surface of the agar, the plates were inverted and placed in an incubator set to 35 °C (±2 °C) within 15 min after the disks were applied. After 24 h of incubation, the inhibition halo was measured.

2.7. Stability Studies

Physicochemical stability studies were performed under accelerated conditions (40, 60 and 80 °C) for one week and long term at 5 ± 3 °C and 25 ± 3 °C. AmB ODF (1 × 1 cm) were placed in sealed vials into Amebis chambers (Amebis Ltd., Dublin, Ireland) at the selected temperature. A sensor cap was used to seal the test chamber and a logger cap connected to the sensor cap was used to collect and transmit the temperature and humidity test conditions wirelessly to the Amebis Control Software [14]. Disintegration time and drug content were quantified at different time points (time zero, day 1, 3 and

7). The degradation rate of AmB was calculated by fitting the percentage of drug degraded at different time points to several degradation kinetic equations (zero order, first order, second order, Avrami and diffusion) and the best fitted degradation kinetic model was selected (i.e., highest R^2). Using the degradation rates at different temperatures, the Arrhenius equation was employed to calculate the activation energy (Equation (1)):

$$K = A\,e^{\frac{-Ea}{RT}} \quad (1)$$

where K is the degradation rate (% drug degraded/day), A is the collision factor, T is the absolute temperature in Kelvin, R is the gas constant (1.985 cal/mol/K) and Ea is the activation energy in cal/mol [14]. Drug stability at room temperature was then predicted using the Arrhenius equation and compared to experimental values.

3. Results

3.1. QbD Studies for Optimisation of AmB-Loaded ODFs

The first-order mathematical model generated for each response variable was found to be statistically significant ($p < 0.05$ in each case). Co-efficients with p values > 0.1 were considered insignificant based on Pareto charts and ANOVA analysis. High R^2 values for the polynomial equations obtained for all the response variables indicate a good fit to experimental data (Table S3). The variables, type and amount of Avicel and number of plasticizers, showed a significant effect on the disintegration time of the ODFs (Figures S1 and S2). ODFs with lower disintegration time were obtained when lower amounts of Avicel and cellulose-derived film formers were used. The disintegration time was reduced when higher percentages of plasticisers were employed and when Avicel 200 was incorporated in the film compared to Avicel CL-611, as the latter acts as a viscosity enhancing agent resulting in thixotropic gels, which retard disintegration (Figure 1A,B).

The choice of dextrose-derived film former, volume of methanol added, type/amount of Avicel and amount of cellulose-derived film formers had a significant impact on burst strength (Figures S3 and S4). The use of maltodextrin and Avicel 200 resulted in films with higher burst strength. The higher the amount of Avicel, HPMC AS/HPC and methanol, the better the mechanical strength of the films (Figure 1C,D).

The appearance of the films was rated as described above (Figure S5). DoE indicated that the main variables that contributed to the appearance of the film were: the type of dextrose-derived film former and the amount of cellulose-derived film formers utilised, followed by type and amount of Avicel and taste masking agent (Figures S6 and S7), although results were not statistically significantly different. The appearance of the film was smoother when maltodextrin was used, although high amounts of maltodextrin increased film tackiness. When higher amounts of Avicel and cellulose-derived film formers were used, appearance was improved. Avicel 200 and sorbitol resulted in smoother film surfaces compared to dextrose films as dextrose can recrystallize resulting in rougher surfaces [19] (Figure 1E,F).

3.2. Manufacturing of Optimised AmB ODF

A trade-off between key CQAs was necessary to attain optimal characteristics, i.e., short disintegration time (which is critical for faster onset of action), maximal burst strength (in order to obtain robust films that can be easily manufactured and packaged without breaking), and good appearance. A closer match to ideal CQAs was obtained with sorbitol, Avicel 200 (10%), 20% of plasticisers (PEG 400:glycerol, 1:1 *w/w*) and 10% of cellulose-derived film formers (HMPC 912 AS:HPC, 1:4 weight ratio). Regarding the type of dextrose-derived film former, maltodextrin conferred better flexibility and faster release from the films compared to those obtained with dextran, as dextran interacts more strongly compared to microcrystalline cellulose or the modified cellulose-derived film formers. However, high amounts of maltodextrin significantly increased adhesion of the films to the release liners. Thus, we decided to optimise the ODF using a mixture of dextran and maltrodextrin (1:1

w/w) (Table 3). The films exhibited a good overall appearance with a dried thickness of 0.14 ± 0.01 mm, a weight of 28.5 ± 1.5 mg/cm^2, a drug content of 0.996 ± 0.045 mg/g (which was uniform with a low standard deviation and a variance coefficient of 4.5%), a burst strength of 2190 mN mm and a disintegration time of ≤60 s in 3 mL of artificial saliva.

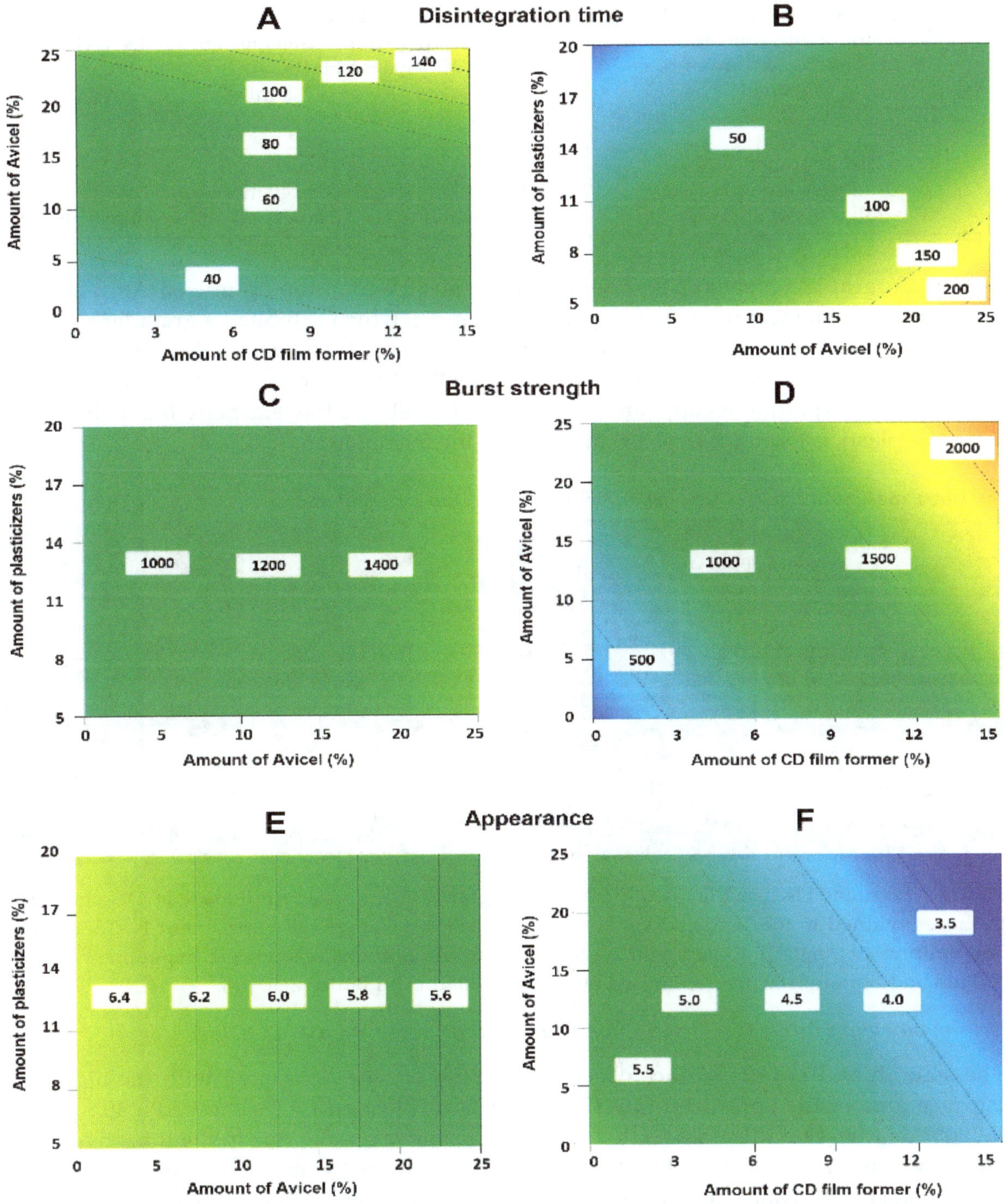

Figure 1. Contour plots showing the influence of the most influential factors affecting the disintegration time (**A**,**B**), the burst strength (**C**,**D**) and the overall appearance (**E**,**F**) of the AmB-loaded orodispersable films (ODFs). Key: CD, cellulose-derived.

Table 3. Composition and properties of the optimised AmB-loaded ODFs.

Composition	
Dextran	25% (0.74 g)
Maltodextrin	25% (0.74 g)
Sorbitol	5% (0.15 g)
Avicel 200	10% (0.3 g)
Plasticisers (PEG 400:Glycerol, 1:1 *w/w*)	20% (0.3 g + 0.3 g)
Simil Fungizone (9)	3 mL (=30 mg AmB + 24.6 mg sodium deoxycholate)
Cellulose-derived film formers	15% (0.09 g HMPC AS + 0.36 g HPC)
Methanol	1.5 mL
Properties	
Disintegration time	60 ± 3 s
Burst strength	2190 ± 140 mN mm
Overall score of appearance	4 = Flexibility (1), tackiness (2) and homogeneity (1)

SEM micrographs revealed a smooth and porous surface of the optimised AmB-loaded ODF compared to films obtained in the DoE experiment 1 and 2, which exhibited a granular rough texture or embedded crystals respectively probably due to the use of dextran in the first film instead of maltodextrin and the presence of dextrose in DoE 2 ODF which tends to crystallise (Figure 2). Films obtained in DoE 6 experiments appeared cracked and exhibited low elasticity likely due to the low percentage of plasticisers and Avicel 200 included in the formulation.

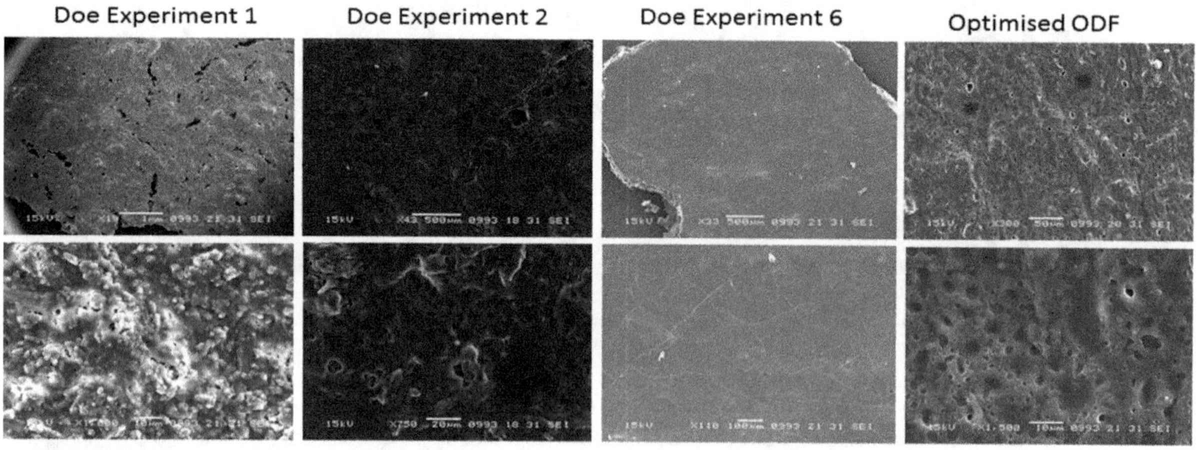

Figure 2. Scanning Electron Microscopy (SEM) micrographs of optimised AmB-loaded ODFs compared to those obtained in the Taguchi DoE before optimization. Bars; DOE Experiment 1—Top: 1 mm and Bottom: 10 μm, DOE Experiment 2—Top: 500 μm and Bottom: 20 μm, DOE Experiment 6—Top: 500 μm and Bottom: 100 μm, Optimised ODF—Top: 50 μm and Bottom: 10 μm.

3.3. Performance and Further Characterisation of the Optimised AmB-Loaded ODF

The smooth and porous surface observed by SEM can be associated with the high 2.3 ± 0.5 m^2/g surface area of the optimized film (Figure 2). AmB-loaded ODFs showed a 40% increase in mass at 90% relative humidity, associated with a large water uptake due to the films hydrophilicity as shown by the water sorption kinetic profile (Figure 3A). No mass loss (associated to phase transformation/crystallization) was observed during the sorption or desorption cycle. The solid state of the film was retained (as demonstrated by post DVS XRD analysis (Figure S8) indicating an overall acceptable physical stability. The FTIR spectra showed a broadening of the peak at 1691 cm^{-1} (C=O stretch) probably attributed to hydrogen bonding between the AmB and excipients such as sodium deoxycholate, sorbitol and acetate succinate groups of the HPMC AS (Figure 3B and Figure S9).

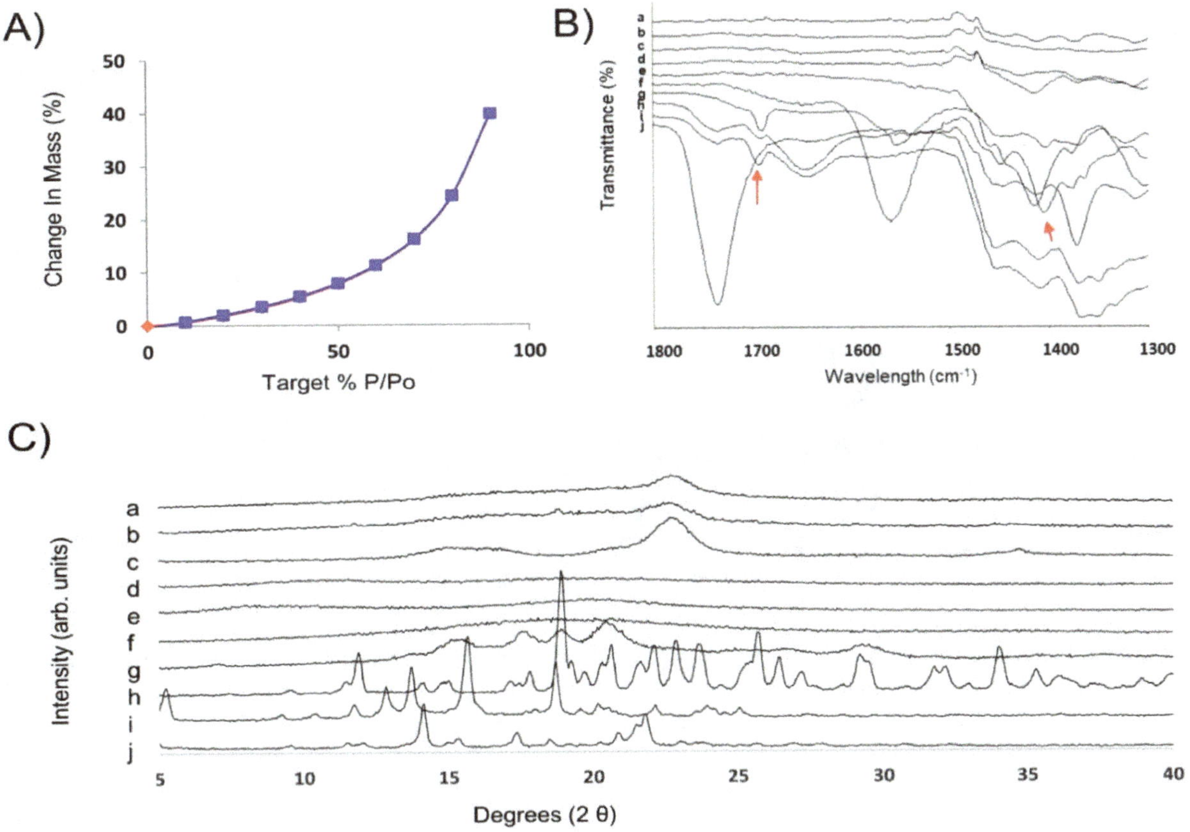

Figure 3. Physicochemical characterization of optimised AmB-loaded ODFs. (**A**) Water sorption kinetic profile. (**B**) FTIR spectra: (a) hydroxypropyl cellulose (HPC), (b) maltodextrin, (c) dextran, (d) Avicel 200, (e) sorbitol, (f) sodium deoxycholate, (g) AmB, (h) AmB-loaded ODF, (i) physical mixture, (j) HPMC 912 AS. (**C**) PXRD patterns: (a) AmB-loaded ODF, (b) Physical mixture of all components, (c) Avicel 200, (d) HPMC 912 AS, (e) HPC, (f) maltodextrin, (g) dextran, (h) sorbitol, (i) sodium deoxycholate, (j) AmB.

The XRD pattern of the physical mixture of all components revealed crystalline Bragg peaks attributed to sorbitol (Figure 3B(b,h)), which are not present in the casted film. However, a characteristic halo attributed to the semi-crystalline nature of the microcrystalline cellulose (Avicel 200) was observed in the optimised ODFs. Lower intensity values at several Bragg peaks (5°, 14.15°, 17.35°, 21.75°) were observed in the diffractogram of the AmB-loaded ODF compared to the physical mixture, which can be attributed to the presence of amorphous AmB-sodium deoxycholate complexes in the films. However, bearing in mind that the AmB content in the ODF is 1%, it is likely that the results obtained from XRD measurements are not conclusive due to the XRD detection limit for crystalline AmB.

3.4. Release and Aggregation State

Aligned with the high porosity of the films, ODF presented a fast-dissolving behaviour (>80% in 10 min) in saliva (Figure 4A). Once disintegrated, particle size and zeta potential of the resulting suspension was measured. Initial particle size was bimodal mainly dominated (>70%) by large particles (>1 μm) due to insoluble excipients. After centrifugation, a white pellet and a transparent yellow supernatant was obtained. The latter demonstrated a bimodal particle size distribution of 8.7 ± 2.5 nm and 918 ± 120 nm with an anionic zeta potential of −14 ± 3 mV, indicating that after disintegration of the ODFs, AmB remained solubilised in the supernatant in equilibrium between micelles and particles close to 1 μm in size. TEM images confirmed the presence of micelles and particles of that size (Figure 4(B1)). Characteristic crystals corresponding to unprocessed AmB (Figure 4(B2)) were not observed after disintegration of the ODF and release of the AmB in the media which supports drug solubilisation within micelles.

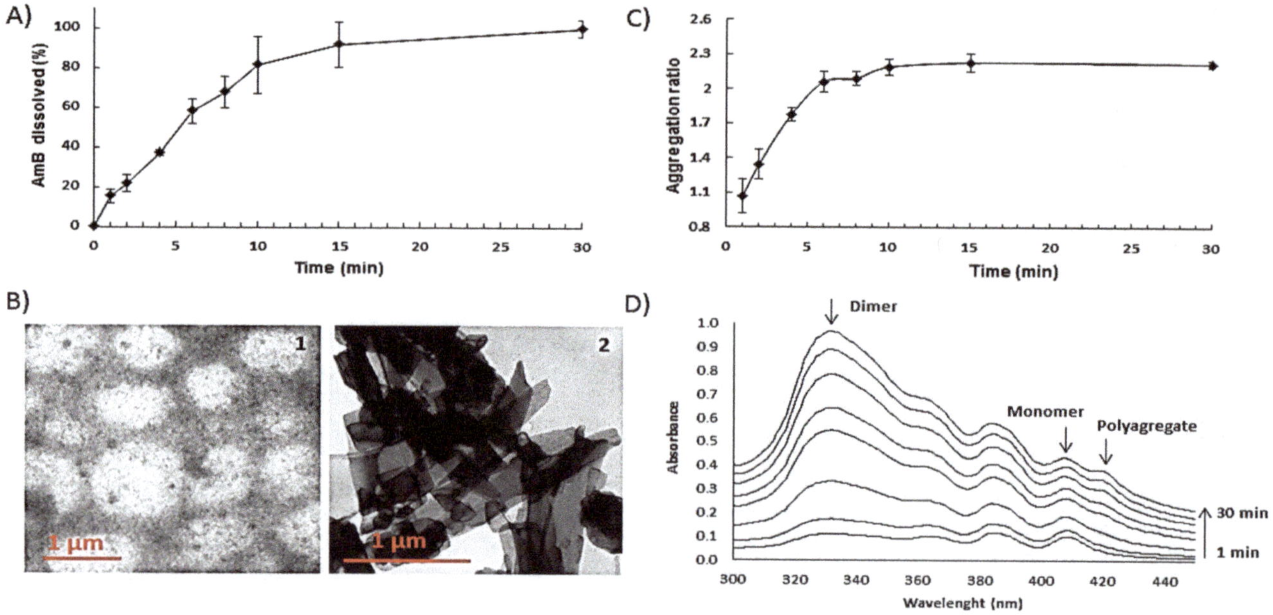

Figure 4. Release profile, morphology and aggregation state of optimised AmB loaded ODFs. Key: (**A**) Release profile of AmB-loaded ODFS in artificial saliva. (**B**) Transmission electron microscopy (TEM) of AmB-loaded ODF after reconstitution in aqueous media (left image) and crystalline unprocessed AmB (right image); (**C**) Aggregation ratio during the release studies; (**D**) Transformation of AmB aggregation states over time.

Regarding the aggregation state of AmB released from the films, UV spectroscopy indicated a shift from the monomeric to dimeric state illustrated by the faster increase in the peak at 332 nm compared to the one at 408 nm corresponding to the monomeric state (Figure 4C,D). At the earlier time points (1–2 min), there is an equilibrium in solution between monomer and dimer. As time progresses and a higher percentage of AmB is released to the media, AmB self-aggregates shifting from monomer to dimer after 2 min and from dimer to polyaggregate after 8 min (peak at 420 nm) [17,20]. AmB solubility can be enhanced by the presence of PEG 400 and sodium deoxycholate in the formulation [21]. Fungizone®, a commercial AmB parenteral formulation, consists of 1:2 AmB:sodium deoxycholate molar fraction that facilitates the solubilisation of AmB in dimeric form within micelles [20]. The presence of nanometric (≈10 nm) spherical single layer particles in solution after ODF disintegration can be explained by the partial solubilisation of the drug within sodium deoxycholate micelles. However, even though initially AmB is incorporated in the solid mixture of excipients solubilised in sodium deoxycholate, the later addition of solvent to produce a pourable castable formulation could destabilise initially formed AmB sodium deoxycholate micelles. Thus, the different aggregation states of released AmB can be a consequence of the initial solubilisation of AmB in the monomer state in the presence of PEG 400 and the formation of ion pairs with sodium deoxycholate, followed by the encapsulation of AmB within micelles resulting in prevalence of the dimeric state. When higher amounts of AmB are released over time in the media, AmB self-aggregates into polyaggregates close to 1 µm in size which are stabilised by the release of dextrose-based polymers, in particular maltodextrin, which has been previously shown to be able to effectively stabilise dispersed systems such as oil-in-water emulsions [22].

3.5. Antifungal Activity

The optimised AmB-loaded ODFs showed good in vitro antifungal activity against the three *Candida* spp. (with an inhibition zone >15 mm) equivalent to that of AmB dissolved in DMSO and the commercially available disks, which indicates good drug release from the film and diffusion across the agar of the solubilised AmB (Figure 5). Bearing in mind the potency of the drug against *C. albicans, C. parapsilopsis* and *C. krusei* (MIC_{50} ranges from 0.25–1 µg/mL) reported in the literature [2], the dose delivered by a 1 × 1 cm film would be adequate to ensure efficacy against buccal candidiasis. Considering that the drug loading is 1% *w/w* and that a 1 cm^2 film weights around 30 mg, each 1 cm^2 film contains approximately 0.3 mg of AmB. Assuming a volume of ~1 mL in the oral cavity [3,23], the concentration of AmB would be 300 μg/mL, which is well above the MIC_{50} reported in literature. Even if the concentration is diluted further with 10 mL or 100 mL i.e., 10 or 100-fold, the AmB concentration would be in range between 3 or 30 μg/mL, which are concentrations still above the MIC_{50} and, for this reason, we believe that the drug levels would be adequate to elicit a pharmacological effect.

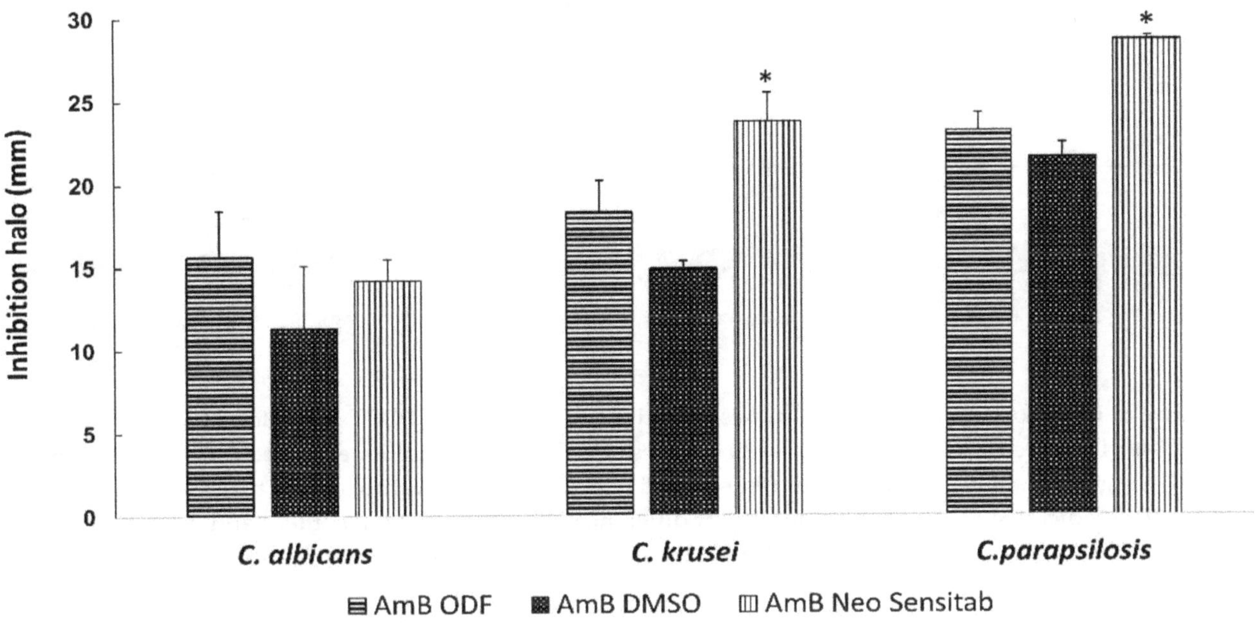

Figure 5. In vitro activity against *C. albicans*, *C. krusei* and *C. parapsilopsis*. The isolates were classified as susceptible (S) to AmB when the inhibition zone was ≥15 mm, resistant (R) when it was ≤10 mm and intermediate (I) or susceptible-dose dependent when the inhibition zone was between 10- and 15-mm. Inhibition zone diameters are expressed as mean ± SD in mm. All experiments were performed in triplicate. * $p < 0.05$ One-way ANOVA test.

3.6. Physicochemical Stability

Stability studies showed that the optimised AmB-loaded ODF was physiochemically stable over a year (>90% drug content) at 5 °C under desiccated conditions. Accelerated stability studies demonstrated a pronounced chemical degradation (80 °C >> 60 °C >> 40 °C), while a change in colour occurred at the highest temperature (Figure 6). The disintegration times of ODFs subject to accelerated stability studies was reduced over time, probably due to the evaporation of bound water within the film and the formation of micropores (Figure 6). However, in all the tested conditions, the disintegration time remained below 2 min as considered appropriate for fast-disintegrating ODFs. The Avrami kinetic model fitted the degradation of AmB from loaded ODFs. This kinetic model is commonly applied to evaluate the growth and formation of crystals [24]. Nevertheless, several authors have also used this model in the stability prediction of nanocomposites [25,26]. The breaking of a 3D network becomes more heterogeneous as the degradation progresses, and thus, the degradation proceeds faster as the combined effects of physical and chemical degradation occur simultaneously, especially at higher temperatures [26]. The activation energy of the AmB-loaded ODFs was 5.71 Kcal/mol, which correlates with the poor physicochemical drug stability observed at high temperatures (Figure 6). Experimental and predicted data from the Arrhenius equation showed that ODFs stored at 25 °C at desiccated conditions remained stable over 15 days (>90% drug content, disintegration time of 55 s). Thus, our AmB ODFs would remain stable for 2 weeks at room temperature in a closed pouch, which is a significant advantage to existing AmB commercialised parenteral formulations that are unstable after 24 h of reconstitution of the lyophilised powder [4] reducing overall cost of treatment and wastage.

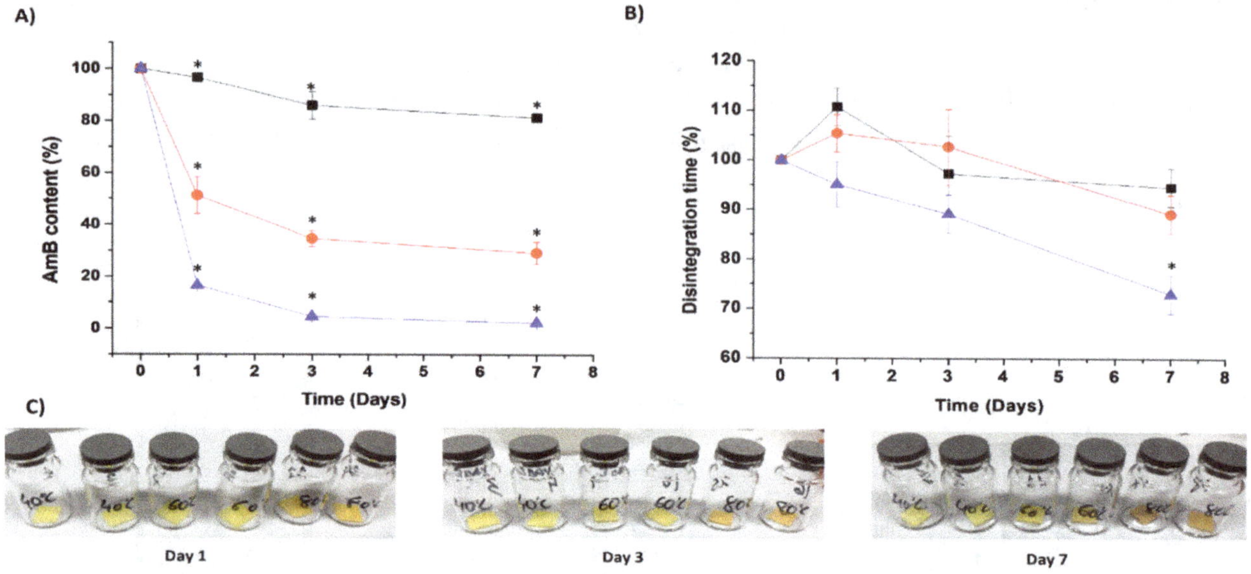

Figure 6. Physicochemical stability studies of optimised AmB-loaded ODFs at different temperatures. Key: -■- 40 degrees, -●- 60 degrees, -▲- 80 degrees. (**A**) Chemical stability expressed as AmB content. (**B**) Change in disintegration time for films stored at different temperatures. (**C**) Physical appearance. * $p < 0.05$ indicative of statistically significant difference compared to AmB content and disintegration time of films at time 0 (One-way ANOVA with a post-hoc Tukey's test, level of significance set at 5%).

4. Discussion

To the best of our knowledge, this is the first report of AmB, a high molecular weight poorly water-soluble antifungal, being formulated as an ODF for the treatment of oropharyngeal candidiasis. The optimised ODF was achieved by combining dextran and maltodrextrin as dextrose-derived polymer film formers with sorbitol for taste masking, microcrystalline cellulose (Avicel 200) for enhancing mechanical strength, PEG 400 and glycerol as plasticizers to ensure faster disintegration and adequate plasticity and HMPC 912 AS /HPC for facilitating film formation. The combination of PEG 400 and glycerol (1:1 weight ratio) was selected based on previous results (data not shown). Glycerol improves mouthfeel, which is a necessity in an ODF formulation, as well as enhancing the viscosity resulting in higher, unacceptable disintegration times. In contrast, PEG 400 decreases disintegration time of ODF and, in combination with HPMC, gives optimal films in terms of tensile strength and flexibility [27].

Currently, nystatin (which has a similar chemical structure to AmB) formulated as a suspension is considered as the reference treatment for oral candidiasis; nevertheless, a recent meta-analysis demonstrated a limited efficacy for nystatin, lower than fluconazole, in treating oral candidiasis in infants, children and HIV patients, which is related to a poor and variable bioavailability in the oral mucosa [28]. AmB has shown 4-fold higher in vitro efficacy than nystatin [29], but its poor aqueous solubility limits its use in clinical practice, and it is only marketed as intravenous formulations. After disintegration of the ODF, AmB is maintained solubilised in the aqueous media in equilibrium between different aggregation states mainly monomer and dimer at earlier times points, which have shown to possess much greater efficacy than polyaggregates against *Candida* [30,31]. Unlike previous studies in which the antifungal activity was tested after disintegration of the films in liquid form [32], enhanced in vitro activity of the AmB-loaded ODF was shown here for the intact film placed on top of the agar, showing that the release and diffusion of the drug across the agar occurs and hence AmB is free to elicit its effect. Excipients utilised in ODFs are used within ranges that are considered GRAS (generally regarded as safe). Sodium deoxycholate, at the concentrations used in optimised the ODFs, has been shown to cause no major morphological changes [10]. Although further toxicological and in vivo efficacy studies are required, we have shown that this technology platform can be a promising AmB formulation for the treatment of oral candidiasis.

5. Conclusions

Fast-dissolving orodispersible films containing a very poorly soluble and unstable drug, AmB, have been successfully engineered and prepared using a solvent casting film method in which the drug is solubilised at a final concentration of 1% *w/w* upon disintegration of the film. The optimised AmB orodispersible flms consisted of a mixture of dextrose-derived polymers (25% dextran and 25% maltodextrin) and cellulose-derived film formers (3% HMPC AS and 12% HPC) with 10% Avicel 200 added to enhance the mechanical strength of the film, 5% sorbitol for taste masking, and 10% PEG 400 and 10% glycerol as plasticizers. The optimised ODF exhibited a fast disintegration time (60 ± 3 s), quick release in artificial saliva (>80% in 10 min), high burst strength (2190 mN mm), good chemical stability (1 year at refrigerated conditions and 2 weeks at room temperature) and high efficacy against several *Candida* spp. (*C. albicans*, *C. parapsilosis* and *C. krusei* with an inhibition halo >15 mm). Although further toxicological and in vivo efficacy studies are required, these novel orodispersible films prepared with GRAS excipients have potential in the treatment of oro-and pharyngeal candidiasis, and hence represent a promising system with wide applications in clinical practice among immunocompromised patients suffering from this disease.

Supplementary Materials
Figure S1: Pareto charts depicting the effect of (C) Type of Avicel, (D) Amount of Avicel, (E) Amount of plasticisers and (G) Amount of cellulose-derived film formers on the disintegration time. Orange colour indicates a positive effect whereas blue colour indicates a negative effect. Figure S2: Effect of the four variables (Type of Avicel, amount of Avicel, amount of plasticizers and amount of cellulose-derived film formers) on the disintegration time. Figure S3: Pareto charts depicting the effect of (A) Type of dextrose-derived film former, (C) Type of Avicel, (D) Amount of Avicel, (F) Volume of methanol and (G) Amount of cellulose-derived film formers on the burst strength of the film (expressed as AUC). Orange colour indicates a positive effect whereas blue colour indicates a negative effect. Figure S4: Effect of the significant variables (Film former, Type of Avicel, amount of Avicel and amount of cellulose-derived film formers) on the burst strength expressed as AUC of the film. Figure S5: Appearance of the eight AmB-loaded films prepared according to Taguchi matrix design. Figure S6: Pareto charts depicting the effect of (A) Type of dextrose-derived film former, (B) Taste masking, (C) Type of Avicel, (D) Amount of Avicel and (G) Amount of cellulose-derived film formers on the appearance of the film. Orange colour indicates a positive effect whereas blue colour indicates a negative effect. Figure S7: Effect of the five variables with higher impact on the final appearance of the film (Type of Avicel, amount of Avicel, taste masking agent, type of dextrose-derived film former and amount of cellulose derived-film formers). Figure S8: PXRD patterns of raw materials and AmB-loaded ODF before and after DVS analyses. Key: AmB ODF post DVS, (b) AmB ODF, (c) physical mixture, (d) Avicel 200, (e) HPMC AS; (f) HPC, (g) maltodextrin, (h) dextran, (i) sorbitol, (j) sodium deoxycholate, (k) AmB. Figure S9: FT-IR spectra. (a) HPC, (b) maltodextrin, (c) dextran, (d) Avicel 200, (e) sodium deoxycholate, (f) sorbitol, (g) HPMC 912 AS, (h) AmB, (i) physical mixture, (j) AmB-loaded. Table S1: Target product profile (TPP) elements for AmB-loaded ODFs. Table S2: Critical quality attributes (CQAs) of AmB-loaded ODFs. Table S3: Co-efficient values and statistical parameters obtained for first order equations for the studied response variables: 1-Type of dextrose-derived-polymer film former, 2-Taste masking agent, 3-Type of Avicel, 4-Amount of Avicel, 5-Amount of plasticisers, 6-Amount of methanol, 7-Amount of cellulose-derived film formers. Results were analysed using a first order equation ($Y = B_0 + B_1X_1 + B_2X_2 + B_3X_3 + B_4X_4 + B_5X_5 + B_6X_6 + B_7X_7$) generated for the response variables investigated in the DoE. Seven coefficients (B1 to B7) were calculated with B0 as the intercept. Only those coefficients which were significant were retained in the simplified equations.

Author Contributions: Conceptualization, D.R.S. and A.L.; methodology: D.R.S. and A.L.; formal analysis, D.R.S., R.F.-G., M.M. and A.L.; resources, A.M.H. and A.L.; software: A.M.H. and A.L.; supervision: D.R.S. and A.L.; validation: A.L.; writing—original draft preparation, D.R.S., A.M.H. and A.L.; writing—review and editing, D.R.S., A.M.H. and A.L., supervision, D.R.S. and A.L.; project administration, A.L.; funding acquisition, A.M.H. and A.L.

References

1. Ruiz, H.K.; Serrano, D.R.; Dea-Ayuela, M.A.; Bilbao-Ramos, P.E.; Bolas-Fernandez, F.; Torrado, J.J.; Molero, G. New amphotericin B-gamma cyclodextrin formulation for topical use with synergistic activity against diverse fungal species and Leishmania spp. *Int. J. Pharm.* **2014**, *473*, 148–157. [CrossRef] [PubMed]
2. Montaga, M.T.; Lovero, G.; Coretti, C.; de Giglio, O.; Mratinelli, D.; Bedini, A.; Delia, M.; Rosato, A.; Codeluppi, M.; Caggiano, C. In vitro activities of amphotericin B deoxycholate and liposomal amphotericin B against 604 clinical yeast isolates. *J. Med. Microbiol.* **2014**, *63*, 1638–1643. [CrossRef] [PubMed]
3. Lagerlof, F.; Dawes, C. The volume of saliva in the mouth before and after swallowing. *J. Dent. Res.* **1984**, *63*, 618–621. [CrossRef] [PubMed]
4. Technical Data Sheet of Fungizone. Available online: https://botplusweb.portalfarma.com/documentos/2003/9/22/F46773%20FUNGIZONA%20IV%20200111.pdf (accessed on 15 January 2019).
5. AmBisome Technical Data Sheet. Available online: https://www.gilead.com/-/media/files/pdfs/medicines/other/ambisome/ambisome_pi.pdf (accessed on 14 March 2019).
6. Reiner, V.; Giarratana, N.; Monti, N.C.; Breitenbach, A.; Klaffenbach, P. Rapidfilm: An innovative pharmaceutical form designed to improve patient compliance. *Int. J. Pharm.* **2010**, *393*, 55–60. [CrossRef] [PubMed]
7. Gijare, C.; Deshpande, A. Orodispersible Films: A Systematic Patent Review. *Recent Patents Drug Deliv. Formul.* **2018**, *12*, 110–120. [CrossRef] [PubMed]
8. Irfan, M.; Rabel, S.; Bukhtar, Q.; Qadir, M.I.; Jabeen, F.; Khan, A. Orally disintegrating films: A modern expansion in drug delivery system. *Saudi Pharm. J.* **2016**, *24*, 537–546. [CrossRef]
9. Choudhary, D.R.; Patel, V.A.; Chhalotiya, U.K.; Patel, H.V.; Kundawala, A.J. Development and characterization of pharmacokinetic parameters of fast-dissolving films containing levocetirizine. *Sci. Pharm.* **2012**, *80*, 779–787. [CrossRef]
10. Dhiman, M.K.; Dhiman, A.; Sawant, K.K. Transbuccal delivery of 5-fluorouracil: Permeation enhancement and pharmacokinetic study. *AAPS Pharm. Sci. Technol.* **2009**, *10*, 258–265. [CrossRef]
11. Rolon, M.; Serrano, D.R.; Lalatsa, A.; de Pablo, E.; Torrado, J.J.; Ballesteros, M.P.; Healy, A.M.; Vega, C.; Coronel, C.; Bolas-Fernandez, F.; et al. Engineering Oral and Parenteral Amorphous Amphotericin B Formulations against Experimental Trypanosoma cruzi Infections. *Mol. Pharm.* **2017**, *14*, 1095–1106. [CrossRef]
12. Okamoto, H.; Taguchi, H.; Iida, K.; Danjo, K. Development of polymer film dosage forms of lidocaine for buccal administration. I. Penetration rate and release rate. *J. Control. Release* **2001**, *77*, 253–260. [CrossRef]
13. Senthilkumar, K.; Vijaya, C. Formulation Development of Mouth Dissolving Film of Etoricoxib for Pain Management. *Adv. Pharm.* **2015**, *2015*, 1–11. [CrossRef]
14. Serrano, D.R.; Walsh, D.; O'Connell, P.; Mugheirbi, N.A.; Worku, Z.A.; Bolas-Fernandez, F.; Galiana, C.; Dea-Ayuela, M.A.; Healy, A.M. Optimising the in vitro and in vivo performance of oral cocrystal formulations via spray coating. *Eur. J. Pharm. Biopharm.* **2018**, *124*, 13–27. [CrossRef] [PubMed]
15. Serrano, D.R.; Persoons, T.; D'Arcy, D.M.; Galiana, C.; Dea-Ayuela, M.A.; Healy, A.M. Modelling and shadowgraph imaging of cocrystal dissolution and assessment of in vitro antimicrobial activity for sulfadimidine/4-aminosalicylic acid cocrystals. *Eur. J. Pharm. Sci.* **2016**, *89*, 125–136. [CrossRef] [PubMed]
16. Serrano, D.R.; Hernandez, L.; Fleire, L.; Gonzalez-Alvarez, I.; Montoya, A.; Ballesteros, M.P.; Dea-Ayuela, M.A.; Miro, G.; Bolas-Fernandez, F.; Torrado, J.J. Hemolytic and pharmacokinetic studies of liposomal and particulate amphotericin B formulations. *Int. J. Pharm.* **2013**, *447*, 38–46. [CrossRef] [PubMed]
17. Torrado, J.J.; Espada, R.; Ballesteros, M.P.; Torrado-Santiago, S. Amphotericin B formulations and drug targeting. *J. Pharm. Sci.* **2008**, *97*, 2405–2425. [CrossRef] [PubMed]
18. Clinical and Laboratory Standards Institute. Method for antifungal disk diffusion susceptibility testing of yeast. In *CLSI document M44-A2*, 2nd ed.; Clinical and Laboratory Standards Institute: Wayne, PA, USA, 2009; Available online: https://clsi.org/media/1634/m44a2_sample.pdf (accessed on 7 July 2019).
19. Markande, A.; Nezzal, A.; Fitzpatrick, J.J.; Aerts, L. Investigation of the Crystallization Kinetics of Dextrose Monohydrate Using In Situ Particle Size and Supersaturation Monitoring. *Part. Sci. Technol.* **2009**, *27*, 373–388. [CrossRef]
20. Serrano, D.R.; Ballesteros, M.P.; Schatzlein, A.G.; Torrado, J.J.; Uchegbu, I.F. Amphotericin B Formulations —The Possibility of Generic Competition. *Pharm. Nanotechnol.* **2013**, *1*, 250–258. [CrossRef]

21. Rajagopalan, N.; Dicken, C.M.; Ravin, L.J.; Sternson, L.A. A study of the solubility of amphotericin B in nonaqueous solvent systems. *J. Parenter. Sci. Technol. Publ. Parenter. Drug Assoc.* **1988**, *42*, 97–102.
22. Pycia, K.; Gryszkin, A.; Berski, W.; Juszczak, L. The Influence of Chemically Modified Potato Maltodextrins on Stability and Rheological Properties of Model Oil-in-Water Emulsions. *Polymers* **2018**, *10*, 67. [CrossRef] [PubMed]
23. Iorgulescu, G. Saliva between normal and pathological. Important factors in determining systemic and oral health. *J. Med. Life* **2009**, *2*, 303–307. [PubMed]
24. Jun, S.; Zhang, H.; Bechhoefer, J. Nucleation and growth in one dimension. I. The generalized Kolmogorov-Johnson-Mehl-Avrami model. *Phys. Rev. E* **2005**, *71*, 011908. [CrossRef] [PubMed]
25. Poletto, M.; Pistor, V.; Zeni, M.; Zattera, A.J. Crystalline properties and decomposition kinetics of cellulose fibers in wood pulp obtained by two pulping processes. *Polym. Degrad. Stab.* **2011**, *96*, 679–685. [CrossRef]
26. Pistor, V.; Soares, B.G.; Mauler, R.S. Influence of the Polyhedral Oligomeric Silsesquioxane n-Phenylaminopropyl—POSS in the Thermal Stability and the Glass Transition Temperature of Epoxy Resin. *Polimeros* **2013**, *23*, 328–331. [CrossRef]
27. Borges, A.F.; Silva, C.; Coelho, J.F.; Simoes, S. Oral films: Current status and future perspectives II Intellectual property, technologies and market needs. *J. Control. Release* **2015**, *206*, 108–121. [CrossRef] [PubMed]
28. Lyu, X.; Zhao, C.; Yan, Z.M.; Hua, H. Efficacy of nystatin for the treatment of oral candidiasis: A systematic review and meta-analysis. *Drug Des. Dev. Ther.* **2016**, *10*, 1161–1171. [CrossRef] [PubMed]
29. Johnson, E.M.; Ojwang, J.O.; Szekely, A.; Wallace, T.L.; Warnock, D.W. Comparison of in vitro antifungal activities of free and liposome-encapsulated nystatin with those of four amphotericin B formulations. *Antimicrob. Agents Chemother.* **1998**, *42*, 1412–1416. [CrossRef] [PubMed]
30. Espada, R.; Valdespina, S.; Alfonso, C.; Rivas, G.; Ballesteros, M.P.; Torrado, J.J. Effect of aggregation state on the toxicity of different amphotericin B preparations. *Int. J. Pharm.* **2008**, *361*, 64–69. [CrossRef] [PubMed]
31. Espada, R.; Valdespina, S.; Molero, G.; Dea, M.A.; Ballesteros, M.P.; Torrado, J.J. Efficacy of alternative dosing regimens of poly-aggregated amphotericin B. *Int. J. Antimicrob. Agents* **2008**, *32*, 55–61. [CrossRef]
32. Singh, S.; Jain, S.; Muthu, M.S.; Tiwari, S.; Tilak, R. Preparation and evaluation of buccal bioadhesive films containing clotrimazole. *AAPS Pharm. Sci. Technol.* **2008**, *9*, 660–667. [CrossRef]

Permissions

All chapters in this book were first published by MDPI; hereby published with permission under the Creative Commons Attribution License or equivalent. Every chapter published in this book has been scrutinized by our experts. Their significance has been extensively debated. The topics covered herein carry significant findings which will fuel the growth of the discipline. They may even be implemented as practical applications or may be referred to as a beginning point for another development.

The contributors of this book come from diverse backgrounds, making this book a truly international effort. This book will bring forth new frontiers with its revolutionizing research information and detailed analysis of the nascent developments around the world.

We would like to thank all the contributing authors for lending their expertise to make the book truly unique. They have played a crucial role in the development of this book. Without their invaluable contributions this book wouldn't have been possible. They have made vital efforts to compile up to date information on the varied aspects of this subject to make this book a valuable addition to the collection of many professionals and students.

This book was conceptualized with the vision of imparting up-to-date information and advanced data in this field. To ensure the same, a matchless editorial board was set up. Every individual on the board went through rigorous rounds of assessment to prove their worth. After which they invested a large part of their time researching and compiling the most relevant data for our readers.

The editorial board has been involved in producing this book since its inception. They have spent rigorous hours researching and exploring the diverse topics which have resulted in the successful publishing of this book. They have passed on their knowledge of decades through this book. To expedite this challenging task, the publisher supported the team at every step. A small team of assistant editors was also appointed to further simplify the editing procedure and attain best results for the readers.

Apart from the editorial board, the designing team has also invested a significant amount of their time in understanding the subject and creating the most relevant covers. They scrutinized every image to scout for the most suitable representation of the subject and create an appropriate cover for the book.

The publishing team has been an ardent support to the editorial, designing and production team. Their endless efforts to recruit the best for this project, has resulted in the accomplishment of this book. They are a veteran in the field of academics and their pool of knowledge is as vast as their experience in printing. Their expertise and guidance has proved useful at every step. Their uncompromising quality standards have made this book an exceptional effort. Their encouragement from time to time has been an inspiration for everyone.

The publisher and the editorial board hope that this book will prove to be a valuable piece of knowledge for researchers, students, practitioners and scholars across the globe.

List of Contributors

Filipa Sousa, Domingos Ferreira and Paulo Costa
UCIBIO, REQUIMTE, Laboratory of Pharmaceutical Technology, Department of Drug Sciences, Faculty of Pharmacy, University of Porto, Rua Jorge Viterbo Ferreira n° 228, 4050-313 Porto, Portugal

Salette Reis
LAQV, REQUIMTE, Department of Chemical Sciences, Faculty of Pharmacy, University of Porto, Rua Jorge Viterbo Ferreira n° 228, 4050-313 Porto, Portugal

Monique L. van Hoek
National Center for Biodefense and Infectious Diseases, and School of Systems Biology, George Mason University, MS1H8, 10910 University Blvd, Manassas, VA 20110, USA

Lilian Sosa, María Rincón and Oscar Domenech
Department of Pharmacy and Pharmaceutical Technology and Physical Chemistry, School of Pharmacy and Food Sciences, University of Barcelona, 08028 Barcelona, Spain

Ana Cristina Calpena and Marcelle Silva-Abreu
Department of Pharmacy and Pharmaceutical Technology and Physical Chemistry, School of Pharmacy and Food Sciences, University of Barcelona, 08028 Barcelona, Spain
Institute de Nanoscience and Nanotechnology (IN2UB), University of Barcelona, 08028 Barcelona, Spain

Lupe Carolina Espinoza
Department of Pharmacy and Pharmaceutical Technology and Physical Chemistry, School of Pharmacy and Food Sciences, University of Barcelona, 08028 Barcelona, Spain
Departamento de Química y Ciencias Exactas, Universidad Técnica Particular de Loja, Loja 1101608, Ecuador

Nuria Bozal
Department of Biology, Healthcare and the Environment, School of Pharmacy and Food Sciences, University of Barcelona, 08028 Barcelona, Spain

María José Rodríguez-Lagunas
Department of Biochemistry and Physiology, Faculty of Pharmacy and Food Sciences, University of Barcelona, 08028 Barcelona, Spain
Institut de Recerca en Nutrició i Seguretat Alimentària (INSA), Universitat de Barcelona, 08921 Barcelona, Spain

Beatriz Clares
Institute de Nanoscience and Nanotechnology (IN2UB), University of Barcelona, 08028 Barcelona, Spain
Department of Pharmacy and Pharmaceutical Technology, School of Pharmacy, University of Granada, 18071 Granada, Spain

Jiajia Wu, Bin Gao and Shunyi Zhu
Group of Animal Innate Immunity, State Key Laboratory of Integrated Management of Pest Insects and Rodents, Institute of Zoology, Chinese Academy of Sciences, 1 Beichen West Road, Chaoyang District, Beijing 100101, China

Guangshun Wang
Department of Pathology and Microbiology, College of Medicine, University of Nebraska Medical Center, 986495 Nebraska Medical Center, Omaha, NE 68198-6495, USA

Diana Berenguer, Magdalena Alcover, Carme Guillén, Roser Fisa and Cristina Riera
Department of Biology, Health and Environment, Laboratory of Parasitology, Faculty of Pharmacy and Food Sciences, University of Barcelona, 08028 Barcelona, Spain

Lilian Sosa, Marcella Sessa, Lyda Halbaut and Ana Cristina-Calpena-Campmany
Department of Pharmaceutical Technology and Physicochemistry, Faculty of Pharmacy and Food Sciences, University of Barcelona, 08028 Barcelona, Spain

Damiana Téllez-Martínez, Deivys Leandro Portuondo, Maria Luiza Loesch, Alexander Batista-Duharte and Iracilda Zeppone Carlos
Department of Clinical Analysis, School of Pharmaceutical Sciences, São Paulo State University (UNESP), Araraquara 14800-903, SP, Brazil

James P. Tam, Ka H. Wong and Wei Liang Tan
School of Biological Sciences, Nanyang Technological University, Singapore

Shujing Wang
Department of Pharmacology and Pharmaceutical Sciences, School of Medicine, Tsinghua University, Beijing 100084, China

Rita Sánchez-Espejo and C. Ignacio Sainz-Díaz
Instituto Andaluz de Ciencias de la Tierra (CSIC-University of Granada), Av. de las Palmeras 4, 18100 Granada, Spain

Pilar Cerezo
Department of Pharmacy and Pharmaceutical Technology, Faculty of Pharmacy, University of Granada, Campus de Cartuja s/n, 18071 Granada, Spain

Ana Borrego-Sánchez and César Viseras
Instituto Andaluz de Ciencias de la Tierra (CSIC-University of Granada), Av. de las Palmeras 4, 18100 Granada, Spain
Department of Pharmacy and Pharmaceutical Technology, Faculty of Pharmacy, University of Granada, Campus de Cartuja s/n, 18071 Granada, Spain

Beatrice Albertini and Nadia Passerini
Department of Pharmacy and BioTechnology, University of Bologna, Via S. Donato 19/2, 40127 Bologna, Italy

Raquel Fernandez-Garcia
Department of Pharmaceutics and Food Technology, School of Pharmacy, Universidad Complutense de Madrid, Plaza Ramon y Cajal s/n, 28040 Madrid, Spain

Dolores R. Serrano
Department of Pharmaceutics and Food Technology, School of Pharmacy, Universidad Complutense de Madrid, Plaza Ramon y Cajal s/n, 28040 Madrid, Spain
Instituto Universitario de Farmacia Industrial (IUFI), School of Pharmacy, Universidad Complutense de Madrid, Avenida Complutense, 28040 Madrid, Spain

Marta Mele and Aikaterini Lalatsa
School of Pharmacy and Biomedical Sciences, University of Portsmouth, St. Michael's Building, White Swan Road, Portsmouth PO1 2DT, UK

Anne Marie Healy
Synthesis and Solid State Pharmaceutical Centre, School of Pharmacy and Pharmaceutical Sciences, Trinity College Dublin, Dublin 2, Ireland

Index